D1287573

# GUT ENVIRONMENT OF PIGS

# Gut Environment of Pigs

Edited by

A Piva
KE Bach Knudsen
JE Lindberg

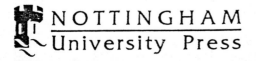
NOTTINGHAM
University Press

Nottingham University Press
Manor Farm, Main Street, Thrumpton
Nottingham, NG11 0AX, United Kingdom

NOTTINGHAM

First published 2001
© The Nottingham University Press 2001

**British Library Cataloguing in Publication Data**
Gut Environment of Pigs:
I. Piva, A., II. Bach Knudsen, K.E., III. Lindberg, J.E.

ISBN   1-897676-778

Typeset by Nottingham University Press, Nottingham
Printed and bound by The Cromwell Press, Trowbridge

# CONTENTS

# PREFACE

This book contains a compilation of papers presented at the workshops entitled "Feed additives and probiotics as an alternative to antibiotics as growth promoters" and "Gut environment: influence of luminar factors" organised on 18 and 19 June 2000, respectively, and in conjunction with the 8th Symposium on Digestive Physiology in Pigs, held at the Swedish University of Agricultural Sciences, Uppsala 20-22 June 2000. In this book the underlying science related to the effect of diet and feeding on the Gut Environment in Pigs is highlighted.

With an increasing awareness amongst politicians and consumers, and in the food industry, of the human health risks of the regular use of feed antibiotics as growth promoters in animal production, this production model has been questioned. In 1986 the Swedish Parliament imposed a ban on antibiotics as growth promoters. In recent years such a ban for the use of antibiotics as growth promoters for pigs has been introduced in several EU countries (Finland, Denmark, Germany) and this will in the future most likely be followed by others. However, in order to make this change in production model possible more knowledge is needed on alternative ways for the prevention of health problems in pigs. The function of the gastrointestinal tract is of major concern in this context.

The gastrointestinal tract is a complex system, which has a number of different functions. It is the site for interaction between feed and the body, and while the main function is digestion and absorption of nutrients the gastrointestinal tract is also a sophisticated defence organ and the body's largest endocrine organ. The interplay between the different functions is carefully modulated by a variety of direct and indirect mechanisms which determines the ability of the gastrointestinal tract to withstand damage that potentially may be aimed against it. Luminal factors are now recognised as having direct (act as nutrients i.e. polyamines or short chain fatty acids) or indirect (i.e. moderated by systemic factors) effects on the gastrointestinal tract.

The workshops attracted delegates from countries worldwide and resulted in fruitful discussions and many interactions between the participants. It is our hope that these proceedings will contribute to develop the science within this area and create a platform for future research that will increase our knowledge on how to prevent diet related gastrointesinal disturbances in pigs.

# ACKNOWLEDGEMENTS

The organisers are grateful to the speakers both for their exellent presentations and for provision of written versions which form the basis of these proceedings. Thanks are also due to the chairs of the two workshops. Finally, thanks are due to the delegates not just because of their precence, which is an essential feature of any meeting, but for their contribution to formal discussions.

Sincere thanks are also due to the following for their financial contributions without which the workshops could not have taken place.

Swedish University of Agricultural Sciences (SLU)
Swedish Council for Forestry and Agricultural Research
JEFO Nutrition Inc
NUTREX NV
Vetagro S.R.L.
AstraZeneca R & D

Essential administrative activities and highly efficient support services were provided by the Conference Service at SLU. The catering services on campus performed to their usual high standard. The editors are particularly grateful to Mr Kristofer Lindberg who with patience and expertise was tested in seeking to obtain a high degree of uniformity throughout this publication.

1

# MORPHOLOGICAL AND FUNCTIONAL CHANGES IN THE SMALL INTESTINE OF THE NEWLY-WEANED PIG

John R. Pluske
*Division of Veterinary and Biomedical Sciences, Murdoch University, Murdoch WA 6150, Australia*

## Abstract

At weaning the young pig experiences a number of abrupt and simultaneous changes such as mixing, moving, and being offered an alien feed type and form. These changes contribute to the post-weaning "growth check". Intimately associated with this growth check are structural and functional changes in the small intestine, such as villous shortening, crypt elongation and reduced specific activities of certain disaccharidase enzymes, which are generally believed to reduce the digestive and absorptive capacity of the small intestine. The population of enterocytes in the small intestine of the young pig is in a dynamic state, with cell turnover being a function of rates of crypt-cell proliferation, migration along the small intestinal crypt-villus axis, and cell renewal. Many factors, such as the withdrawal of immunoglobulins and growth factors at weaning, the presence of antigenic feed components and proliferation of certain bacteria in the gut, influence these processes. It is evident, however, that enteral nutrient availability is a potent regulator of growth and mucosal regeneration. Furthermore, recent evidence points to a compromising influence of luminal nutrient deprivation on both immunologic and non-immunologic components of the intestinal immune system. A major objective of feeding programs after weaning should be to encourage maximum levels of voluntary food intake to avoid deleterious changes in gut structure and function.

## Introduction

Low voluntary food intake, poor growth, expression of enteric diseases and, in some cases, morbidity and mortality, are well recognised features occurring in the period after weaning that impose major limitations to the efficiency of pig production worldwide. However, and despite the large volume of research that has been conducted endeavoring to reduce the deleterious impact of the post-weaning "growth check", it is apparent that the growth check still represents a major production penalty. With the (impending) withdrawal of numerous growth promotant additives for weanling pig diets in some countries, it is evident that more research directed at overcoming poor performance after weaning will continue in the future, as it is this phase of the pig's growth where large production gains are still possible due to the enormous growth potential of the young pig (Pluske and Dong, 1998).

The small intestine serves as an interface between the external and the internal environments of the pig, with its primary functions being to digest and absorb feed and to provide a physical and immunological barrier against harmful materials such as microbes and allergenic macromolecules. Enterocytes populating the mucosa of the small bowel are in a dynamic state. They are constantly being replaced by cells arising from the crypts of Lieberkühn, with the rate of regeneration matching the normal loss of villous epithelium (Tang, Laarveld, Van Kessel, Hamilton, Estrada and Patience, 1999; Van Dijk, Mouwen and Koninkx, 1999). However the mucosal epithelium of the small intestine is regarded as anatomically and functionally immature in neonatal pigs (Gaskins and Kelley, 1995), a feature that is exacerbated at weaning where there are dramatic changes in gut morphology and function. The marked changes that occur after weaning, such as villous atrophy and crypt hyperplasia, are generally associated with the poor performance observed as they are thought to cause a temporary decrease in digestive and absorptive capacity of the small intestine.

Many factors are thought responsible for changes in gut structure and function, and Pluske, Hampson and Williams (1997) have described many of these previously. In addition, the reader is directed to more recent reviews regarding some of these factors, for example that by Dréau and Lallès (1999) detailing the contribution of allergenic dietary proteins to gut hypersensitivity reactions in young pigs, and Ziegler, Estívariz, Jonas, Gu, Jones and Leader (1999) describing interactions between nutrients and growth factors in intestinal growth and repair. The focus of this particular review is to reiterate some of the changes that occur in gut architecture and function around the time of weaning, with particular attention paid to the role of 'luminal nutrition' (Diamond and Karasov, 1983) on these small intestinal indices. Other sections covered in this review include the role of colostrum- and milk-derived products on gut structure and function. Furthermore, exciting new studies point to a compromising influence of luminal nutrient deprivation on both immunologic and non-immunologic components of the intestinal immune system and interactions with gut morphology. Finally, the anatomy and physiology of the small intestine has been described many times before (eg, Friedrich, 1989; Kelly, Begbie and King, 1992; Cranwell, 1995) so will not be covered in this review.

## Structure and function of the small intestine after weaning

### VILLOUS HEIGHT AND CRYPT DEPTH

The dynamic process of small intestinal cell turnover is a function of the rates of crypt cell proliferation, migration along the crypt-villus axis, and cell extrusion from the villous apex via apoptosis and sloughing (Ziegler *et al.*, 1999). Villous atrophy after weaning can be caused either by an increased rate of cell loss or a reduced rate of cell renewal. If villous shortening occurs via an increased rate of cell loss, then this is associated with increased crypt-cell production and, generally, increased crypt depth. However, villous atrophy might also be due to a decreased rate of cell renewal that is the result of reduced cell division in the crypts, such as that which occurs as a consequence of fasting (Altmann, 1972; Goodlad and Wright, 1984; Goodlad, Plumb and Wright, 1988). While both these events are likely to operate after weaning to reduce the villous height:crypt depth ratio, it is likely that the former will have the most profound effect on gut structure.

A large number of authors have reported that there is a reduction in villous height and either an increase or decrease in crypt depth after weaning (see Pluske *et al.*, 1997, for list of references; also van Beers-Schreurs, Nabuurs, Vellenga, Kalsbeek-van der Valk, Wensing and Breukink, 1998; McCracken, Spurlock, Roos, Zuckermann and Gaskins, 1999; Tang *et al.*, 1999). These morphological changes are more conspicuous when weaning occurs earlier at 14 days rather than later at 28 days of age. In a detailed study of changes in small intestinal structure occurring after weaning, Hampson (1986a) reported that villous height was reduced to 75% of pre-weaning values within 24 hours of weaning at 21 days of age. Subsequent reductions in villous height were smaller but continued to decline until the fifth day after weaning, at which point villous height at most sites along the gut was approximately 50% of initial values found at weaning (Figure 1). Additionally, Cera, Mahan, Cross, Reinhart and Whitmoyer (1988) reported a reduction in the length of microvilli three to seven days after weaning. From five to eight days after weaning villous height generally begins to recover. In contrast, pigs that continue to suckle the sow show only slight reductions in villous height. The longer villi present in the proximal part of the small intestine decrease in height proportionally more than villi towards the distal part of the gut. Hampson (1986a) reported that villous atrophy was caused by a reduction in the number of enterocytes lining the villus and was not due to villous contraction, a phenomenon suggested to represent either an increased rate of cell loss from the villous apex or a brief reduction in the rate of cell production in the crypts.

A decrease in crypt cell production rate associated with villous atrophy was also reported by Hall and Byrne (1989), a mechanism attributed to sub-optimal intakes of energy and protein. Since crypt depth was reduced at three days after weaning, Hall and Byrne (1989) suggested that villous stunting was due to a slowed production of new cells and not an accelerated rate of loss of mature enterocytes from the surface of the villi. Hampson (1986a) reported that the number of cells in the crypts was not increased two days after weaning, but increased steadily thereafter until the eleventh day. Crypt elongation also occurred in unweaned pigs, but the extent of the increase was greater in weaned animals.

As a result of these changes in villous height and crypt depth after weaning, the villous height:crypt depth ratio in weaned pigs is markedly reduced compared to unweaned animals. Hampson (1986a) suggested that this represented a balance of cell production in the crypts and cell loss from the villi that began on the fifth day after weaning and persisted for at least five weeks. This is manifested in a change from the longer, finger-like villi seen in newborn and sucking pigs to wider leaf-like or tongue-like villi. These changes only occur after weaning if there is continuous absence from the sow, since pigs weaned for two days and then returned to the dam for three days showed crypt elongation only equivalent to that of pigs weaned for two days (Hampson, 1983). These changes also occur at a time when growth *per se* of the small intestine is extremely rapid. Goodlad and Wright (1990) and Kelly (1994) suggested that this could be explained by the young animal devoting a considerable part of its intestinal cell differentiation to cryptogenesis rather than the influx of new cells onto the villi, an event likely to be under a degree of genetic control.

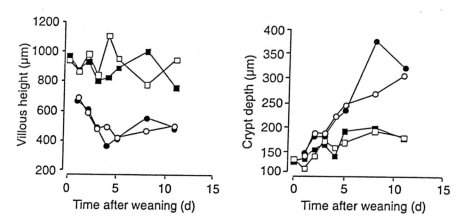

Figure 1 Villous height and crypt depth at a site 25% along the length of the small intestine of weaned and unweaned pigs killed between 21 and 32 days of age: ○———○ pigs weaned at 21 days of age and offered creep food prior to weaning; ●———● pigs weaned at 21 days of age but not offered creep food prior to weaning; □———□ pigs unweaned and offered creep food; ■———■ pigs unweaned but not offered creep food. Values are means for between two and seven pigs killed per treatment combination per day (redrawn from Hampson, 1986a).

## DIGESTIVE AND ABSORPTIVE CAPACITY OF THE SMALL INTESTINE AFTER WEANING

Reduction in villous height and increases in crypt depth in the small intestine after weaning have been associated with reductions in the specific activity of the brush-border enzymes lactase and sucrase (Hampson, 1986b), although the large variation associated with assay techniques and the variability between studies has not always resulted in a statistical decline in activity. Hampson and Kidder (1986) reported large, rapid reductions in the specific activity of lactase and sucrase that reached minimum values four to five days after weaning and occurred regardless of whether creep food was offered prior to weaning or not. Whereas lactase continued to decline at all but the most distal sites along the gut, sucrase activity had recovered by 11 days after weaning. The greater loss in lactase than sucrase activity was most likely due to the more apical distribution of lactase activity along the villus (Tsuboi, Kwong, Neu and Sunshine, 1981; Tsuboi, Kwong, D'Harlingue, Stevenson, Kerner, Jr. and Sunshine, 1985). In unweaned pigs there was an age-dependent fall in lactase activity that paralleled the ontogenetic decline in villous height (Kelly, King, McFadyen, and Travis, 1991a). Miller, James, Smith and Bourne (1986) reported that sucrase, isomaltase and lactase specific activities fell by at least 50% by five days after weaning in pigs weaned at 28 or 42 days of age. Activities of maltase II and maltase III showed no change in four-week-old pigs but increased in response to weaning at six weeks of age. Similarly, McCracken (1984), McCracken and Kelly (1984) and Kelly, Smyth and McCracken (1990, 1991b, c) reported increases in the activities of maltase and glucoamylase when pigs were weaned onto solid diets at 14 days of age.

In several studies the decrease in villous height, increase in crypt depth, and loss of digestive enzyme activity after weaning coincided with a reduced ability of weaned pigs to absorb a standard dose of D-xylose. D-xylose is a pentose sugar that is absorbed across the brush-border membrane and, as with alanine, is thought to provide an assessment of the absorptive capacity of the enterocytes. However, some authors (Kelly *et al.*, 1990; Kelly *et al.*, 1991b; Pluske, Williams and Aherne, 1996c) failed to detect a reduction in the ability of villi to absorb xylose after weaning. Miller *et al.* (1986) concluded that problems induced by weaning are caused more by changes in intestinal structure and specific loss of digestive enzymes rather than any gross change in absorptive function, although the data of Nabuurs, Hoogendoorn and Zijderveld (1994) showing differences between weaned and suckling pigs in net fluid absorption across isolated loops of small intestine would appear to be in contrast to this notion.

Reasons for the inconsistencies between studies are not clear, but may be attributable to the timing of the first introduction of creep food, the quantity of diet presented and amount consumed, dietary composition, age at weaning, and differences in villous height, all of which varied between the various reports. The failure to demonstrate this in every study may not only be a reflection of the factors mentioned previously, but may also indicate that some existing tests (eg, the xylose absorption test) are unreliable measures of absorptive function in the small intestine.

## AN ALTERNATIVE APPROACH TO ASSESSING DIGESTIVE AND ABSORPTIVE CAPACITY AFTER WEANING

Sufficient evidence now exists in the literature to question the suitability of measurements *in vitro* of digestive and absorptive function in the weaned pig. Determinations of specific activities of brush-border membrane lactase and sucrase, for example, have been assumed to provide an indication of digestive capacity *in vivo* (Kidder and Manners, 1980). Some authors (Berg, Dahlqvist, Lindberg and Nordén, 1973; Hampson, 1983) have commented that lactase and sucrase are 'markers' of enterocyte maturity and functional capacity, while others have advocated the use of total gut enzyme activity as a more meaningful measure of digestion *in vivo* (Kelly *et al.*, 1991c). However, the inadequacy of these measurements is borne out in the data of Kelly *et al.* (1991c). These authors demonstrated that irrespective of the basis of expression, measurements of digestive enzyme activities *in vitro* can only provide a crude assessment of digestive capacity and are of little value unless supported by findings *in vivo* of digestion and absorption.

In an attempt to alleviate this biological disparity, research at The University of Western Australia (Bird and Hartmann, 1994; Bird, Atwood and Hartmann, 1995; Pluske, Thompson, Atwood, Bird, Williams, and Hartmann, 1996a) has focused on an alternative means for estimating digestive and absorptive capacity *in vivo*. Full details of the procedures involved are outlined in the above publications, but briefly, a physiological solution containing lactose and fructose (LAC + FRU) and a physiological solution containing sucrose and galactose (SUC + GAL) are prepared and piglets are then dosed orally with 25 ml of each solution. Ear veins of the piglets are pricked using a finger lancet, and blood samples (~ 60 µl) collected into heparinised capillary tubes. Samples are taken at regular intervals (3-5 minutes) for 60 min and then again at 75 and 90 minutes after dosing. After samples from this first dose (eg, LAC + FRU) are completed, the alternative solution (eg, SUC + GAL) is administered and blood samples are collected again for 90 minutes. The concentrations of glucose, galactose and fructose in the blood versus time after oral dosing are plotted and the area under the curve (AUC) for each piglet calculated by the trapezoid method reported by Williams, Philips and Macdonald (1983), which was derived from Yeh and Kwan (1978). Galactose and fructose indexes both before and after weaning are calculated from an adjusted AUC value. By dividing the adjusted AUC values for galactose and fructose ingested as components of lactose and sucrose, respectively, by the values obtained for galactose and fructose ingested as monosaccharides, respectively, and then expressing the ratio as a percentage, an index equivalent to the glycaemic index used in human nutrition (Brand Miller Holt, Thomas, Byrnes, Denyer, and Truswell, 1994) can be obtained. The "Galactose Index" and the "Fructose Index", therefore, provide an index of efficiency *in vivo* of disaccharide digestion and monosaccharide absorption in the small intestine. If, for example, the GI was 50%, then the AUC for galactose consumed as lactose was half that observed when the same quantity of galactose was ingested as the monosaccharide. The GI and FI therefore provide a qualitative index of the capacity of lactase and sucrase *in vivo* to digest lactose and sucrose, and the capacity *in vivo* of enterocytes to absorb their monosaccharide products.

Using this approach, Pluske *et al.* (1996a) found that when pigs were fed cows' fresh milk for five days after weaning there was an enhancement in the capacity of lactase and sucrase to digest physiological boluses of lactose and sucrase, respectively. Despite these increases in apparent digestive and absorptive capacity of the small intestine, a decrease in the efficiency of absorption of galactose and fructose after weaning (ie, the 'galactose index' and 'fructose index' respectively, which provide efficiency estimates *in vivo* of disaccharide digestion and monosaccharide absorption) was found. This apparent anomaly may be explained by increased growth, and hence total surface area, of the small intestine after weaning such that total digestion and absorption were increased despite seeming decreases in the efficiency at which they occurred (Pluske *et al.*, 1996a). Information such as this is impossible to obtain using current *in vitro* methods of assessment.

Furthermore, Pluske *et al.* (1996a) reported a positive linear correlation between villous height and the 'galactose index' at a site 25% along the small intestine from the duodenum (Figure 2). These data *in vivo* concur with those *in vitro* of Kelly *et al.* (1991a) that maximum lactase activity occurs further along (ie, more apically) the crypt:villous axis. The failure to detect relationships between lactose digestion and villous height at sites 50% and 75% along the small intestine supports earlier research that lactase activity in the young pig is maximal in the more proximal region of the small intestine (Manners and Stevens 1972; Kidder and Manners, 1980; Shulman, Henning and Nicholls, 1988; Kelly *et al.* 1991a, b, c). These data also support the findings of Puchal and Buddington (1992) who reported proximal to distal gradients in the rate and extent of galactose (and glucose) transport in sucking piglets. These findings illustrate the role of luminal nutrition in determining gradients of disaccharidase activity along the small intestine of the young pig.

To date, this approach has only been conducted in pigs either sucking the sow or fed cows' milk after weaning. To fully assess its worth as a measure of digestive and absorptive function *in vivo*, experiments need to be conducted in pigs consuming other feeds or in which the small intestine has been compromised in some way, such as total parenteral nutrition. Additionally, only lactose and sucrose have been used as disaccharide 'markers' of the efficacy of lactase and the sucrase-isomaltase complex. From a practical point of view, it may be more beneficial to dose pigs with starch, since the enzymes responsible for their hydrolysis are more important to digestion in the weaned pig than lactase and sucrase given the high starch content of starter feeds.

## The influence of substances contained in colostrum and milk

There is increasing interest in the important role that colostrum- and milk-borne growth factors, hormones and other bioactive substances may play in postnatal differentiation and development of the small intestine of the pig. The nutritional benefits of, for example, bovine colostrum, bovine milk and milk-related products (eg, whey-derived protein concentrates) have been acknowledged for hundreds of years, although the potential of these products to directly influence physiological function, such as the mammalian immune system and gastrointestinal structure, has only recently been identified (Newby, Stokes and Bourne, 1982). This is especially pertinent to the weaned pig because the source of some of these compounds, ie, sow's milk, is removed abruptly at weaning, leaving the small intestinal epithelium devoid of these products. This is likely to have marked effects on the processes regulating cell growth, cell differentiation, cell function and immune function in the gastrointestinal tract. A host of compounds have been implicated in small intestinal development, function and the prevention of enteric disease in young mammals, including the pig. These have been the subject of numerous reviews that include those by Donovan and Odle (1994), Froetschel (1996), Odle, Ziljstra and Donovan (1996), Xu (1996), Pakkanen and Aalto (1997), Seare and Playford (1998) and Pluske and Dong (1998).

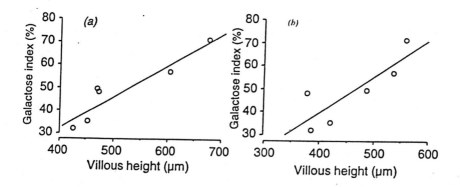

**Figure 2** Relationships between *(a)* villous height at a site 25% along the small intestine (y = -20.8 + 0.14x, *P* = 0.007, R² = 0.87) and *(b)* mean villous height along the entire length of the small intestine (y = -23.3 + 0.16x, *P* = 0.037, R² = 0.70), and the GI assessed five days after weaning. Each point represents an individual pig (redrawn from Pluske *et al.*, 1996a).

With respect to bovine dairy components, recent work from Massey University in New Zealand suggests that bovine IgG may have a positive influence on structure and function in the small intestine, in addition to enhancing pig performance both after weaning and to market weight. Work by Morel, Schollum, Buwalda and

Pearson (1995) showed that oral provision of bovine IgG increased the local concentration of this immunoglobulin in the gastrointestinal tract, particularly the proximal portion of the small intestine. Further work by King, Morel, Revell, James, Birtles and Pluske (1999) showed that provision to sucking piglets of a colostrum-based dairy product ('Immulac') for 14 days during lactation that contained either 75 g/kg (Im1) or 150 g/kg (Im2) bovine IgG enhanced gut structure at weaning. Compared to a control diet of whey-protein concentrate (6 g/kg IgG), piglets offered Immulac had higher villi and a higher epithelial cell height (Table 1). Pigs offered Im1 had higher villi than those offered Im2, a result most likely caused by a significantly greater dry matter intake of this particular supplement during lactation. No differences were observed in the crypts, and a significant proximal to distal reduction in villous height and crypt depth along the small intestine was also observed (Table 1). A significant interaction occurred between treatments Im1 and Im2 with site along the small intestine, whereby villous height was greatest in the jejunum compared to piglets offered the whey-protein concentrate product. These data show a significant effect of a bovine colostrum-based product containing IgG, which incidentally also contained growth factors such as IGF-1 and IGF-II, on intestinal structure. Subsequent work has shown a similar effect even when intakes between experimental treatments are equal (King *et al.*, unpublished data).

**Table 1** Least squares means of small intestinal morphological measurements in piglets fed supplementary liquid diets containing whey protein concentrate (WPC) or colostrum powder (Immulac) (after King *et al.*, 1999).

| | Treatment[1] | | | | P-value | | |
|---|---|---|---|---|---|---|---|
| | WPC | Im1 | Im2 | SE | T | S[5] | TxS |
| VH[2] (µm) | 503[a] | 601[b] | 545[c] | 8.1 | 0.03 | 0.001 | 0.08 |
| CD[3] (µm) | 196 | 195 | 190 | 2.8 | 0.92 | 0.001 | 0.88 |
| ECH[4] (µm) | 22.6[a] | 24.9[b] | 24.4[b] | 0.22 | 0.09 | 0.003 | 0.56 |

[a,b,c] Values within treatment or site with different superscripts are significantly different ($P < 0.01$). [1]Treatment (T): WPC: whey-protein concentrate, Im1, Immulac with 75 g/kg IgG, Im2: Immulac with 150 g/kg IgG; [2]VH, villous height; [3]CD, crypt depth; [4]ECH, epithelial cell height; [5]Site (S) along small intestine; proximal to distal gradient in indices (data not shown).

The possible mechanism(s), however, whereby a dairy product may cause such an effect, which may or may not be specific, is unknown, and is currently the focus of further work. Numerous workers have reported an enhancement of immune function by feeding bovine whey protein products (Gill and Rutherfurd, 1998; Cross and Gill, 1999) and, in young pigs, it has been reported that porcine immunoglobulins or bovine colostrum are satisfactory sources of immunoglobulins for survival and growth (eg, Gomez, Phillips and Goforth, 1998). Given this, and the fact that passive protection of piglets against post-weaning colibacillosis can be provided by egg IgG immunised against enterotoxigenic strains of *Escherichia coli* (Mroz, Grela, Matras, Krasucki, Kichura and Shipp, 1999), it appears that there may be a role for colostrum- and (or) milk-derived immunoglobulins in diets for young pigs to enhance overall gut structure and function, especially if incorporation of antibiotics into diets becomes redundant.

Furthermore, both Vanavichial, Morel, Revell, James, Camden and Schollum (1997) and Pluske, Pearson, Morel, King, Skilton and Skilton (1999b) reported reduced number of days to slaughter in pigs offered commercial products containing IgG, both during lactation (Vanavichial *et al.*, 1997) and if offered for seven days after weaning at 28 days of age (Pluske *et al.*, 1999b). Similarly, Grinstead, Goodband, Dritz, Tokach, Nelssen, Woodworth and Molitor (2000) reported comparable performance in nursery-aged pigs when a whey-protein product containing 730 g/kg crude protein, 68 g/kg lysine and 128 g/kg fat (IgG content not reported) was substituted for spray-dried animal plasma in diets fed for 14 days after weaning. Given that spray-dried animal plasma also contains immunoglobulins, it is conceivable that enhanced performance in young pigs fed bovine IgG products may be an overall consequence of an improved gut environment, such as enhanced intestinal immunity, reduced proliferation of enteric bacteria, or any combination of these factors.

## Dietary changes at weaning

Newly-weaned piglets are subjected to nutritional (eg, loss of sow's milk), psychological (eg, mixing and moving) and environmental (eg, change in pen design, change in feeder location) stressors that are imposed simultaneously. Weaning, therefore, presents several unique problems not experienced in other phases of pig growth. With reference to dietary change, the feed offered to the young pig changes from one that is based on liquid milk and is therefore rich in fat to one that is relatively low in fat but high in complex carbohydrates and proteins. In addition, piglets receive 20-24 regular meals per day that they are conditioned to drink simultaneously and only when the sow allows them to. At weaning there is a transformation from a complete nutritional and behavioural dependence on the dam to complete independence requiring very different adult feeding and drinking patterns (Epstein, 1986). In this regard, numerous authors (eg, Funderburke, 1985; Bark, Crenshaw and Leibbrandt, 1986; P. H. Brooks, personal communication) have considered that low food intake and poor performance following weaning has a very strong behavioural component, such that it takes several days for pigs to make the necessary behavioural adaptations to the change in both the form and presentation of the diet in order to eat and grow. Recent advances in feeding technology and management, such as liquid feeding and offering "small but often" amounts of feed in trays on a pen floor, have helped to alleviate some of these difficulties that the weaned pig encounters.

Despite this, voluntary food intake in the post-weaning period is both low and variable, with pigs often failing to eat enough food to cover their energy requirement for maintenance (Leibbrandt, Ewan, Speer and Zimmerman, 1975; Robertson, Clark and Bruce, 1985; Bark *et al.*, 1986; Pluske, 1993; Le Dividich and Herpin, 1994). Interpretation of the data of Bark *et al.* (1986) shows that the estimated energy requirement for maintenance was not met until the fifth day after weaning, while Robertson *et al.* (1985) found that maximum estimated energy intake was not achieved until 14 days after weaning. Le Dividich and Herpin (1994) and Pluske (1993) summarised several data sets and concluded that the metabolisable energy (ME) requirement for maintenance was not met until the fifth day after weaning, with pre-weaning ME intake not being attained until the end of the second week following weaning (Figure 3). Although advances in nutritional and feeding management have most likely shifted this curve to the left, it is apparent that low food intake after weaning remains a serious production problem.

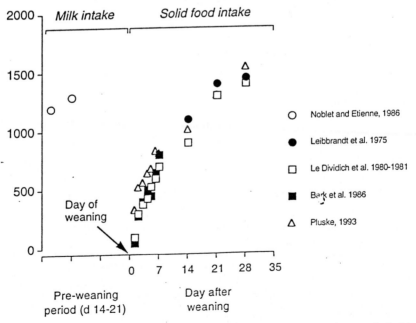

**Figure 3** The voluntary food intake of pigs before and after weaning (expressed as metabolisable energy (ME) intake per metabolic kilogram) (adapted from Le Dividich and Herpin, 1994).

## The role of 'luminal nutrition' in gut structure and function

One of the most powerful stimuli for proliferation of the gastrointestinal tract is the presence of food in the lumen or, more specifically, nutrient flow along the gut (Diamond and Karasov, 1983). The absence of nutrients from the lumen of the small intestine such as that which occurs after weaning will have marked effects on the rate of cell differentiation and cell turnover. It is well established that the oral intake of food and its physical presence in the gut *per se* are necessary for structural and functional maintenance of the intestinal mucosa (see Kelly *et al.*, 1992). The presence of food in the gastrointestinal tract has direct and indirect effects on epithelial cell proliferation (Johnson, 1987). For example, the exclusion of nutrients from the lumen of the small intestine either by starvation (eg, McNeill and Hamilton, 1971; Altmann, 1972), dietary restriction (eg, Núñez Bueno, Ayudarte, Almendros, Ríos, Suárez and Gil, 1995), or intravenous feeding (eg, Goodlad, Lee and Wright, 1992), results in villous atrophy and a decrease in crypt-cell production rate. Since these changes have been reported in the gut of the newly-weaned pig, it is likely that luminal nutrition plays a strong role in the integrity of the structure and function of the small intestine after weaning.

The major effect of starvation and then re-feeding is to increase and decrease, respectively, the duration of the cell-cycle time, or $T_c$, in the crypts of Lieberkühn (Al-Dewachi, Wright, Appleton and Watson, 1975). Numerous workers have also reported an increase in cell-cycle time, or a decrease in the production of crypt cells, associated with starvation (eg, Altmann, 1972; Clarke, 1975; Al-Mukhtar, Sagor, Ghatei, Polak, Koopmans, Bloom and Wright, 1982; Goodlad *et al.*, 1988). Re-feeding an animal for as little as 9-12 hours causes a reduction in cell-cycle time and a general increase in cell proliferation in the crypts (Al-Dewachi *et al.*, 1975; Goodlad and Wright, 1984). Goodlad and Wright (1984) concluded that after re-feeding, cell migration from crypt to villus is not immediately dependent upon cell proliferation, but may be a response to the presence of nutrients in the lumen stimulating cell migration directly to produce an immediate increase in digestive and absorptive capacity.

Concomitantly, the reduction in liveweight gain caused by decreased food intake after weaning reduces fasting heat production (Koong, Nienaber, Pekas and Yen, 1982). Since heat production is associated with protein synthesis (Webster, 1980, 1981), and this is most active in the digestive tract (Pekas and Wray, 1991), the lack of food in the small intestine would be expected to reduce cell production and decrease cell renewal. Furthermore, Koong and Ferrell (1990) and Pekas and Wray (1991) demonstrated that the energy expenditure of the small intestine varies directly with fasting heat production in the growing pig under different nutritional regimens. If the gut mucosa responds directly to the level of energy intake it is likely, therefore, that the structure and function of the small intestine also depends on the level of intake.

## TYPE OF DIET FED AFTER WEANING

It is possible that the form of diet fed after weaning may influence gut architecture, although this has received surprisingly little attention in the literature. Deprez, Deroose, Van den Hende, Muylle and Oyaert (1987) compared a pelleted diet with the same diet fed in slurry form, and recorded higher villi on days eight and 11 after weaning when pigs were fed the slurry. Villous height may have been maintained after weaning because the digesta from a pelleted diet may be more abrasive than that from liquid diets, which could decrease villous height by increasing the shedding of enterocytes. Alternatively, the higher villi recorded by these workers in pigs fed the slurry diet may be a reflection of their higher level of energy intake. Partridge, Fisher, Gregory and Prior (1992) showed that weaned pigs fed a dry, solid diet in slurry form consumed 13% more food ($P < 0.05$) and grew 11% faster ($P < 0.01$) than pigs fed the same diet in pelleted form. Selby, Cadogan, Campbell and Choct (1999) and Toplis, Blanchard and Miller (1999) showed similar results. Recent work from The University of Plymouth (Moran, Miller and Brooks, unpublished data) has shown that newly-weaned pigs fed either a fermented liquid feed (FLF) or a non-fermented liquid feed (NFLF) had villi the same height, and crypts the same depth, as pigs offered the same diet in dry form when pigs were killed 14 days after weaning. Interestingly, when either FLF or NFLF was offered every 12 hours instead of on an hourly or four-hourly basis, mean villous height was lower, suggesting a negative effect of increased feeding interval on gut structure in pigs fed via a liquid feeding system.

## VOLUNTARY FOOD INTAKE AFTER WEANING – IS IT IMPORTANT?

In some experiments, however, the likely contribution of food intake *per se* on morphological and biochemical alterations in the gut after weaning could not be gauged because researchers have not quantified the amount of food consumed. The first workers to recognise that low food intake in the period immediately after weaning may be responsible for changes in gut structure and function in the pig were Kelly, Greene, O'Brien and McCracken (1984) and McCracken and Kelly (1984). These authors adopted the technique of gastric intubation as a means of regulating food consumption and reducing the variation in food intake after weaning. Commensurate with a similar report by McCracken (1984), these workers suggested that mucosal atrophy after weaning may be related more to the lack of a continuous supply of substrate than to any antigenicity in the diet or to inherently low levels of digestive enzyme activity.

Kelly *et al.* (1991c), Pluske *et al.* (1996c) and van-Beers Schreurs *et al.* (1998) have since studied the effects of different levels of food intake on the digestive and absorptive development of the weaned piglet. Kelly *et al.* (1991c), for example, fed by stomach tube a low or high amount of a cereal-based diet to pigs weaned at 14 days of age for the first five days after weaning. Pigs fed less food showed villous atrophy and decreased crypt depth at all sites along the small intestine compared to pigs fed a higher quantity of food. Moreover, the authors' estimates of brush-border enzyme activity and xylose absorption failed to corroborate the marked changes in gut structure that occurred (Table 2), since there was no association between the amount of food gavage-fed to pigs and hence villous height to any greater lactase and sucrase activities. Kelly *et al.* (1991c) also reported that feeding more food increased the total activities of maltase and glucoamylase in accordance with substrate-induction of these carbohydrases (Table 2).

Table 2 Mean values measured over five sites along the small intestine for lactase (*EC* 3.2.1.23), sucrase (*EC* 3.2.1.48), maltase (*EC* 3.2.1.20) and glucoamylase (*EC* 3.2.1.3) activities, and serum xylose concentration, of pigs weaned at 14 days of age and given either continuous or restricted nutrient supply for five days (after Kelly *et al.*, 1991c).

| | *Feeding level*[1] | | | |
| | *Continuous* | *Restricted* | *SEM*[2] | *P* -value |
|---|---|---|---|---|
| Lactase | | | | |
| µmol/min/g protein | 66 | 86 | 9.9 | 0.15 |
| µmol/min/g mucosa | 10 | 11 | 1.3 | 0.80 |
| mol/day | 0.8 | 0.7 | 0.09 | 0.60 |
| Sucrase | | | | |
| µmol/min/g protein | 74 | 100 | 9.7 | 0.08 |
| µmol/min/g mucosa | 12 | 13 | 1.2 | 0.65 |
| mol/day | 0.9 | 0.9 | 0.10 | 0.75 |
| Maltase | | | | |
| µmol/min/g protein | 24 | 23 | 2.2 | 0.71 |
| µmol/min/g mucosa | 4 | 3 | 0.4 | 0.04 |
| mol/day | 0.3 | 0.2 | 0.03 | 0.01 |
| Glucoamylase | | | | |
| µmol/min/g protein | 63 | 61 | 5.0 | 0.40 |
| µmol/min/g mucosa | 9 | 7 | 0.7 | 0.06 |
| mol/day | 0.8 | 0.5 | 0.06 | 0.01 |
| Serum xylose (mmol/L) | 0.7 | 0.7 | 0.08 | 0.72 |

[1]Amount of food given per piglet from day 1-5 after weaning: *continuous* (150, 175, 200, 225 and 250 g/day); *restricted* (0, 25, 50, 75 and 100 g/day). [2]SEM: standard error of the mean.

Using an alternative approach, Pluske (1993) reasoned that if the nutritional stress of interrupted intake at weaning could be overcome, then the transition from sow's milk to solid food would be less traumatic and piglet growth would increase. Since an increase in food intake in the immediate post-weaning period is likely to exert potent stimulatory effects on mucosal growth and function, this may preserve the integrity of the small intestine and promote growth through an enhancement and (or) preservation of digestive and absorptive capacity.

By coaxing pigs to drink either ewes' or cows' fresh milk immediately after weaning at two-hourly intervals, Pluske *et al.* (1996b, c) demonstrated that, in comparison to unweaned piglets, villous height and crypt depth could be maintained after weaning by feeding a milk liquid diet. Since villous height can be correlated to the number of enterocytes on the villous column in 'normal' villi (Wright, 1982; Hampson, 1986a), maintenance of food intake after weaning must have preserved enterocyte number commensurate with a maintenance, or even enhancement (eg, James, Smith and Tivey, 1988), of digestive and absorptive capacity of each enterocyte. Indeed, pigs fed on an *ad libitum* basis in the study of Pluske *et al.* (1996c) grew at rates in excess of 500 g/d suggesting that digestive and absorptive capacity was not impaired. An alternative reason for preservation of villous height, as suggested by Goodlad *et al.* (1988), is that villous cell population might increase by means of cell migration from the crypts without a concomitant increase in crypt-cell production rate. However this has only been observed in rats re-fed after a period of short-term starvation (Altmann, 1972; Clarke, 1975), and so this mechanism is unlikely to be responsible for the maintenance of villous height seen after weaning in the present investigation.

Pluske *et al.* (1996c) also demonstrated that when pigs were weaned onto cows' fresh milk and offered three levels of energy intake (ie, estimated maintenance, 2.5 times estimated maintenance and *ad libitum* intake) every two hours for five days, there was a linear relationship between total dry matter intake and mean villous height along the length of the small intestine (Figure 4a). In turn, mean villous height explained 47% of the total variation in empty body-weight gain in the first five days after weaning (Figure 4b). Similar relationships have been reported by Li, Nelssen, Reddy, Blecha, Klemm, and Goodband (1991) and Moran *et al.* (unpublished data). These data highlight the interdependence between absorbed nutrients, intestinal structure and growth rate in the immediate post-weaning period, and underline the importance of stimulating food intake after weaning.

In contrast, pigs consuming a pelleted starter diet at the same level of energy intake as pigs consuming cows' whole milk at 2.5 maintenance (M) showed villous atrophy and crypt hyperplasia, although linear relationships similar to those described above were also evident (Pluske *et al.*, 1996c). This finding shows an independent effect of diet *per se* on gut structure after weaning that is uncomplicated by any differences in the level of voluntary energy intake. Despite these marked histological changes between pigs fed milk and solid diets, and the fact that pigs consuming the solid diet grew at similar rates to pigs drinking milk at 2.5 M, no differences in gut function as assessed by brush-border enzyme activity and xylose were detected.

Van-Beers-Schreurs *et al.* (1998) reported that pigs fed a commercial diet and sows' milk at the same level of energy intake had similar villous heights and crypt depths. However the average energy intake of pigs fed these two diets was approximately 2.8 and 2.5 MJ DE/day, respectively, which was about half the daily energy intake achieved by the pigs in the study of Pluske *et al.* (1996c). This difference most likely explains the differences observed between the two studies.

This discussion has focused primarily on the direct effects of a reduction in energy intake *per se* on gut structure and function. It is likely also that factors other than a dietary shortage of energy and (or) protein may contribute to gut architecture and function after weaning. In this regard, Williams, Rumsey and Powers (1996) found that feeding a riboflavin-deficient diet for eight weeks to weanling rats caused a significantly lower villous number, a significant increase in villous length, and an increased rate of enterocyte migration along the villus, in comparison to weight-matched controls. In pigs, Jiang, Chang, Stoll, Fan, Arthington, Weaver, Campbell and Burrin (2000) investigated the effects of a diet containing spray-dried porcine plasma (SDPP) on small intestinal growth and mucosal morphology in 14-day-old weaned pigs. Pigs offered SDPP and pair-fed to pigs receiving a control diet without SDPP for 16 days had reduced jejunal and ileal protein and DNA masses together with a reduced intravillous lamina propria cell density in the jejunum. Although SDPP stimulates food intake immediately after weaning (Ermer, Miller and Lewis, 1994), in this study *ad libitum*-fed pigs offered SDPP failed to have higher villi at any stage after weaning compared to pair-fed pigs fed SDPP. In conclusion, Jiang *et al.* (2000) speculated that dietary SDPP might suppress local intestinal proinflammatory responses associated with weaning, as will be discussed in the following section.

## Immunological and non-immunological consequences of luminal nutrition after weaning

McCracken, Gaskins, Ruwe-Kaiser, Klasing and Jewell (1995) demonstrated that pigs weaned at three weeks of age onto either a milk replacer or a solid (corn-soy) diet showed both diet-independent (ie, increased glucagon, decreased glucose, increased IL-1 and increased fibrinogen concentrations) and diet-dependent (ie, decreased insulin levels and decreased villous height in corn-soy-fed pigs) responses associated with weaning. Of particular interest were the increase in IL-1 and fibrinogen that occurred, as these are considered general indicators of inflammation and weaning-associated intestinal inflammation has been reported in other species, such as the rat (Cummins, Steele, LaBrooy and Shearman, 1988).

In a subsequent study, McCracken *et al.* (1999) evaluated inflammatory responses in the small intestine in association with the morphological changes that occur after weaning. Cumulative food intake averaged less than 100 g per pig immediately after weaning, which is most probably less than that required to meet the pigs' daily maintenance requirement for energy. Low voluntary food intake immediately after weaning was associated with increased numbers of inflammatory T-cells and local expression of the matrix metalloproteinase stromelysin, while jejunal villous height and crypt depth, CD8+ T-cell numbers and major histocompatibility complex (MHC) class I RNA expression decreased. In addition, McCracken *et al.* (1999) postulated that aberrant upregulation of stromelysin in response to low food intake after weaning may increase the breakdown of the extracellular matrix, resulting in compromised changes to the intestinal integrity such as villous atrophy. Pluske, Gaskins, Morel, Revell, King and James (1999a) also reported increased numbers of CD4+ cells in the jejunum of pigs measured 24 hours after weaning. Furthermore, Cunha Ferreira, Forsyth, Richman, Wells, Spencer and MacDonald (1990) showed that activation of T cells in the lamina propria of explants of fetal human small intestine caused villous atrophy and crypt hyperplasia, in the absence of damage to surface enterocytes. Similarly, Lionetti, Breese, Braegger, Murch, Taylor and MacDonald (1993), using a similar model of fetal human small intestinal explants, demonstrated that large numbers of activated macrophages can result in villous atrophy, crypt hyperplasia and, in some cases, complete mucosal destruction.

To confirm the role of luminal nutrition in the alteration of intestinal immune function in the young pig, Ganessunker, Gaskins, Zuckermann and Donovan (1999) used a piglet total parenteral nutrition (TPN) model to compare immune cell composition within the intestinal epithelium and lamina propria in intravenously-fed and orally-fed piglets. Intestinal atrophy in piglets fed parenterally was evidenced by decreased width of intestinal villi and reduced crypt depth, along with a threefold increase in the number of CD4+ and CD8+ T lymphocytes in the lamina propria of jejunal and ileal villi. In addition, MHC class II mRNA expression and goblet cell numbers were increased in villi isolated from the jejunum and ileum. Of particular interest were relationships found between T-lymphocyte numbers, intestinal morphology indices and goblet cell numbers, with highly negative correlations being observed between villous height and villous width to CD4+ and CD8+ T-cell numbers (Ganessunker *et al.*, 1999). However, whether compromised villous morphology preceded intestinal T-cell expansion or vice versa could not be ascertained from the study. Collectively, these data demonstrate that both immunologic and non-immunologic components of the gastrointestinal immune

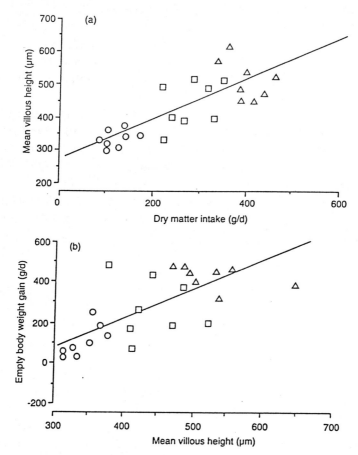

**Figure 4** Relationship between (a) daily dry matter intake and mean villous height along the small intestine [y = 286.10 + 0.54x, $R^2$ = 0.68 (RSD = 56.91); $P$ < 0.001], and (b) mean villous height along the small intestine and daily empty body-weight gain [y = -325.69 + 1.39x, $R^2$ = 0.4 8 (RSD = 127.10); $P$ = 0.002], in pigs offered cow's liquid milk at maintenance ( O ), 2.5 times maintenance ( □ ), or *ad libitum* ( △ ) energy intake for five days after weaning (8 pigs per treatment). Each point represents a single piglet killed on the fifth day following weaning at 28 days of age (redrawn from Pluske *et al.*, 1996c).

system associated with intestinal inflammation are associated with nutrient deprivation in the intestines.

## Conclusions

This review describes only a small number of reported factors that cause changes to the structure and function of the small intestine in the weaned pig. Although I have described these factors individually, it must be reiterated that many of these factors interact with each other to effect the alterations seen. Emphasis in this review was paid to the morphological and biochemical changes that are commonly seen in weaned pigs, although it is evident that there is often a lack of agreement between histological measurements and *in vitro* estimates of digestive and absorptive capacity. Weaning is characterised by an abrupt dietary change coupled with the sudden withdrawal of specialised components contained in sows' milk that may afford a degree of protection, stimulation and cellular differentiation to the small intestinal mucosa. Weaning is also distinguished by a period of low voluntary food intake that deprives the gut of 'luminal nutrition', which in turn has a hypotrophic effect on epithelial growth, development and differentiation. Accumulated evidence now exists demonstrating the importance of food *per se* in the maintenance of small intestinal structure and function after weaning, which in turn impacts upon the rate of growth of the young pig. Finally, recent research has shown that both immunologic and non-immunologic components of the immune system associated with inflammation of the small intestine are associated with nutrient deprivation in the intestines. This is clearly an exciting area of future research.

## References

Al-Dewachi, H.S., Wright, N.A., Appleton, D.R. and Watson, A.J. (1975) The effect of starvation and refeeding on cell population kinetics in the rat small bowel mucosa. *Journal of Anatomy*, **119**, 105-121.

Al-Mukhtar, M.Y.T., Sagor, G.R., Ghatei, M.A., Polak, J.M., Koopmans, H.S., Bloom, S.R. and Wright, N.A. (1982) The relationship between endogenous gastrointestinal hormones and cell proliferation in models of adaptation. In *Mechanisms of Intestinal Adaptation*, pp. 243-254. Edited by J.W.L. Robinson, R.H. Dowling and E.-O. Riecken. MTP Press Limited, Lancaster.

Altmann, G.G. (1972) Influence of starvation and refeeding on mucosal size and epithelial renewal in the rat small intestine. *American Journal of Anatomy*, **133**, 391-400.

Bark, L.J., Crenshaw, T.D. and Leibbrandt, V.D. (1986) The effect of meal intervals and weaning on feed intake of early weaned pigs. *Journal of Animal Science*, **62**, 1233-1239.

Berg, N.O., Dahlqvist, A., Lindberg, T. and Nordén, Å. (1973) Correlation between morphological alterations and enzyme activities in the mucosa of the small intestine. *Scandinavian Journal of Gastroenterology*, **8**, 703-712.

Bird, P.H. and Hartmann, P.E. (1994) The response in the blood of piglets to oral doses of galactose and glucose and intravenous administration of galactose. *British Journal of Nutrition*, **71**, 553-561.

Bird, P.H., Atwood, C.S. and Hartmann, P.E. (1995) The response of blood galactose to oral doses of lactose, galactose plus glucose and milk to piglets. *British Journal of Nutrition*, **73**, 753-761.

Brand Miller, J., Holt, S., Thomas, D., Byrnes, S., Denyer, G. and Truswell, A.S. (1994) Glycaemic index: Is it a useful tool in human health and disease? *Proceedings of the Nutrition Society of Australia*, **18**, 15-22.

Cera, K.R., Mahan, D.C., Cross, R.F., Reinhart, G.A. and Whitmoyer, R.E. (1988) Effect of age, weaning and postweaning diet on small intestinal growth and jejunal morphology in young swine. *Journal of Animal Science*, **66**, 574-584.

Clarke, R.M. (1975) The time-course of changes in mucosal architecture and epithelial cell production and cell shedding in the small intestine of the rat after fasting. *Journal of Anatomy*, **120**, 321-327.

Cranwell, P.D. (1995) Development of the neonatal gut and enzyme systems. *In The Neonatal Pig: Development and Survival*, pp. 99-154. Edited by M.A. Varley. CAB International, Wallingford.

Cross, M.L. and Gill, H.S. (1999) Modulation of immune function by modified bovine whey protein concentrate. *Immunology and Cell Biology*, **77**, 345-350.

Cummins, A.G., Steele, T.W., LaBrooy J.T. and Shearman, D.J.C. (1988) Maturation of the rat small intestine at weaning: Changes in the epithelial cell kinetics, bacterial flora, and mucosal immune activity. *Gut*, **29**, 1672-1679.

Cunha Ferreira, R. da, Forsyth, L.E., Richman, P.I., Wells, C., Spencer, J. and MacDonald, T.T. (1990) Changes in the rate of crypt epithelial cell proliferation and mucosal morphology induced by a T-cell-mediated response in human small intestine. *Gastroenterology*, **98**, 1255-1263.

Deprez, P., Deroose, P., Van den Hende, C., Muylle, E. and Oyaert, W. (1987) Liquid versus dry feeding in weaned piglets: The influence on small intestinal morphology. *Journal of Veterinary Medicine and Biology*, **34**, 254-259.

Diamond, J.M. and Karasov, W.H. (1983) Trophic control of the intestinal mucosa. *Nature (London)*, **304**, 18.

Donovan, S.M. and Odle, J. (1994) Growth factors in milk as mediators of infant development. *Annual Review of Nutrition*, **14**, 147-167.

Dréau, D. and Lallès, J.P. (1999) Contribution to the study of gut hypersensitivity reactions to soybean proteins in preruminant calves and early-weaned piglets. *Livestock Production Science*, **60**, 209-218.

Epstein, A.A. (1986) The ontogeny of ingestive behaviour: control of milk intake by suckling rats and the emergence of feeding and drinking at weaning. *In Feeding Behaviour, Neural and Hormonal Controls*, pp.1-26. Edited by R.C. Ritter, S. Ritter and C.D. Barnes. Academic Press, Florida.

Ermer, P.M., Miller, P.S. and Lewis, A.J. (1994) Diet preference and meal patterns of weanling pigs offered diets containing either spray-dried porcine plasma or dried skim milk. *Journal of Animal Science*, **72**, 1548-1554.

Friedrich, M. (1989) Physiology of intestinal digestion and absorption. *In Protein Metabolism in Farm Animals: Evolution, Digestion, Absorption, and Metabolism*, pp. 218-272. Edited by H.-D. Bock, B.O. Eggum, A.G. Low, O. Simon and T. Zebrowska. Oxford University Press, Oxford.

Froetschel, M.A. (1996) Bioactive peptides in digesta that regulate gastrointestinal function and intake. *Journal of Animal Science*, **74**, 2500-2508.

Funderburke, D.W. (1985) Physiological changes in the weanling pig resulting from nutritional, environmental and psychological stressors. PhD Thesis, University of Georgia.

Ganessunker, D., Gaskins, R.H., Zuckermann, F.A. and Donovan, S.M. (1999) Total parenteral nutrition alters molecular and cellular indices of intestinal inflammation in neonatal piglets. *Journal of Parenteral and Enteral Nutrition*, **23**, 337-344.

Gaskins, H.R. and Kelley, K.W. (1995) Immunology and neonatal mortality. *In The Neonatal Pig: Development and Survival*, pp. 39-55. Edited by M.A. Varley. CAB International, Wallingford.

Gill, H.S. and Rutherfurd, K.J. (1998) Immunomodulatory properties of bovine milk. *International Dairy Federation Bulletin*, **336**, 31-35.

Gomez, G.G., Phillips, O. and Goforth, R.A. (1998) Effect of immunoglobulin source on survival, growth, and hematological and immunological variables in pigs. *Journal of Animal Science*, **76**, 1-7.

Goodlad, R.A., Lee, C.Y. and Wright, N.A. (1992) Cell proliferation in the small intestine and colon of intravenously fed rats: effects of urogastrone-epidermal growth factor. *Cell Proliferation*, **25**, 393-404.

Goodlad, R.A., Plumb, J.A. and Wright, N.A. (1988) Epithelial cell proliferation and intestinal absorptive function during starvation and refeeding in the rat. *Clinical Sciences*, **74**, 301-306.

Goodlad, R.A. and Wright, N.A. (1984) The effects of starvation and refeeding on intestinal cell proliferation in the mouse. *Virchows Archives [Cell Pathology]*, **45**, 63-73.

Goodlad, R.A. and Wright, N.A. (1990) Changes in intestinal cell proliferation, absorptive capacity and structure in young, adult and old rats. *Journal of Anatomy*, **173**, 109-118.

Grinstead, G.S., Goodband, R.D., Dritz, S.S., Tokach, M.D., Nelssen, J.L., Woodworth, J.C. and Molitor, M. (2000) Effects of a whey protein product and spray-dried animal plasma on growth performance of weanling pigs. *Journal of Animal Science*, **78**, 647-657.

Hall, G.A. and Byrne, T.F. (1989) Effects of age and diet on small intestinal structure and function in gnotobiotic piglets. *Research in Veterinary Science*, **47**, 387-392.

Hampson, D.J. (1983) Post-weaning changes in the piglet small intestine in relation to growth-checks and diarrhoea. PhD Thesis, University of Bristol.

Hampson, D.J. (1986a) Alterations in piglet small intestinal structure at weaning. *Research in Veterinary Science*, **40**, 32-40.

Hampson, D.J. (1986b) Attempts to modify changes in the piglet small intestine after weaning. *Research in Veterinary Science*, **40**, 313-317.

Hampson, D.J. and Kidder, D.E. (1986) Influence of creep feeding and weaning on brush border enzyme activities in the piglet small intestine. *Research in Veterinary Science*, **40**, 24-31.

James, P.S., Smith, M.W. and Tivey, D.R. (1988) Single-villus analysis of disaccharidase expression by different regions of the mouse intestine. *Journal of Physiology*, **393**, 583-594.

Jiang, R., Chang, X., Stoll, B., Fan, M.Z., Arthington, J., Weaver, E., Campbell, J. and Burrin, D.G. (2000) Dietary plasma protein reduces small intestinal growth and lamina propria cell density in early weaned pigs. *Journal of Nutrition*, **130**, 21-26.

Johnson, L.R. (1987) Regulation of gastrointestinal growth. *In Physiology of the Gastrointestinal Tract*, 2nd edition, pp. 301-333. Edited by L.R. Johnson, J. Christensen, E.D. Jacobson, M.J. Jackson and J.H. Walsh. Raven Press, New York.

Kelly, D. (1994) Colostrum, growth factors and intestinal development in pigs. *In VIth International Symposium on Digestive Physiology in Pigs*, pp. 151-166. Edited by W.-B. Souffrant and H. Hagemeister. EAAP Publication N° 80, Forschungsinstitut für die Biologie landwirtschaftlicher Nutztiere (FBN), Dummerstorf.

Kelly, D., Begbie, R. and King, T.P. (1992) Postnatal intestinal development. *In Neonatal Survival and Growth*, pp. 63-79. Edited by M.A. Varley, P.E.V. Williams and T.L.J. Lawrence. British Society of Animal Production, Occasional Publication No. 15, Edinburgh.

Kelly, D., Greene, J., O'Brien, J.J. and McCracken, K.J. (1984) Gavage feeding of early-weaned pigs to study the effect of diet on digestive development and changes in intestinal microflora. *In Proceedings of the VIIIth International Pig Veterinary Society Congress*, p. 317. Edited by M. Tensaert, J. Hoorens, P.H. Lampo, P.B. Onte, W. Coussement and P. Debouck. Faculty of Veterinary Medicine, State University of Ghent, Belgium.

Kelly, D., King, T.P., McFadyen, M. and Travis, A.J. (1991a) Effect of lactation on the decline of brush border lactase activity in neonatal pigs. *Gut*, **32**, 386-392.

Kelly, D., Smyth, J.A. and McCracken, K.J. (1990) Effect of creep feeding on structural and functional changes of the gut of early weaned pigs. *Research in Veterinary Science*, **48**, 350-356.

Kelly, D., Smyth, J.A. and McCracken, K.J. (1991b) Digestive development in the early-weaned pig. I. Effect of continuous nutrient supply on the development of the digestive tract and on changes in digestive enzyme activity during the first week post-weaning. *British Journal of Nutrition*, **65**, 169-180.

Kelly, D., Smyth, J.A. and McCracken, K.J. (1991c) Digestive development in the early-weaned pig. II. Effect of level of food intake on digestive enzyme activity during the immediate post-weaning period. *British Journal of Nutrition*, **65**, 181-188.

Kidder, D.E. and Manners, M.J. (1980) The level and distribution of carbohydrases in the small intestine mucosa of pigs from 3 weeks of age to maturity. *British Journal of Nutrition*, **43**, 141-153.

King, M.R., Morel, P.C.H., Revell, D.K., James, E.A.J., Birtles, M.J. and Pluske, J.R. (1999) Bovine colostrum supplementation increases villous height in sucking pigs. *In Manipulating Pig Production VII*, p. 255. Edited by P.D. Cranwell. Australasian Pig Science Association, Werribee.

Koong, L.-J. and Ferrell, C.L. (1990) Effects of short term nutritional manipulation on organ size and fasting heat production. *European Journal of Clinical Nutrition*, **44 (Suppl.1)**, 73-77.

Koong, L.-J., Nienaber, J.A., Pekas, J.C. and Yen, J.-T. (1982) Effects of plane of nutrition on organ size and fasting heat production in pigs. *Journal of Nutrition*, **112**, 1638-1642.

Le Dividich, J. and Herpin, P. (1994) Effects of climatic conditions on the performance, metabolism and health status of weaned piglets: a review. *Livestock Production Science*, **38**, 79-90.

Leibbrandt, V.D., Ewen, R.C., Speer, V.C. and Zimmerman, D.R. (1975) Effect of weaning and age at weaning on baby pig performance. *Journal of Animal Science*, **40**, 1077-1080.

Li, D.F., Nelssen, J.L., Reddy, P.G., Blecha, F., Klemm, R.D. and Goodband, R.D. (1991) Interrelationship between hypersensitivity to soybean proteins and growth performance in early-weaned pigs. *Journal of Animal Science*, **69**, 4062-4069.

Lionetti, P., Breese, E., Braegger, C.P., Murch, S.H., Taylor, J. and MacDonald, T.T. (1993) T-cell activation can induce either mucosal destruction or adaptation in cultured human fetal small intestine. *Gastroenterology*, **105**, 373-381.

Manners, M.J. and Stevens, J.A. (1972) Changes from birth to maturity in the pattern of distribution of lactase and sucrase activity in the mucosa of the small intestine of pigs. *British Journal of Nutrition*, **28**, 113-127.

McCracken, B.A., Gaskins, R.H., Ruwe-Kaiser, P.J., Klasing, K.C. and Jewell, D.E. (1995) Diet-dependent and diet-independent metabolic responses underlie growth stasis of pigs at weaning. *Journal of Nutrition*, **125**, 2838-2845.

McCracken, B.A., Spurlock, M.E., Roos, M.A., Zuckermann, F.A. and Gaskins, R.H. (1999) Weaning anorexia may contribute to local inflammation in the piglet small intestine. *Journal of Nutrition*, **129**, 613-619.

McCracken, K.J. (1984) Effect of diet composition on digestive development of early-weaned pigs. *Proceedings of the Nutrition Society*, **43**, 109A.

McCracken, K.J. and Kelly, D. (1984) Effect of diet and post-weaning food intake on digestive development of early-weaned pigs. *Proceedings of the Nutrition Society*, **43**, 110A.

McNeill, L.K. and Hamilton, J.R. (1971) The effect of fasting on disaccharidase activity in the rat small intestine. *Pediatrics*, **47**, 65-72.

Miller, B.G., James, P.S., Smith, M.W. and Bourne, F.J. (1986) Effect of weaning on the capacity of pig intestinal villi to digest and absorb nutrients. *Journal of Agricultural Science, Cambridge*, **107**, 579-589.

Morel, P.C.H., Schollum, L.M., Buwalda, T.R. and Pearson, G. (1995) Digestibility of bovine immunoglobulin in the piglet. *In Manipulating Pig Production V*, p. 181. Edited by D.P. Hennessy and P.D. Cranwell. Australasian Pig Science Association, Werribee.

Mroz, Z., Grela, E.R., Matras, J., Krasucki, W., Kichura, T. and Shipp, T.E. (1999) Passive protection of piglets against diarrhoea with specialized egg immunoglobulins (Protimax). *In Manipulating Pig Production VII*, p. 238. Edited by P.D. Cranwell. Australasian Pig Science Association, Werribee.

Nabuurs, M.J.A., Hoogendoorn, A. and Zijderveld, F.G. van (1994) Effects of weaning and enterotoxigenic *Escherichia coli* on net absorption in the small intestine of pigs. *Research in Veterinary Science*, **56**, 379-385.

Newby, T.J., Stokes, C.R. and Bourne, F.J. (1982) Immunological activity of milk. *Veterinary Immunology and Immunopathology*, **3**, 67-94.

Núñez, M.C., Bueno, J.D., Ayudarte, M.V., Almendros, A., Ríos, A., Suárez, M.D., and Gil, A. (1995) Dietary restriction induces biochemical and morphometric changes in the small intestine of nursing piglets. *Journal of Nutrition*, **126**, 933-944.

Odle, J., Zijlstra, R.T. and Donovan, S.M. (1996) Intestinal effects of milkborne growth factors in neonates of agricultural importance. *Journal of Animal Science*, **74**, 2509-2522.

Pakkanen, R. and Aalto, J. (1997) Growth factors and antimicrobial factors of bovine colostrum. *International Dairy Journal*, **7**, 285-297.

Partridge, G.G., Fisher, J., Gregory, H. and Prior, S.G. (1992) Automated wet feeding of weaner pigs versus conventional dry feeding: effects on growth rate and food consumption. *Animal Production*, **54**, 484 (Abstr.).

Pekas, J.C. and Wray, J.E. (1991) Principal gastrointestinal variables associated with metabolic heat production in pigs: Statistical cluster analyses. *Journal of Nutrition*, **121**, 231-239.

Pluske, J.R. (1993) Psychological and nutritional stress in pigs at weaning: Production parameters, the stress response, and histology and biochemistry of the small intestine. PhD Thesis, The University of Western Australia.

Pluske, J.R. and Dong, G.Z. (1998) Factors influencing the utilisation of colostrum and milk. *In The Lactating Sow*, pp. 45-70. Edited by M.W.A. Verstegen, P.J. Moughan and J.W. Schrama. Wageningen Pers, Wageningen.

Pluske, J.R., Gaskins, R.H., Morel, P.C.H., Revell, D.K., King, M.R. and James, E.A.J. (1999a) The number of villus and crypt CD4+ cells in the jejunum of piglets increases after weaning. *In Manipulating Pig Production VII*, p. 244. Edited by P.D. Cranwell. Australasian Pig Science Association, Werribee.

Pluske, J.R., Hampson, D.J. and Williams, I.H. (1997) Factors influencing the structure and function of the small intestine in the weaned pig: a review. *Livestock Production Science*, **51**, 215-236.

Pluske, J.R., Pearson, G., Morel, P.C.H., King, M.R., Skilton, G. and Skilton, R. (1999b) A bovine colostrum product in a weaner diet increases growth rate and reduces days to slaughter. *In Manipulating Pig Production VII*, p. 256. Edited by P.D. Cranwell. Australasian Pig Science Association, Werribee.

Pluske, J.R., Thompson, M.J., Atwood, C.S., Bird, P.H., Williams, I.H. and Hartmann, P.E. (1996a) Maintenance of villous height and crypt depth, and enhancement of disaccharide digestion and monosaccharide absorption, in piglets fed cows' whole milk after weaning. *British Journal of Nutrition*, **76**, 409-422.

Pluske, J.R., Williams, I.H. and Aherne, F.X. (1996b) Maintenance of villous height and crypt depth in piglets by providing continuous nutrition after weaning. *Animal Science*, **62**, 131-144.

Pluske, J.R., Williams, I.H. and Aherne, F.X. (1996c) Villous height and crypt depth in piglets in response to increases in the intake of cows' milk after weaning. *Animal Science*, **62**, 145-158.

Puchal, A.A. and Buddington, R.K. (1992) Postnatal development of monosaccharide transport in pig intestine. *American Journal of Physiology*, **262**, G895-G902.

Robertson, A.M., Clark, J.J. and Bruce, J.M (1985) Observed energy intake of weaned piglets and its effect on temperature requirements. *Animal Production*, **40**, 475-479.

Seare, N.J. and Playford, R.J. (1998) Growth factors and gut function. *Proceedings of the Nutrition Society*, 57, 403-408.

Selby, E., Cadogan, D.J., Campbell, R.G. and Choct, M. (1999) The effect of steeping and enzyme supplementation on the performance of liquid-fed weaner pigs. *In Manipulating Pig Production VII*, p. 38. Edited by P.D. Cranwell. Australasian Pig Science Association, Werribee.

Shulman, R.J., Henning, S.J. and Nicholls, B.L. (1988) The miniature pig as an animal model for the study of intestinal enzyme development. *Pediatric Research*, 23, 311-315.

Tang, M., Laarveld, B., Van Kessel, A.G., Hamilton, D.L., Estrada, A. and Pateience, J.F. (1999) Effect of segregated early weaning on postweaning small intestinal development in pigs. *Journal of Animal Science*, 77, 3191-3200.

Toplis, P., Blanchard, P.J. and Miller, H.M. (1999) Creep feed offered as a gruel prior to weaning enhances performance of weaned piglets. *In Manipulating Pig Production VII*, p. 129. Edited by P.D. Cranwell. Australasian Pig Science Association, Werribee.

Tsuboi, K.K., Kwong, L.K., D'Harlingue, A.E., Stevenson, D.K., Kerner, Jr., J.A. and Sunshine, P. (1985) The nature of maturational decline of intestinal lactase activity. *Biochimical and Biophysical Acta*, 840, 69-78.

Tsuboi, K.K., Kwong, L.K., Neu, J. and Sunshine, P. (1981) A proposed mechanism of normal intestinal lactase decline in the postweaned mammal. *Biochemical and Biophysical Research Communications*, 101, 645-652.

Vanavichial, B., Morel, P.C.H., Revell, D.K., James, E.A.J., Camden, B.J. and Schollum, L.M. (1997) Provision of immunoglobulins to sucking pigs can enhance post-weaning growth performance. *In Manipulating Pig Production VII*, p. 308. Edited by P.D. Cranwell. Australasian Pig Science Association, Werribee.

Van Beers-Schreurs, H.M.G., Nabuurs, M.J.A., Vellenga, L., Kalsbeek-van der Valk, H.J., Wensing, T. and Breukink, H.J. (1998) Weaning and the weanling diet influence the villous height and crypt depth in the small intestine of pigs and alter concentrations of short-chain fatty acids in the large intestine and blood. *Journal of Nutrition*, 128, 947-953.

Van Dijk, J.E., Mouwen, J.M.V.M. and Koninkx, J.F.J.G. (1999) Review on histology and absorptive capacity of the gastrointestinal epithelium. *In Nutrition and gastrointestinal physiology – today and tomorrow*, pp. 1-9. Edited by A.J.M. Jansman and B.P.M. Janszen. TNO Nutrition and Food Research Institute, Wageningen.

Webster, A.J.F. (1980) The energetic efficiency of growth. *Livestock Production Science*, 7, 243-252.

Webster, A.J.F. (1981) The energetic efficiency of metabolism. *Proceedings of the Nutrition Society*, 40, 121-128.

Williams, C.A., Philips, T. and Macdonald, I. (1983) The influence of glucose on serum galactose levels in man. *Metabolism*, **32**, 250-256.

Williams, E.A., Rumsey, R.D.E. and Powers, H.J. (1996) Cytokinetic and structural responses of the rat small intestine to riboflavin depletion. *British Journal of Nutrition*, **75**, 315-324.

Wright, N.A. (1982) The experimental analysis of changes in proliferative and morphological status in studies on the intestine. *Scandinavian Journal of Gastroenterology*, **17** (**Suppl. 74**), 3-10.

Xu, R.-J. (1996) Development of the newborn GI tract and its relation to colostrum/milk intake: a review. *Reproduction, Fertility and Development*, **8**, 35-48.

Yeh, K.C. and Kwan, K.C. (1978) A comparison of numerical integrating algorithms by trapezoidal, lagrange and spline approximation. *Journal of Pharmacokinetics and Biopharmaceutics*, **6**, 79-98.

Ziegler, T.R., Estívariz, C.F., Jonas, C.R., Gu, L.H., Jones, D.P. and Leader, L.M. (1999) Interactions between nutrients and peptide growth factors in intestinal growth, repair, and function. *Journal of Parenteral and Enteral Nutrition*, **23**, S174-S183.

# 2

# THE ROLE OF POLYAMINES IN INTESTINAL FUNCTION AND GUT MATURATION

Susan Bardocz, Ann White, George Grant, Tracey J. Walker, David S. Brown and Arpad Pusztai
*The Rowett Research Institute, Bucksburn, Aberdeen AB21 9SB Scotland, UK*

## Summary

In the gut, putrescine can be used as an immediate energy source either to fuel adaptational gut growth or to supply energy to the fasting gut. Therefore, changes in the polyamine pool size of the gut and its uptake capacity, as well as the polyamine content of the milk and serum, were measured in rats from birth to weaning. The putrescine content of milk increased between days 1-7, but thereafter remained constant. During suckling, the spermidine and spermine content remained constant. The polyamine content of milk, compared with solid food, was low. Polyamines were continuously absorbed from the gut. At 7 days of age about 74-90% of spermidine and spermine was absorbed. By day 14, the percentage was 80-82% and on the day of weaning only 32-57% was absorbed. By day 28, absorption was at the values measured in adult rats. Serum spermidine content increased between days 18 and 19 and reflected the changes in dietary intake and capacity of absorption. Spermine content showed an increase between days 19 and 20 only, when suckling stopped. Weaning also coincided with a drop in serum putrescine content. The polyamine content of blood did not reflect any of the dietary changes.

## Introduction

Growth requires nutrients and energy, provided by the food/feed and components of the diet. These are fully or partially degraded and absorbed by the gut to be made available for the rest of the body. The distribution of nutrients between the internal organs is under the strict control of hormones, growth factors and cytokines.

   The natural polyamines (the diamine putrescine and the polyamines spermidine and spermine; Figure 1) are essential for cell growth and proliferation, although their exact function in cellular metabolism is still unclear (Jänne, Pösö and Raina,

1978; Pegg, 1986; Tabor and Tabor, 1984). However, it is well established that whenever hormones, growth factors or cytokines act on cells there is an immediate increase in cellular polyamine concentrations and the activity of the enzyme ornithine decarboxylase (ODC, EC 4.1.1.17), the first enzyme of polyamine biosynthesis (Figure 1), indicating that polyamines act as possible second messengers. When cells in culture are restricted in their ability to either synthetise or take up polyamines from the medium, proliferation stops after the second or third cell division (Heby and Persson, 1990). Removal of the inhibitor or adding polyamines to the culture medium restores the ability of the cells to divide.

Contrary to earlier reports that all the polyamines required by the cell are formed by *de novo* synthesis, we found that the biosynthetic capacity of some organs is not always sufficient to satisfy their polyamine requirement (Bardocz, Grant, Brown, Ewen and Pusztai, 1989; Bardocz, Grant, Brown, Wallace, Ewen and Pusztai, 1989; Pusztai, Grant, Brown, Ewen and Bardocz, 1988). This is especially true for the gut. In several models, such as the fasting-refeeding (Bardocz, Grant, Brown, Ewen, Stewart and Pusztai, 1991) or the lectin-induced adaptational growth of the gut, most of the polyamines originated from other, external sources (Bardocz, Brown, Grant and Pusztai, 1990).

## Polyamine pools of the gut and the body

When studying the phytohaemagglutinin (PHA) induced gut growth model in the rat, it became evident, that most of the polyamines necessary for cell proliferation in the crypts of the Lieberkuhn came from the systemic circulation via the basolateral membrane of the cells. Only this uptake system is stimulated during gut growth, with the polyamine body pool being the supplier via systemic circulation (Figure 2; Bardocz *et al.*, 1990). During gut growth, polyamine absorption from the gut lumen remains unchanged. Although dietary polyamines are absorbed from the gut lumen, probably using free diffusion as an uptake mechanism, at least under normal physiological conditions (Bardócz, Grant, Hughes, Brown and Pusztai, 1999), they do not directly contribute to the gut polyamine pool. The absorbed polyamines are distributed between the organs according to their need (Figure 3) and converted to the most preferred form using the interconversion pathway (Figure 1). Excess luminal polyamines are metabolised by gut bacteria or excreted with faeces.

The polyamine body pool is depleted according to the demands of the different organs and replenished by polyamines originating from food and biosynthesis (Ralph, Englyst and Bardócz, 1999; White and Bardócz, 1999). The exact location of the "body pool" has not been studied in detail, but the main organs of biosynthesis are the liver and the kidneys. From there, the polyamines can re-enter the circulation,

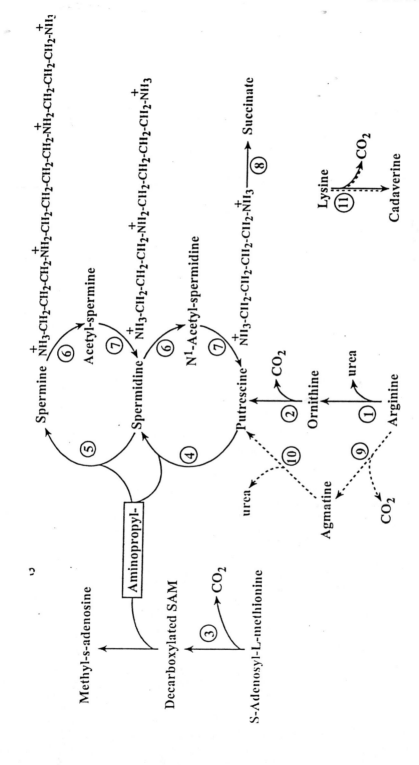

Figure 1. Structure, biosynthesis and 'interconversion' of polyamines. Dotted lines mark alternative pathways in bacteria and plants. 1=arginase (EC 3.5.3.1); 2=ornithine decarboxylase (EC 4.1.1.17); 3= S-adenosyl-L-methionine decarboxylase (EC 4.1.1.50); 4=spermidine synthase (EC 2.5.1.16); 5=spermine synthase (EC 2.5.1.22); 6=spermidine/spermine N¹-acetyltransferase activity (EC 2.3.1.57); 7=polyamine oxidase (EC 1.5.3.11); 8=diamine oxidase (EC 1.4.3.6); 9=arginine decarboxylase (EC 4.1.1.19); 10=agmatinase (EC 3.5.3.11); 11=lysine decarboxylase (EC 4.1.1.18).

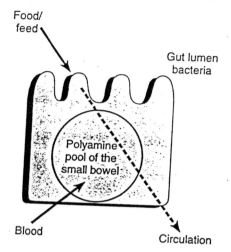

Figure 2. Novel model for gut polyamine uptake.

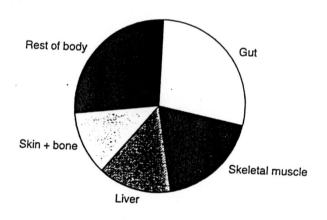

Figure 3. Distribution of spermidine between the internal organs.

in a similar manner to the semi-indispensable amino acids. The origin and usage of the body polyamine pool and terminal catabolism is shown in Figure 4.

## Polyamine content of food/feed and contribution by the bacterial flora

Since polyamines are ubiquitous to every living cell, it is not surprising that the food or feed contains large amounts of polyamines. In an adult rat, dietary polyamines can contribute half of the body pool daily (Figure 4). As an example, the composition of two industrial creep meal and piglet diets is given in Table 1.

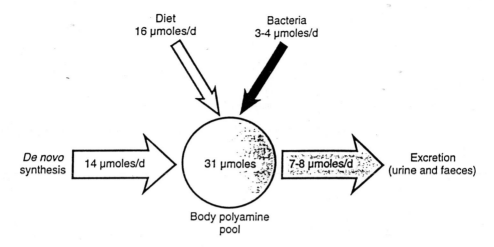

**Figure 4.** Possible daily contribution of *de novo* biosynthesis, diet and gut bacteria to the body polyamine pool of a 100 g rat.

**Table 1.** Polyamine composition of piglet rations.

| Feed | Polyamines (nmoles/g feed) | | |
| --- | --- | --- | --- |
| | *Putrescine* | *Spermidine* | *Spermine* |
| Creep meal | 212 ± 26 | 207 ± 28 | 59 ± 1 |
| Creep pellet | 214 ± 12 | 245 ± 27 | 52 ± 1 |
| Feed 1 | 388 ± 38 | 276 ± 25 | 60 ± 10 |
| Feed 2 | 562 ± 59 | 312 ± 33 | 76 ± 2 |
| Rat chow | 223 ± 26 | 570 ± 50 | 110 ± 28 |

Data are the mean analysis of 3 rations of the same diet ± SD except for rat chow

There is a continuing discussion about the contribution of bacterial flora to the polyamine body pool. In rats, this contribution appears minimal. In healthy, well-fed rats, the bacterial numbers in the small bowel, which is the major site of polyamine absorption, are minimal. However, in animals treated with antibiotics, killed bacteria may liberate their polyamine and biogenic amine contents for absorption from the bowel.

## Biogenic amines

The biogenic amines (cadaverine, histamine, tyramine, tryptamine) are formed by bacterial decarboxylases from free amino acids under acidic conditions. Animal feed, especially if it is prepared from starting materials of low hygienic standards, can contain large amounts of biogenic amines with detrimental effect on young animals (Bardocz, 1995). Of the biogenic amines, cadaverine and histamine are also substrates of the enzyme diamine oxidase (DAO, EC 1.4.3.6). The pig rations in Table 1 also contained large amounts of cadaverine (399±64; 431±27; 847±49 and 1236±16) and histamine (37±30; 61±1; 164±31 and 277±21 nmoles/g feed), respectively. When high amounts of diamines and histamine occur in food, the gut is unable to degrade them. If these amines enter systemic circulation they are able to exert their biological effect on the hormonal and immune system. This is most likely to happen in young animals whose gut is immature: their DAO activity is low compared with adults since they are unable to metabolise all the diamines (histamine). Therefore, it is important to keep the cadaverine, histamine and diamine content of the feed low allowing the gut to oxidise putrescine effectively.

## Diamine and polyamine oxidases in the gut

Both the terminal catabolism of polyamines and their interconversion is based on the presence of oxidases (Morgan, 1999). The above mentioned enzyme DAO is responsible for putrescine degradation (γ-aminobutyric acid and succinate formation, see below) and this enzyme is considered to be a marker for gut maturation (Luk, Vaughan, Burke and Baylin, 1981; Sessa, Tunici, Ewen, Grant, Pusztai, Bardocz and Perin, 1995). In immature animals or during intensive crypt cell proliferation/villus cell turnover the activity of this enzyme decreases, while the activity of polyamine oxidase (PAO, EC 1.5.3.11) increased. This enzyme converts acetylated spermidine to putrescine or acetylated spermine to spermidine (Figure 1), and also acts on spermine when present at high concentrations (Sessa et al., 1995). The consequences of these changes are that, in an animal with a less mature gut, more putrescine escapes oxidation and less of the acetyl-polyamines are oxidised. PAO also adapts to polyamine consumption: when rats are fed exclusively on spermidine- or spermine-containing diets the activity of the enzyme increases in their gut (Sessa, Tunici, Rabellotti, Bardocz, Grant and Pusztai, 1996).

## Role of putrescine in the gut

It has been suggested that putrescine acts as a growth factor for the gut (Seidel, Haddox and Johnson, 1985) although the mechanism of this is still unclear. Putrescine is a precursor of the polyamines spermidine and spermine (Figure 1) and when catabolised by acetylation and oxidation, or just oxidised to γ-aminobutyric acid (GABA), it can act as a direct growth factor.

The localisation of putrescine and ODC in the small intestinal mucosa is surprising. ODC activity is higher and more putrescine is found in the non-proliferating epithelial cells at the tip of the villi than in the crypts where putrescine would be needed for polyamine synthesis to support cell proliferation. If the role of ODC is to produce polyamines via putrescine locally, it is unreconcilable with the low concentration of spermidine and spermine and with the localization of DAO in the same cells. Although DAO might be present in the plasma membrane of the cells, it can either oxidise luminal putrescine, probably during uptake into the cells, or the putrescine formed by ODC. If one considers the concentration of polyamines, especially of putrescine, in the gut compartments with different functions and relates that to the activities of enzymes responsible for biosynthesis and metabolism (Figure 5; Luk and Baylin, 1983), the correlation suggests a role for putrescine as an instant energy source to kick start the growth process or supplying energy for the fasting gut (Bardócz, Grant, Brown and Pusztai, 1998). This is supported by the fact that, in fasting animals, the uptake of putrescine is stimulated but upon refeeding it returns to basal levels, and during adaptational gut growth the uptake of putrescine is stimulated within the first hour (Bardocz *et al.*, 1990). Therefore, the gut can use putrescine as an instant energy source when the nutrient supply is limited or there is a need to kick start growth. There is an intricate metabolic connection between ornithine, α-ketoglutarate, glutamine, putrescine, GABA and succinate (Figure 6).

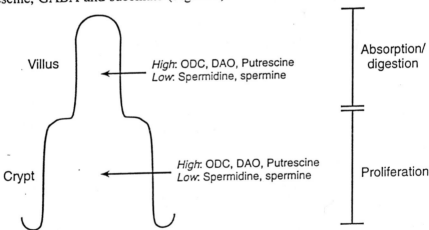

**Figure 5.** Distribution of ODC, DAO and polyamines along the villus-cryptases.

## Role of spermidine and spermine

In the cells at the tip of the villus the concentration of spermidine and spermine is lower than in the crypt. In the crypt compartment, where the actual cell division

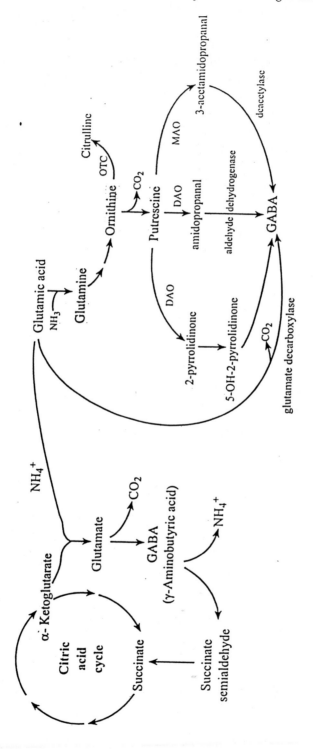

**Figure 6.** Metabolic relationship between ornithine, α-ketoglutarate, glutamine, putrescine, GABA and succinate. (MAO: monoamine oxidase; OTC: ornithine transcarbamoylase)

happens the activities of ODC and DAO are lower, but the concentration of spermidine and spermine are higher (Figure 4). This can only be explained by a continual uptake of these molecules from the circulation via the basolateral membrane. A very special role for spermine, and to some extent spermidine, in the gut of young rats has been suggested by Dandrifosse and colleagues (Dufour, Dandrifosse, Forget, Vermesse, Romain and Lepoint, 1988). They observed that if rat pups are intubated with doses of spermidine or spermine before weaning, precocious maturation of their gut, pancreas and liver occurs (Dandrifosse, Deloyer, El Khefif and Peulen, 1999). This process is more specific to spermine than to spermidine, but glucocorticoids and other hormones are implicated in exerting some of these effects.

## Polyamine metabolism and uptake of young rats

From birth, the small bowel grows and develops continuously with age. The gut of new born rat pups is immature and only reaches its full maturity after weaning. The protein content and polyamine pool increases steadily in the rat, parallel with its growth with the biggest increases occurring in all parameters measured between days 1 and 7 (Table 2).

**Table 2.** Changes in growth and composition of the rat small intestine at different ages.

| | Ages (days) | | | |
| --- | --- | --- | --- | --- |
| | *1* | *7* | *14* | *28* |
| *Small bowel* | | | | |
| Weight (g) | $0.16 \pm 0.01$ | $0.65 \pm 0.07$ | $1.38 \pm 0.06$ | $3.21 \pm 0.69$ |
| Length (cm) | $20 \pm 0$ | $30 \pm 0$ | $58 \pm 1$ | $76 \pm 2$ |
| Protein (mg) | $13.8 \pm 1.5$ | $49.0 \pm 5.8$ | $93.7 \pm 3.3$ | $306.4 \pm 60.5$ |
| RNA (mg) | $0.67 \pm 0.11$ | $2.64 \pm 0.34$ | $7.45 \pm 0.68$ | $26.55 \pm 1.94$ |
| DNA (mg) | $0.42 \pm 0.02$ | $4.54 \pm 0.14$ | $3.88 \pm 0.16$ | $11.08 \pm 0.33$ |
| *Polyamines (nmoles)* | | | | |
| Putrescine | $3.7 \pm 0.3$ | $9.6 \pm 2.0$ | $16.6 \pm 0.4$ | $27.8 \pm 4.2$ |
| Spermidine | $13.9 \pm 2.3$ | $31.9 \pm 3.6$ | $98.2 \pm 17.9$ | $165.8 \pm 7.8$ |
| Spermine | $4.6 \pm 0.8$ | $15.3 \pm 1.8$ | $39.5 \pm 0.2$ | $77.8 \pm 5.2$ |
| *Polyamine uptake (nmoles/h)* | | | | |
| Putrescine* | ND | $0.85 \pm 0.03$ | $1.15 \pm 0.04$ | $9.04 \pm 2.1$ |
| Spermidine** | ND | $2.15 \pm 0.45$ | $2.93 \pm 0.12$ | $0.60 \pm 0.19$ |
| Spermine** | ND | $1.52 \pm 0.31$ | $1.96 \pm 0.79$ | $0.41 \pm 0.13$ |

Data represent means ± SD for 5 male rats; ND: not determined; Total amount intubated: *8.5 nmoles; **9.9 nmoles

**Table 3.** Polyamine composition of rat milk/feed and stomach content at different ages.

| | Ages (days) | | | | | |
|---|---|---|---|---|---|---|
| | *1* | *7* | *14* | *18* | *19* | *28* |
| Body weight (g) | 6.3 ± 0.3 | 16.1 ± 0.6 | 24.7 ± 1.6 | 34.5 ± 1.6 | 38.5 ± 1.3 | 69.5 ± 2.7 |
| *Milk/feed Polyamines (nmoles/g)* | | | | | | |
| Putrescine | 16.95 ± 10.16 | 47.28 ± 20.43 | 55.65 ± 9.61 | 30.77 ± 24.28 | 33.60 ± 9.73 | 156 ± 12 |
| Spermidine | 86.47 ± 29.99 | 118.85 ± 22.52 | 118.85 ± 15.85 | 110.9 ± 32.85 | 51.6 ± 8.09 | 461 ± 35 |
| Spermine | 45.38 ± 30.34 | 55.53 ± 20.96 | 58.30 ± 20.51 | 57.50 ± 11.65 | 53.05 ± 7.11 | 78 ± 9 |
| *Polyamines in stomach content (nmoles/g)* | | | | | | |
| Putrescine | 2.0 ± 0.9 | 13.9 ± 6.8 | 24.8 ± 12.2 | 13.9 ± 10.1 | 63.5 ± 19.4 | 13.1 ± 8.0 |
| Spermidine | 12.1 ± 2.7 | 42.8 ± 10.2 | 49.5 ± 13.8 | 45.5 ± 4.6 | 97.7 ± 10.5 | 168 ± 39 |
| Spermine | 6.2 ± 1.7 | 16.7 ± 5.8 | 12.9 ± 2.3 | 8.1 ± 1.6 | 102.3 ± 13.1 | 38 ± 1 |
| *Polyamine uptake (% of intubated)* | | | | | | |
| Putrescine | ND | 74 ± 2 | 79 ± 2 | ND | 71 ± 3 | 62 ± 9 |
| Spermidine | ND | 88 ± 1 | 73 ± 1 | ND | 32 ± 4 | 37 ± 8 |
| Spermine | ND | 93 ± 1 | 80 ± 3 | ND | 57 ± 6 | 41 ± 9 |

Data represent means ± SD for 5 males rats

Pups after a period of suckling were removed from their mother and their stomach content analysed 1 h later

8.5 nmoles putrescine, or 9.9 nmoles spermidine or spermine were intubated intragastrically and uptake was measured after 1 h

However, there is a growth check between days 19-20, when the animals are weaned (Table 4). Up to 14 days of age all nutrients are derived from maternal milk (thereafter the pups nibble on their mother's food and faeces). The polyamine composition of rat milk up to 28 days after birth is given in Table 3. The putrescine content of maternal milk increased between days 1 and 7, but thereafter remained constant within experimental errors. During the suckling period the spermidine content remained constant but dropped on day 19, whereas the spermine content did not change. Compared with solid food, the putrescine, spermidine and spermine content of rat milk is much lower (day 28, Table 3).

**Table 4.** Changes in small bowel and serum/blood polyamine content during weaning.

| | Ages (days) | | | |
|---|---|---|---|---|
| | *18* | *19* | *20* | *21* |
| Body weight (g) | 34.7 ± 1.6 | 38.5 ± 1.3 | 39.8 ± 2.6 | 42.8 ± 1.4 |
| *Small bowel* | | | | |
| Weight (g) | 1.28 ± 0.08 | 1.66 ± 0.06 | 1.67 ± 0.21 | 2.17 ± 0.13 |
| Length (cm) | 52 ± 0 | 60 ± 1 | 60 ± 1 | 70 ± 2 |
| Protein (mg) | 185 ± 14 | 197 ± 19 | 200 ± 25 | 186 ± 11 |
| RNA (mg) | 8.1 ± 0.9 | 10.4 ± 1.2 | 12.1 ± 2.6 | 12.7 ± 0.8 |
| DNA (mg) | 5.2 ± 0.8 | 4.9 ± 0.4 | 5.1 ± 0.9 | 4.7 ± 0.5 |
| *Stomach polyamine content (nmoles)* | | | | |
| Putrescine | 12 ± 1 | 46 ± 11 | 29 ± 4 | 28 ± 4 |
| Spermidine | 68 ± 9 | 191 ± 38 | 191 ± 21 | 168 ± 8 |
| Spermine | 46 ± 11 | 83 ± 13 | 86 ± 92 | 78 ± 5 |
| *Serum polyamines (pmoles/ml)* | | | | |
| Putrescine | 858 ± 110 | 874 ± 214 | 547 ± 109 | 678 ± 189 |
| Spermidine | 2264 ± 586 | 4123 ± 758 | 3927 ± 1045 | 3136 ± 1512 |
| Spermine | 200 ± 148 | 186 ± 107 | 358 ± 121 | 337 ± 41 |

Data represent means ± SD for 5 male rats

Pups were removed from their mothers an hour after a period of suckling and their stomach content was analysed for polyamine concentrations. It was evident that by 7 days of age approximately 74-90% of the polyamines from their stomach was absorbed. By day 14, it was 80-82%. At the time of weaning, spermidine and spermine absorption was only 32-57% and by day 28 the absorption levels had reached the values measured in adult rats (Bardocz *et al.*, 1990). The changes observed in polyamine uptake capacity indicate that the immature gut absorbs more polyamines on a per weight basis than after weaning (day 28, Table 2). This capacity is sufficient to utilise all polyamines present in the rat milk or feed (Table 3).

The changes in the milk/stomach polyamine content around weaning are reflected in serum spermidine levels (Table 4) which increased between days 18 and 19. Spermine content showed an increase between days 19 and 20 only, when suckling completely stopped, co-incidently with a drop in serum putrescine content. The polyamine content of blood did not reflect the changes.

In summary, the gut of the pups developed continuously and reached maturity by 28 days of age. The milk polyamine content was reasonably constant between days 7 and 18 and most of the polyamines could be absorbed from the small bowel. Polyamine content of solid food/feed is much higher than that of milk. Therefore, at the time of weaning, there is a dramatic increase in dietary polyamines.

## Acknowledgements

This work was supported by the Scottish Executive Rural Affairs Department.

## References

Bardocz, S. (1995) Polyamines in food and their consequences for food quality and human health. *Trends in Food Science and Technology*, **6**, 341-346.

Bardocz, S., Brown, D.S., Grant, G. and Pusztai, A. (1990) Luminal and basolateral polyamine uptake by rat small intestine stimulated to grow by Phaseolus vulgaris lectin phytohaemagglutinin in vivo. *Biochimica et Biophysica Acta*, **1034**, 46-52.

Bardocz, S., Grant, G., Brown, D.S., Ewen, S.W.B. and Pusztai, A. (1989) Involvement of polyamines in *Phaseolus vulgaris* lectin induced growth of rat pancreas *in vivo*. *Medical Science Research*, **17**, 309-311.

Bardocz, S., Grant, G., Brown, D.S., Ewen, S.W.B., Stewart, J.C. and Pusztai, A. (1991) Effect of fasting and refeeding on basolateral polyamine uptake and metabolism by the rat small bowel. *Digestion*, **50**, 28-35.

Bardocz, S., Grant, G., Brown, D.S., Wallace, H.M., Ewen, S.W.B. and Pusztai, A. (1989) Effect of a-difluoromethylornithine on *Phaseolus vulgaris* lectin-induced growth of the rat small intestine. *Medical Science Research*, **17**, 143-145.

Bardócz, S., Grant, G., Brown, D.S. and Pusztai, A. (1998) Putrescine as a source of instant energy in the small intestine of the rat. *Gut*, **42**, 24-28.

Bardócz, S., Grant, G., Hughes, E.L., Brown, D.S. and Pusztai, A. (1999) Uptake, inter-organ distribution and metabolism of dietary polyamines in the rat. *In Polyamines in Health and Nutrition*, pp. 241-258. Edited by S. Bardócz and A. White. Kluwer Academic Publishers, Boston, USA.

Dandrifosse, G., Deloyer, P., El Khefif, N. and Peulen, O. (1999) Dietary polyamines during lactation. *In Polyamines in Health and Nutrition*, pp. 213-231. Edited by S. Bardócz and A. White. Kluwer Academic Publishers, Boston, USA.

Dufour, C., Dandrifosse, G., Forget, P., Vermesse, F., Romain, N. and Lepoint, A. (1988) Spermine and spermidine induce intestinal maturation in the rat. *Gastroenterology*, **95**, 112-116.

Heby, O. and Persson, L. (1990) Molecular genetics of polyamine synthesis in eukaryotic cells. *Trends in Biochemical Sciences*, **15**, 153-158.

Jänne, J., Pösö, H. and Raina, A. (1978) Polyamines in rapid growth and cancer. *Biochimica et Biophysica Acta*, **473**, 241-293.

Luk, G.D. and Baylin, S.B. (1983) Polyamines and intestinal growth - increased polyamine biosynthesis after jejumectomy. *American Journal of Physiology*, **245**, G656-G660.

Luk, G.D., Vaughan, W.P., Burke, P.J. and Baylin, S.B. (1981) Diamine oxidase as a plasma marker of rat intestinal mucosal injury and regeneration after administration of 1-b-D-arabinofuranosylcytosine. *Cancer Research*, **41**, 2334-2337.

Morgan, D.M.L. (1999) Polyamine biosynthesis, catabolism and homeostasis: an overview. *In Polyamines in Health and Nutrition*, pp. 3-26. Edited by S. Bardócz and A. White. Kluwer Academic Publishers, Boston, USA.

Pegg, A.E. (1986) Recent advances in the biochemistry of polyamines in eukaryotes. *Biochemical Journal*, **234**, 249-262.

Perin, A. and Sessa, A. (1993) Polyamine acetylation in rat liver following long-term ethanol ingestion. *Biochimica et Biophysica Acta*, **1156**, 113-116.

Pusztai, A., Grant, G., Brown, D.S., Ewen, S.W.B. and Bardocz, S. (1988) *Phaseolus vulgaris* lectin induces the growth and increases the polyamine content of rat small intestine *in vivo*. *Medical Science Research*, **16**, 1283-1284.

Ralph, A., Englyst, K. and Bardócz, S. (1999) Polyamine content of the human diet. *In Polyamines in Health and Nutrition*, pp. 123-137. Edited by S. Bardócz and A. White. Kluwer Academic Publishers, Boston, USA.

Seidel, E.R., Haddox, M.K. and Johnson, L.R. (1985) Ileal mucosal growth during intraluminal infusion of ethylamine or putrescine. *American Journal of Physiology*, **249**, G434-G438.

Sessa, A., Tunici, P., Ewen, S.W.B., Grant, G., Pusztai, A., Bardocz, S. and Perin, A. (1995) Diamine and polyamine oxidase activities in phytohaemagglutinin-induced growth of rat small intestine. *Biochimica et Biophysica Acta*, **1244**, 198-202.

Sessa, A., Tunici, P., Rabellotti, E., Bardocz, S., Grant, G. and Pusztai, A. (1996) Response of intestinal transglutaminase activity to dietary phytohemag-glutinin. *Biochimica et Biophysica Acta*, **1314**, 66-70.

Tabor, C.W. and Tabor, H. (1984) Polyamines. *Annual Review of Biochemistry*, 53, 747-790.

White, A. and Bardócz, S. (1999) Estimation of the polyamine body pool: contribution by *de novo* biosynthesis, diet and luminal bacteria. *In Polyamines in Health and Nutrition*, pp. 117-122. Edited by S. Bardócz and A. White. Kluwer Academic Publishers, Boston, USA.

**3**

# GLUTAMINE IN GUT METABOLISM

Pierzynowski S.G. [1,2], Valverde Piedra J.L [3]., Hommel-Hansen T. [4], Studzinski T [3].
[1]R&D Gramineer International AB, Lund, Sweden. [2]Department of Animal Physiology, Lund University, Sweden. [3]Department of Animal Physiology, Faculty of Veterinary Medicine, Lublin Agricultural University, Poland. [4] Gramineer Feed A/S, Taastrup, Denmark.

## Summary

Glutamine and its derivatives seem to be indispensable as a metabolic fuel to be oxidised by the intestinal mucosa and consequently are an important nitrogen source for the synthesis of protein in gut mucosa. Thus, administration of glutamine should prove beneficial for piglets at the time of weaning when the immune system is compromised by stress situations as well as during intensive growth or lactation.

## Introduction

Studies during the last decades have demonstrated that glutamine is an amino acid of special importance determining and guarding normal metabolic processes of the cell (Brooks, Hall, Wagstaff and Michell, 1998; Den Hond, Hiele, Peeters, Ghoos and Rutgeerts, 1999; Graham, Sgro, Friars and Gibala, 2000). This amino acid is indispensable for the optimal growth of most cells and tissues. Although glutamate is considered to be a nonessential amino acid, numerous recent studies have demonstrated that endogenous glutamine storage and synthesis capabilities may not be sufficient to meet the needs of the organism during long-term stress, hypercatabolic and hypermetabolic states or during prolonged starvation (Elia and Lunn, 1997; Griffiths, Jones and Palmer, 1997; Hammarqvist, Wernerman, Von der Decken and Vinnars, 1990; Hammarqvist, Westman, Leijonmarck, Andersson and Wernerman, 1996; Pierzynowski and Sjödin, 1998; Tremel, Kienle, Weilemann, Stehle and Fürst, 1994). This has led to a redesignation of glutamine as a "conditionally essential" amino acid.

Glutamine is the most abundant amino acid found in extracellular fluid and in the free amino acid pool of the body. It constitutes about 25 % of the total amino acids in extracellular fluid and more than 60 % of the free amino acid pool in

43

skeletal muscle (Neu, Shenoy and Chakrabarti, 1996). The transmembrane concentration gradient of glutamine across the muscle cell membrane is over 30 times greater than in extracellular fluid. Being not only a precursor for protein synthesis glutamine functions as an intermediate in various metabolic pathways and takes part in the regulation of acid-base balance (Nissim, 1999). Glutamine donates nitrogen for the synthesis of purines, pyrimidines, nucleotides and amino sugars. Presenting the highest concentration in the extracellular fluid glutamine serves as a nitrogen transporter between various cells and tissues in the body. Due to its diverse participation in transamination reactions, glutamine can be classified as true regulator of amino acid homeostasis (Nissim, 1999).

The human gastrointestinal tract (GIT) is a major site of glutamine utilisation accounting for more than half of the net splanchnic utilisation (approximately 15 g/day) of glutamine obtained from the systemic circulation. Dietary glutamine (approximately 5 g/day) is less important than circulating glutamine. However, especially in disease conditions associated with substantial reductions in food intake, which in any case is a source of all amino acids including glutamine, the food/feed pool of glutamine/glutamate can be critical for gut function and other organ function. Considering the necessity of glutamine for intestinal function and also the "aggressive" metabolic behaviour of enterocytes to obtain glutamine one can easily predict a critical stress scenario in which whole body - but especially muscle - metabolism is set up for the production/release of glutamine for gut energy and protein synthesis. The GIT distribution of enzymes involved in glutamine metabolism is varied. Apart from the stomach in man and upper stomach in the rat, there is very little and weak activity of glutamine synthetase, suggesting that the gut derives glutamine formed in other tissues and from the diet. The activity of glutaminase, which is a key-flux generating enzyme involved in glutaminolysis, is very weak in mucosa with stratified squamous epithelium such as the oesophagus, while intermediate in the upper intestine, and highest in the small intestinal mucosa which accounts for about 80% of the total glutaminase in the entire human GIT mucosa (Elia and Lunn, 1997). However, young enterocytes display marked activity of glutamine synthetase (Neu *et al.*, 1996).

Emerging data from both animal and human studies indicate that combinations of selected growth factors and specific nutrients may improve the growth, adaptation, and repair of the intestinal mucosa (Ziegler, Estívariz, Jonas, Gu, Jones and Leader, 1999).

Glutamine has received considerable interest as a gut-targeted nutrient due to its proposed key role in the maintenance of intestinal structure and function. Glutamine seems to be indispensable as a metabolic fuel to be fully oxidised by the intestinal mucosa (Li, Li, Jiang, Liu, Li, Qin and Zhu, 1999) and an important nitrogen source for the enterocytes. It plays a key role in maintaining mucosal cell integrity and gut barrier function (Den Hond *et al.*, 1999). The role of intestinal glutamine metabolism seems to be threefold: a- provides sufficient amounts of nitrogen precursors for mucosal anabolic pathways to maintain intestinal structure and function, b- supplies the liver with an optimal substrate mix, and c- provides citrulline - and thereby arginine- for the whole organism (Plauth, Raible, Vieillard Baron, Bauder Gross and Hartmann, 1999).

Glutamine depletion results in immuno-suppression and there is a great deal of evidence that the key functions of cells of the immune system are dependent upon the provision of glutamine (Graham *et al.*, 2000). Thus, administration of glutamine can be beneficial for piglets at the time of weaning when the immune system is compromised by stress situations.

## Effects of Glutamine and its derivatives on intestine and animal performance

The luminal surface of the small intestine is composed of a single layer of columnar epithelium overlaying mucosal projections (i.e. villi) that serve to increase the surface area of the gastrointestinal tract. The intestinal epithelium has two conflicting functions: it must serve as a protective barrier against luminal bacteria and toxins yet also absorbs solutes necessary to maintain the well being of the host (Jankowski, Goodlad and Wright, 1994). This conflict is notable at the intercellular space, which acts as a sieve that theoretically allows passage of selected solutes and water (Pappenheimer, 1990; Soergel, 1993) but prevents passage of bacterial toxins (Madara, 1990). The intercellular space is regulated by the tight junction (Madara, 1990), which, in turn, fluctuates in size depending on the degree to which the attached cytoskeleton contracts (Madara, Moore and Carlson, 1987). Intestinal injury, such as that caused by intestinal ischemia or inflammatory cell infiltration, results in enlargement of the intercellular space, initially caused by loosening of tight junction (Madara, 1990; Madara, 1989) and subsequently caused by disruption of epithelial continuity (Madara, 1990).

## GLUTAMINE

Glutamine is the principal metabolic fuel of the small intestine enterocytes, compared with glucose in other cells (Wu, Knabe, Yan and Flynn, 1995), and it may aid enterocyte proliferation as a cellular energy source (Ko, Beauchamp, Townsend and Thompson, 1993) since part of the mitogenic effect is glutamine dependent (i.e. DNA, RNA, and protein synthesis).

Some 94% of the enteral [U-$^{13}$C] glutamine but only 6% of the enteral [U-$^{13}$C] glucose was utilised in the first pass by the portal drained viscera (PDV) in fed piglets, which extracted 6.5% of the arterial flux of [U-$^{13}$C] glucose and 20.4% of the arterial flux of [U-$^{13}$C] glutamine (Stoll, Burrin, Henry, Yu, Jahoor and Reeds, 1999).

The activity of TGF-$\alpha$ on epithelial proliferation in cell culture appears to be most effective in the presence of glutamine (Blikslager, Bristol, Rhoads, Roberts and Argenzio, 1996). However, glutamine appears to possess proliferative actions of its own. For example, in the IPEC-J2 cell line from neonatal pigs, glutamine enhances gene transcription by increasing mitogen activated protein kinase activity (Blikslager and Roberts, 1997). Additionally, glutamine significantly improves structure (i.e. mucosal villus height, surface area) in a rat model of total parenteral nutrition (TPN) and transplanted small intestine (Frankel, Zhang, Afonso, Klurfeld, Don, Laitin, Deaton, Furth, Pietra, Naji and Rombeau, 1993).

Dietary glutamine supplementation prevented an increase in jejunal lamina propria depth (LPD) (an indicator of crypt depth and increased number of less mature cells) on day 14 postweaning. Because the intestinal LPD consists of less mature cells compared with villus enterocytes (Lipkin, 1985), these data suggest that glutamine enhances maturation of intestinal crypt cells. Glutamine supplementation had no effect on duodenal villi height on day 7 postweaning. This may reflect difference in glutamine metabolism and cell proliferation between porcine duodenum and jejunum (Wu, Meier and Knabe, 1996).

Glutamine oxidation to $CO_2$ in enterocytes, from 29 day old weaned pigs compared with 21 day old suckling piglets, progressively increases ($P<0.05$) with the piglet's age (Wu, Knabe and Flynn, 1994) rather than being induced by diet or weaning. There is further evidence (Watford, 1994) that metabolically significant quantities of glutamine (and presumably glutamate) carbon are transformed to lactate and alanine in enterocytes and that its oxidation is thereby incomplete.

## GLUTAMATE

It was found that glutamate is rapidly removed from the intestine and partly enters the circulation, in agreement with the amino acid homeostasis of mature enterocytes. In contrast, ornithine can be accumulated by mucosal cells, as well as by virtually all tissues, to high levels (Daune-Anglard, Bonaventure and Seiler, 1993).

## ORNITHINE $\alpha$-KETOGLUTARATE (OKG)

Raul, Gosse, Galluser, Hasselmann and Seiler (1995) observed an adaptive hyperplasia of the villi and an increase in the brush-border hydrolase activities in rats receiving ornithine $\alpha$-ketoglutarate (OKG). $\gamma$-aminobutyric acid is formed in suckling piglets, the capacity of enterocytes to utilise glutamine was high (2.5 – 3.8 nmol/ min/10$^6$ cells) and the major products from glutamine were ammonia, glutamate, $CO_2$, and aspartate. The effect of glutamine was more marked in piglet enterocytes as compared with rat or chicken enterocytes, but remained smaller than in human enterocytes (Watford, Lund and Krebs, 1979; Ashy, 1988; Porteous, 1980).

Enteral labeled measuring of amino acid concentration in portal and arterial blood over an hour after feeding of piglets, Reeds, Burrin, Jahoor, Wykes, Henry and Frazer (1996) found that there was a significant ($P<0.05$) net absorption of the indispensable amino acids as well as arginine, proline, serine, and alanine. There was no portal uptake of glutamate, aspartate or glycine, and arterial glutamine was removed by the portal drained viscera ($P<0.05$). In piglets the gut metabolises virtually all of the enteral glutamate during absorption. Therefore, glutamate and glutamine in the body as a whole must derive almost entirely from synthesis *de novo*.

Although the intestine utilised approximately 35% of the dietary protein, the fractional portal tracer balance exceeded the fractional mass balance, suggesting that the portal drained viscera continued to utilise arterial amino acids. This result also shows that no more than 20% of the measured first pass metabolism was recovered in mucosal constitutive protein. Taken together, the results imply that amino acid catabolism accounted for approximately 80% of the total $CO_2$ production by the portal drained viscera and of this about 50% could be ascribed to the oxidation of glutamate and aspartate. It is not certain whether the results reflect an obligatory utilisation of amino acids. The results of Reeds *et al.* (1996) shows, that in piglets, the capacity of the small intestine to catabolise, in the first pass, enteral glutamate is very high.

Stoll, Henry, Reeds, Yu, Jahoor and Burrin (1998a) found that on average 56% of the essential amino acid (EAA) intake appeared in the portal blood, and that the net outflow of ammonia accounted for 18% of the total amino acid nitrogen intake. Roughly one third of dietary intake of EAA is consumed in first pass metabolism by the intestine, and amino acid catabolism by the mucosal cells is qualitatively greater than amino acid incorporation into mucosal protein. This implies that differences in the apparent digestibility of protein among diets are largely a function of differences in the rate of endogenous protein loss (Stoll *et al.*, 1998a).

Stoll *et al.* (1998a) also argues, that even though there is substantial metabolism of dietary amino acids in the enterocytes, it has been known for many years, that some dietary amino acids, with glutamate and aspartate as notable examples (Reeds *et al.*, 1996; Windmueller and Spaeth, 1980), are catabolised extensively in the gut.

Stoll *et al.* (1998a) found, that the catabolism of glutamine, glutamate, and aspartate alone amounted to 660 mmol N/(kg·h). However, on the basis of the measurement of tracer balance and incorporation into mucosal protein, it would appear that at least 60% of the first pass metabolism of the EAA was also catabolised. The quantities of dietary amino acids that were utilised in the first pass by the intestine were closely related to the mucosal mass of the piglets, implying that environmental conditions affecting intestinal mass have an important effect on the overall nutritional efficiency of dietary protein utilisation.

There were major differences between the portal balance of other amino acids (Stoll *et al.*, 1998a), confirming previous observations (Windmueller and Spaeth 1975, 1980) of the almost complete first pass removal of dietary glutamate and aspartate as well as the substantial net synthesis of alanine by the intestinal tissues.

Stoll *et al.*, (1999) found, that the exit of nitrogen in newly synthesised alanine (338 mmol/kg/h) accounted for only 47% of the nitrogen generated from the estimated catabolism of glutamate, aspartate, and glutamine (715 mmol/kg/h). The remainder apparently exited as ammonia produced by portal drained viscera (PDV). The rate of ammonia production exceeds glutamine deamidation (190 mmol/kg/h) by a factor of five. The total sum of alanine synthesis and ammonia production exceeds the quantity of nitrogen that would have been generated from aspartate, glutamate, and glutamine catabolism. This finding implies that 1) there is metabolically significant glutamate deamidation (i.e., an active glutamate dehydrogenase) in the mucosa and, 2) other dietary amino acids are catabolised in first pass by the mucosa.

Jahoor, Wykes, Reeds, Henry, Del Rosario and Frazer, 1995 showed that in piglets, both the concentration and turnover rate of mucosal reduced glutathione are high. Additionally, Reeds, Burrin, Stoll, Jahoor, Wykes, Henry and Frazer, (1997) suggest that the glutamate and glycine in the mucosal glutathione pool of fed piglets derive directly from the diet.


## ENERGY GENERATION

Studies (Kight and Fleming, 1993) imply that the selection of substrates for oxidation by mucosal enterocytes appears to depend on their relative concentrations rather than on extracellular regulators.

The intestinal tissues make a disproportional contribution to whole body energy expenditure and variations in mucosal mass have a measurable effect on maintenance of energy needs (Burrin, Ferrell, Britton and Bauer, 1990). The first pass metabolism of enteral amino acids (e.g. Matthews, Marano and Campbell, 1993b), may well reflect intestinal rather than hepatic metabolism.

Stoll *et al.* (1999) found that *in vivo*, three-fourths of the energy needed by the PDV is supplied by the oxidation of glucose, glutamate, and glutamine, and that dietary glutamate is the most important single contributor to mucosal oxidative energy generation.

The findings by Windmueller and Spaeth (1975, 1980) that the metabolism of enteral glutamic acid was of much more quantitative importance to mucosal energy generation than that of glutamine has been largely overlooked. Also among humans Battezzati, Brillon and Matthews (1995); Matthews, Marano and Campbell (1993a) have shown that the splanchnic extraction of enteral glutamate exceeds that of glutamine.

Even though the removal of luminal glutamate (both free and protein bound) is efficient, little dietary glutamate appears in the portal circulation (Reeds *et al.*, 1997; Reeds *et al.*, 1996; Rérat, Jung and Kandé, 1988). Also Windmueller and Spaeth (1975) explicitly commented on the fact that luminal glutamate appeared to be a more important oxidative substrate than glutamine. The fact that such similar results have been obtained in different species, at different stages of development, and under quite different experimental circumstances, strongly suggests that this reflects a specific feature of mucosal metabolism, i.e., a critical role of amino acids as energy sources.

## The effect of glutamine or derivatives on growth and feed conversion in pigs

Weaning is associated with increasing plasma concentrations of stress hormones such as glucocorticoids in pigs (Worsaae and Schmidt, 1980). Interestingly, glucocorticoid administration to dogs increases intestinal glutamine metabolism (Souba, Smith and Wilmore, 1985).

The increased rate of polyamine synthesis from ornithine (Seiler, 1990) may stimulate anabolic processes in tissues (i.e. DNA, RNA, and protein synthesis).

### IMPROVED DIGESTIBILITY

Enterally administered OKG induced an adaptive process in the intestinal mucosa. This is characterised by an increase in the length of the villi and the enhanced activity of sucrase and aminopeptidase in the brush-border membranes of the enterocytes. These changes suggest an improved digestive capacity in healthy animals treated with OKG, which in part might be due to the accumulation of ornithine in the intestinal mucosa (Raul *et al.*, 1995).

## Intestinal atrophy and total parenteral nutrition (TPN)

Intestinal atrophy may be explained as a decrease in the dietary supply of nutrients due to minimal feed intake during the first week postweaning (Wu, 1996). Thus, the minimal supply of glutamine from the diet during the first week postweaning is unlikely to support the high metabolic activity of enterocytes as well as the proliferation, maturation and migration of crypt cells or to maintain the function of intestinal lymphocytes (Alverdy, 1990).

Glutamine supplementation (1.0%) prevented jejunal atrophy (as indicated by villus height) during the first week postweaning and increased the gain/feed ratio by 25% during the second week postweaning. This supplementation also increased plasma concentrations of aspartate, glutamate and alanine and reduced the extent to which plasma taurine concentration fell in postweaning pigs (Wu, 1996). Studies in rats indicate that glutamine supplemented to TPN solutions significantly improved recovery of the intestine from starvation atrophy and dysfunction that accompanies starvation (Inoue, Grant and Snyder, 1993; Souba and Austgen, 1990a) and long-term TPN (Platell, McCauley, McCulloch and Hall, 1993).

## Effects of glutamine and its derivatives on gestating and lactating sows

In pigs, amino acid patterns changed between colostrum and mature milk; glutamate, proline, methionine, isoleucine, and lysine increased; cystine, glycine, serine, threonine, and alanine decreased. The total amino acid concentration decreases 75% between colostrum and mature milk. Because most milk amino acid is derived from milk proteins, the change in milk amino acid pattern during the course of lactation can probably be ascribed to a change during the course of lactation in the relative distribution of milk protein containing different amino acid patterns (Davis, Nguyen, Garcia-Bravo, Fiorotto, Jackson and Reeds, 1994). In this regard, it is noteworthy that glutamine is the most abundant free amino acid in sow's milk on day 21 of lactation (1.93 mmol l$^{-1}$) (Wu *et al.*, 1995).

## Effects of L-alanyl-L-glutamine (Ala-Gln) dipeptide administration on general growth, GIT growth and certain blood parameters and immunological indices in postnatal pigs

Experiments (Valverde, Piedra and Studzinski, unpublished data) were conducted on piglets between the 23$^{rd}$ and the 52$^{nd}$ day of postnatal life. The piglets were divided into three groups: one control group and two experimental groups. The piglets of the first experimental group were administered L-alanyl-L-glutamine (Ala-Gln) *per os* (0.4 mg/kg/b.w.), while of the second experimental group Ala-Gln at the same dose subcutaneously. At the end of the experiment blood samples and cerebro-spinal fluid were taken and the piglets were sacrificed. Higher body weight values were noted in the piglets receiving L- alanyl - L- glutamine orally. Although body weight gain was higher in this group of piglets compared to the controls these changes were not significant. L- alanyl - L- glutamine administration resulted in higher stomach weight, showing the highest values in piglets supplemented orally, while pancreas weight showed quite the opposite, that is lower values in the orally supplemented piglets. After 21 days of oral L-alanyl-L-glutamine administration an increase in proteolytic activity of the slow moving fraction belonging to pepsinogen A was observed.

The development of a stable and highly soluble synthetic dipeptide L-alanyl-L-glutamine (Ala-Gln) shows great promise as a route for the provision of this amino acid - otherwise difficult to deliver. This substrate presents the unique possibility of providing the organism with readily available glutamine. Considerable high hydrolase activity in body compartments and organs facilitates rapid liberation of glutamine from Ala-Gln. During parenteral administration of Ala-Gln only trace amounts of dipeptide are measurable in blood plasma, while it is not detectable in tissues and not excreted in urine. These combined observations indicate a readily quantitative hydrolysis of the administered Ala-Gln and subsequent utilisation in body fluids, thus avoiding the risk of undesirable pharmacological and physiological side effects. Alanine is readily metabolised via the gluconeogenic pathway, thereby sparing endogenous body proteins. This effect is of great importance during weaning, when the stress of separation of piglets from the sow and the change of diet negatively affect feed intake and body weight gain. An additional factor indicating higher demand for energy is the high metabolic rate at that time and immunosuppression affecting GIT immunity as well. Therefore glutamine administration in the form of dipeptide (Ala-Gln) seems to be reasonable for theoretical and practical purposes.

These results indicate that after 21 days of oral Ala-Gln administration significantly higher values in body weight gain occurred in piglets supplemented orally. Similar but short lasting effects of body weight gain increase occurred in the experimental group of piglets that were given Ala-Gln subcutaneously.

It should be stressed that glutamine and its metabolites serve as obligatory nutrients necessary for normal maintenance of the integrity of the intestinal mucosa requiring sufficient supplies to cover the demand for metabolic energy as a fuel and presumably for proliferating cells (Steginak, Filer and Baker, 1973).

Although the experiment was conducted on a limited number of piglets the results indicate that Ala-Gln dipeptide stimulated the increase of stomach mass by about 25.8% when administered orally. The tendency toward a stimulating effect (14%) in the other group of piglets which were injected with the same amount of Ala-Gln subcutaneously shows that this dipeptide can determine postnatal organ development of GIT. According to these results there are additional effects such as the stimulatory influence of Ala-Gln on the activity of stomach and duodenal proteases in the group of piglets that received this dipeptide orally.

When the concentration of the intracellular glutamine pool decreases, the body supply becomes depleted rapidly. This depletion of the glutamine pool leads to epithelial atrophy in the small intestine, which is associated with a breakdown of the gut barrier and facilitated bacterial translocation (Scheppach, Loges, Bartram, Christl, Richter, Dusel, Stehle, Fuerst and Kasper, 1994). Both glutamine and Ala-Gln stimulate crypt cell proliferation in the ileum, proximal colon and rectosigmoid colon in humans (Scheppach *et al.*, 1994). These results indicate that the trophic effect of Ala-Gln can be confined to a much larger area of GIT, including the stomach in the pig.

The results of research published in recent years indicate that GIT secretory functions can be graded in the pattern of gradients and on the other hand are strictly interdependent as is liver ureogenesis which depends on glutamine deamidation in the cells of the intestinal tract (Tan and Hooi, 2000; Yang, Hazey, David, Singh, Rivchum, Streem, Halperin and Brunengraber, 2000).

The intestinal mucosal barrier is composed of a single layer of epithelial cells anchored to one another by series of interepithelial junctions (Blikslager, Roberts, Young, Rhoads and Argenzio, 2000; O'Riordain, Fearon, Ross, Rogers, Falconer, Bartolo, Garden and Carter, 1994). The apically situated tight junction regulates the paracellular flux of solutes and bacterial toxins. Breakdown of the intestinal barrier is observed during total parenteral nutrition (TPN) intestinal ischemia and reperfusion injury (Blikslager *et al.*, 2000).

Ala-Gln supplementation stops bacteria translocation similarly to genistein derived from dietary sources such as soybean meal and enhances recovery of trasmucosal resistance (Blikslager *et al.*, 2000).

The resident microflora present a highly varied profile of antigenic material to the mucosal immune system. Mucosal integrity which depends on normal intestinal microflora can be illustrated by structural and functional alterations seen in germ free environments such as reduction of epithelial turnover, motility and smooth muscle function, and diminished anatomic and functional development of gut-associated lymphoid tissue GALT (Shanahan, 2000). Innate or natural immunity is characterised by ready and rapid response and is modulated by glutamine (Skubitz and Anderson, 1996). Elements of innate immunity include macrophages, natural killer cells, defensins, lysozyme, cecropines and the complement cascade (Shanahan, 2000). During normal healthy conditions the upper part of the small intestine contains few bacteria. Below the duodenum, the concentration of bacteria progressively increases until it achieves maximum, which is reached in the large intestine (Lee, Boman, Chuanxin, Andersson, Jörnvall, Mutt and Boman, 1989; Boman, Agerberth and Boman, 1983). It is remarkable that the collective mass of bacteria contained in the human gut ranges from 1-2 kg. Such masses of bacteria coexist with a delicate host organ. Thus one might predict that the intestine could produce antibacterial factors that regulate the bacterial concentration in the upper part of the intestine and protect the mucosa of the large intestine (Lee *et al.*, 1989). The pig small intestine contains several potent antibacterial factors, cecropins among them. In addition, such known endocrine peptides as VIP seem to be antibacterial in their natural or modified forms. This seems expedient if the protection of the intestine is based on small peptides, easily secreted and with a broad specificity. It is worth emphasising that an antibacterial defence based on protein synthesis is faster, easier and not as energy demanding as mechanisms depending on cell proliferation. It is worth mentioning and hypothesising that small peptides released from protein digestion can possess antibacterial functions. Ala-Gln seems to modulate general defence mechanisms but precise pathways of these reactions should be researched in the future.

## Implications

Glutamine/glutamate are the most abundant forms of amino acid in proteins and protein is the most desired component of feed or food stuffs, even though nutritional patterns in farm animals and humans have recently changed because of cultural reasons (fast food) or economy (animal feed). Considering evolutionary history it should not be surprising that all living creatures (and their organs) are well adapted to utilise proteins and their most abundant component - glutamine/glutamate as a main source for energy (intestine) and structure (muscle building).

Gut metabolism and energy requirements are proof of this fact. Glutamine and its derivatives independently of our wishes, remain major factors affecting intestinal function, growth and development.

## Acknowledgements

Grants from SJFR, Dr A Påhlsson Foundation and The Visby Programme (Sweden), and grant from the State Committee for Scientific Research (Poland) supported this work.

## References

Alverdy, J.C., Aoys, E. and Moos, G.S. (1988) Total Parenteral nutrition promotes bacterial translocation from the gut. *Surgery*, **104**, 185-190.

Alverdy, J.C. (1990) Effects of Glutamine-Supplemented Diets on Immunology of the Gut. *Journal of Parenteral and Enteral Nutrition*, **14**, 109S-113S.

Ardawi, M.S.M. and Newsholme, E.A. (1982) Maximum activities of some enzymes of glycolysis, the tricarboxylic acid cycle and ketone-body and glutamine utilisation pathways in lymphocytes of the rat. *Biochemical Journal*, 208, 743-748.

Ashy, A.A. and Ardawi, S.M. (1988) Glucose, Glutamine and Ketone-Body Metabolism in Human Enterocytes. *Metabolism*, 37, 602-609.

Barbul, A. (1990) Arginine and immune function. *Nutrition*, 6, 53-57.

Battezzati, A., Brillon, D.J. and Matthews, D.E. (1995) Oxidation of glutamic acid by the splanchnic bed in humans. *American Journal of Physiology - Endocrinology and Metabolism*, 269, E269-E276.

Blikslager, A.T., Bristol, D.G., Rhoads, J.M., Roberts, M.C. and Argenzio, R.A. (1996) Glutamine and transforming growth factor alpha enhance repair of intestinal ischemia/reperfusion injury. *(Abstr)* – *Gastroenterology*, 110, A313.

Blikslager, A.T. and Roberts, M.C. (1997) Mechanisms of intestinal mucosal repair. *Journal of the American Veterinary Medical Association*, 211, 1437-1441.

Blikslager, A.T., Roberts, M.C., Young, K.M., Rhoads, J.M. and Argenzio, R.A. (2000) Genistein augments prostaglandin-induced recovery of barrier function in ischemia-injured procine ileum. *American Journal of Physiology - Gastrointestinal and Liver Physiology*, 278, G207-G216.

Boman, H.G., Agerberth, B., and Boman, A. (1993) Mechanisms of action on *Escherichia coli* of cecropin P1 and PR-39, two antibacterial peptides from pig intestine. *Infection and Immunity*, 61, 2978-2984.

Brooks, H.W., Hall, A.G., Wagstaff, A.J. and Michell, A.R. (1998) Detrimental effects on villus form during conventional oral rehydration therapy for diarrhoea in calves; alleviation by a nutrient oral rehydration solution containing glutamine. *The Veterinary Journal*, 155, 263-274.

Burke, D.J., Alverdy, J.C., Aoys, E. and Moss, G.S. (1989) Glutamine-Supplemented Total Parenteral Nutrition Improves Gut Immune Fuction. *Archives of Surgery*, 124, 1396-1399.

Burrin, D.G., Ferrell, C.L., Britton, R.A. and Bauer, M. (1990) Level of nutrition and visceral organ size and metabolic activity in sheep. *British Journal of Nutrition*, 64, 439-448.

Coffey, J.A., Milhoan, R.A., Abdullah, A., Herndon, D.N., Townsend, C.M. and Thompson, J.C. (1988) Bombesin inhibits bacterial translocation from the gut in burned rats. *Surgical Forum*, 39, 109-110.

Cynober, L. (1991) Ornithine alpha-ketoglutarate in nutritional support. *Nutrition*, 7, 313-320.

Darcy-Vrillon, B., Posho, L., Morel, M-T., Bernard, F., Blachier F., Meslin, J-C. and Duée, P-H. (1994) Glucose, Galactose and Glutamine Metabolism in Pig Isolated Enterocytes during Development. *Pediatric Research*, 36, 175-181.

Daune-Anglard, G., Bonaventure, N. and Seiler, N. (1993) Some Biochemical and Pathophysiological Aspects of Long-Term Elevation of Brain Ornithine Concentrations. *Pharmacology & Toxicology*, **73**, 29-34.

Davis, T.A., Nguyen, H.V., Garcia-Bravo, R., Fiorotto, M.L., Jackson, E.M. and Reeds, P.J. (1994) Amino acid composition of the milk of some mammalian species changes with stage of lactation. *British Journal of Nutrition*, **72**, 845-853.

Den Hond, E., Hiele, M., Peeters, M., Ghoos, Y. and Rutgeerts, P. (1999) Effect of long-term oral glutamine supplements on small intestinal permeability in patients with Crohn's disease. *Journal of Parenteral and Enteral Nutrition*, **23**, 7-11.

Donaldson, R.M. (1964) Normal Bacterial Populations of the Intestine and Their Relation to Intestinal Fuction. *The New England Journal of Medicine*, **30**, 938-945.

Elia, M. and Lunn, PG. (1997) The use of glutamine in the treatment of gastrointestinal disorders in man. *Nutrition*, **13**, 743-747.

Fox, A.D., Kripke, S.A., De Paula, J., Berman, J.M., Settle, R.G. and Rombeau J.L. (1988) Effect of a Glutamine-Supplemented Enteral Diet on Methotrexate-Induced Enterocolitis. *Journal of Parenteral and Enteral Nutrition*, **12**, 325-331.

Frankel, W.L., Zhang, W., Afonso, J. Klurfeld, D.M., Don, S.H., Laitin, E., Deaton, D., Furth, E.E., Pietra, G.G., Naji, A. and Rombeau, J.L. (1993) Glutamine Enhancement of Structure and Function in Transplanted Small Intestine in the Rat. *Journal of Parenteral and Enteral Nutrition*, **17**, 47-55.

Frisell, W.R. (1982) Synthesis and catabolism of nucleotides. In: Frisell (ed). *Human Biochemistry*. MacMillan, New York, pp. 292-304.

Graham, T.E., Sgro, V., Friars, D. and Gibala, M.J. (2000) Glutamate ingestion: the plasma and muscle free amino acid pools of resting humans. *American Journal of Physiology - Endocrinology and Metabolism*, **278**, E83 – E 89.

Griffiths, R.D., Jones, Ch. and Palmer, A.T.E. (1997) Six-month outcome of critically III patients given glutamine-supplemented parenteral nutrition. *Nutrition*, **13**, 295-302.

Hammarqvist, F., Wernerman, J., Von der Decken, A. and Vinnars, E. (1990) Alanyl-glutamine counteracts the depletion of free glutamine and the postoperative decline inprotein synthesis in skeletal muscle. *Annals of Surgery*, **212**, 637-644.

Hammarqvist, F., Westman, B., Leijonmarck, C.E., Andersson, K. and Wernerman, J. (1996) Decrease in muscle glutamine, ribosomes, and the nitrogen losses are similar after laparoscopic compared with open cholecystectomy during the immediate postoperative period. *Surgery*, **119**, 417-423.

Inoue, Y., Grant, J.P. and Snyder, P.J. (1993) Effect of Glutamine-Supplemented Total Parenteral Nutrition on Recovery of the Small Intestine After Starvation Atrophy. *Journal of Parenteral and Enteral Nutrition*, **17**, 165-170.

Jahoor, F., Wykes, L.J., Reeds, P.J., Henry, J.F., Del Rosario, M.P. and Frazer, M.E. (1995) Protein-Deficient Pigs Cannot Maintain Reduced Glutathione Homeostasis When Subjected to the Stress of Inflammation. *Journal of Nutrition*, **125**, 1462-1472.

Jankowski, J.A., Goodlad, R.A. and Wright, N.A. (1994) Maintenance of normal intestinal mucosa: function, structure and adaptation. *Gut*, **1**, S1-S4.

Kalfarentzos, F., Spiliotis, J., Melachrinou, M., Katsarou, C.H., Spiliopoulou, I., Panagopoulos, C. and Alexandrides, T.H. (1996) Oral ornithine "-ketoglutarate accelerates healing of the small intestine and reduces bacterial translocation after abdominal radiation. *Clinical Nutrition*, **15**, 29-33.

Karatzas, T., Scopa, S., Tsoni, I., Panagopoulos, K., Spiliopoulou, I., Moschos, S., Vagianos, K. and Kalfarentzos, F. (1991) Effect of glutamine on intestinal mucosal integrity and bacterial translocation after abdominal radiation. *Clinical Nutrition*, **10**, 199-205.

Kight, C.E. and Fleming, S.E. (1993) Nutrient Oxidation by Rat Intestinal Epithelial Cells Is Concentration Dependent. *Journal of Nutrition*, **123**, 876-882.

Klimberg, V.S., Salloum, R.M., Kasper, M., Plumley, D.A., Dolson, J.D., Hautamaki, D., Mendenhall, W.R., Bova, F.C., Bland, K.I., Copeland, E.M. and Suoba, W.W. (1990) Oral Glutamine Accelerates Healing of the Small Intestine and Improves Outcome After Whole Abdominal Radiation. *Archives of Surgery*, **125**, 1040-1045.

Ko, T.C., Beauchamp, R.D., Townsend, C.M. and Thompson, J.C. (1993) Glutamine is essential for epidermal growth factor – stimulated intestinal cell proliferation. *Surgery*, **114**, 147-154.

Lee, J.-Y., Boman, A., Chuanxin, S., Andersson, M., Jörnvall, H., Mutt, V. and Boman, H.G. (1989) Antibacterial peptides from pig intestine: Isolation of a mammalian cecropin. *Proceedings of the National Academy of Sciences of the United States of America*, **86**, 9159-9162.

Li, Y.S., Li, J.S., Jiang, J.W., Liu, F.N., Li, N., Qin, W.S. and Zhu, H. (1999) Glycyl-glutamine-enriched long-term total parenteral nutrition attenuates bacterial translocation following small bowel transplantation in the pig. *Journal of Surgical Research*, **82**, 1, 106-111.

Lipkin, M. (1985) Growth and Development of Gastrointestinal Cells. *Annual Review of Physiology*, **47**, 175-197.

Madara, J.L. (1989) Loosing tight junctions: lessons from the instesine. *Journal of Clinical Investigation*, **83**, 1089-1094.

Madara, J.L. (1990) Pathobiology of the Intestinal Epithelial Barrier. *American Journal of Pathology*, **137**, 1273-1281.

Madara, J.L., Moore, R. and Carlson, S. (1987) Alteration of intestinal tight junction structure and permeability by cytoskeletal contraction. *American Journal of Physiology - Cell Physiology*, **253**, C854-C861.

Matthews, D.E., Marano, M.A. and Campbell, R.G. (1993a) Splanchnic bed utilization of leucine and phenylalanine in humans. *American Journal of Physiology – Endocrinology and Metabolism*, **264**, E109-E118.

Matthews, D.E., Marano, M.A. and Campbell, R.G. (1993b) Splanchnic bed utilization of glutamine and glutamic acid in humans. *American Journal of Physiology – Endocrinology and Metabolism*, **264**, E848-E854.

Neu, J., Shenoy, V. and Chakrabarti, R. (1996) Glutamine nutrition and metabolism: Where do we go from here? *FASEB Journal*, **10**, 829-837.

Nissim, I. (1999) Newer aspects of glutamine/glutamate metabolism: the role of acute pH changes. *American Journal of Physiology – Renal Physiology*, **277**, F493-F497.

O'Riordain, M.G., Fearon, K.C.H., Ross, J.A., Rogers, P., Falconer, J.S., Bartolo, D.C.C., Garden, O.J. and Carter, D.C. (1994) Glutamine-supplemented total parenteral nutrition enhances T-lymphocyte response in surgical patients undergoing colorectal resection. *Annals of Surgery*, **220**, 212-221.

Pappenheimer, J.R. (1990) Paracellular intestinal absorption of glucose, creatinine and mannitol in normal animals: relation to body size. *Gastrointestinal Liver Physiology*, **22**, G290-G299.

Pierzynowski, S.G. and Sjödin, A. (1998) Perspectives of glutamine and its derivatives as feed additives for farm animals. *Journal of Animal and Feed Sciences*, **7**, 79-91.

Platell, C., McCauley, R., McCulloch, R. and Hall, J. (1993) The Influence of Parenteral Glutamine and Branched-Chain Amino Acids on Total Parenteral Nutrition – Induced Atrophy of the Gut. *Journal of Parenteral and Enteral Nutrition*, **17**, 348-354.

Plauth, M., Raible, A., Vieillard Baron, D., Bauder Gross, D. and Hartmann, F. (1999) Is glutamine essential for the maintenance of intestinal function? A study in the isolated perfused rat small intestine. *International Journal of Colorectal Disease*, **14**, 86-94

Porteous, J.W. (1980) Glutamate, Glutamine, Aspartate, Asparagine, Glucose and Ketone-Body Metabolism in Chick Intestinal Brush-Border Cells. *Biochemal Journal*, **188**, 619-632.

Posho, L., Darcy-Vrillon, B., Blachier, F. and Duée, P.-H. (1994) The contribution of glucose and glutamine to energy metabolism in newborn pig enterocytes. *Journal of Nutritional Biochemistry*, **5**, 284-290.

Raul, F., Gosse, F., Galluser, M., Hasselmann, M. and Seiler, N. (1995) Functional and Metabolic Changes in Intestinal Mucosa of Rats After Enteral Administration of Ornithine "-Ketoglutarate Salt. *Journal of Parental and Enteral Nutrition*, **19**, 145-150.

Reeds, P.J., Burrin, D.G., Jahoor, F., Wykes, L., Henry, J. and Frazer, E.M. (1996) Enteral glutamate is almost completely metabolized in first pass by the gastrointestinal tract of infant pigs. *American Journal of Physiology - Endocrinology and Metabolism*, 270, E413-E418.

Reeds, P.J., Burrin, D.G., Stoll, B., Jahoor, F., Wykes. L., Henry, J. and Frazer, E.M. (1997) Enteral glutamate is the preferential source for mucosal glutathione synthesis in fed piglets. *American Journal of Physiology*, 273, E408-415.

Rérat, A., Jung, J. and Kandé, J. (1988) Absorption kinetics of dietary hydrolysis products in conscious pigs given diets with different amounts of fish protein. *British Journal of Nutrition*, 60, 105-120.

Saito, H., Trocki, O., Wang, S., Gonce, S.J., Joffe, S.N. and Alexander, J.W (1987) Metabolic and Immune Effects of Dietary Arginine Supplementation After Burn. *Archives of Surgery*, 122, 784-789.

Scheppach, W., Loges, Ch., Bartram, P., Christl, S.U., Richter, F., Dusel, G., Stehle, P., Fuerst, P. and Kasper, H. (1994) Effect of free glutamine and Alanyl-glutamine dipeptide on mucosal proliferation of the human ileum and colon. *Gastroenterology*, 107, 429-436.

Seiler, N. (1990) Polyamine Metabolism. *Digestion*, 46, Supplement 2, 319-330.

Shanahan, T. (2000) Nutrient tasting and signaling in the gut. V. Mechanisms of immunologic sensation of intestinal contents. *American Journal of Physiology - Gastrointestinal and Liver Physiology*, 278, G191-G196.

Skubitz, K.M. and Anderson, P.M. (1996) Oral glutamine to prevent chemotherapy induced stomatitis: A pilot study. *Journal of Laboratory and Clinical Medicine*, 127, 223-238.

Soergel, K.H. (1993) Showdown at the Tight Junction. *Gastroenterology*, 105, 1247-1250.

Souba, W.W., Smith, R.J. and Wilmore, D.W. (1985) Effects of Clucocorticoids on Glutamine Metabolism in Visceral Organs. *Metabolism*, 34, 450-456.

Souba, W.W. and Austgen, T.R. (1990a) Interorgan Glutamine Flow Following Surgery and Infection. *Journal of Parenteral and Enteral Nutrition*, 14, 90S-93S.

Souba, W.W., Herskowitz, K., Salloum, R.M., Chen, M.K. and Austgen, T.R. (1990b) Gut Glutamine Metabolism. *Journal of Parenteral and Enteral Nutrition*, 14, 45S-50S.

Souba, W.W., Klimberg, V.S., Hautamaki, R.D., Mendenhall, W.H., Bova, F.C., Howard, R.J., Bland, K.I. and Copeland, E.M. (1990c) Oral Glutamine Reduces Bacterial Translocation following Abdominal Radiation. *Journal of Surgical Research*, 48, 1-5.

Stegink, L.D., Filer, L.J., Jr. and Baker, G.L. (1973) Monosodium glutamate metabolism in the neonatal pig: effect of load on plasma, brain, muscle and spinal fluid free amino acid levels. *Journal of Nutrition*, **103**, 1138-1145.

Stoll, B., Henry, J., Reeds, P.J., Yu, H., Jahoor, F. and Burrin, D.G. (1998a) Catabolism Dominates the First-Pass Intestinal Metabolism of Dietary Essential Amino Acids in Milk Protein-Fed Piglets. *Journal of Nutrition*, **128**, 606-614.

Stoll, B., Burrin, D.G., Henry, J., Yu, H., Jahoor, F. and Reeds, P.J. (1998b) Dietary Amino Acids Are the Preferential Source of Hepatic Protein Synthesis in Piglets. *Journal of Nutrition*, **128**, 1517-1524.

Stoll, B., Burrin, D.G., Henry, J. Yu, H., Jahoor, F. and Reeds, P.J. (1999) Substrate oxidation by the portal drained viscera of fed piglets. *American Journal of Physiology – Endocrinology and Metabolism*, **277**, 40, E168-E175.

Swords, W.E., Wu, C.-C., Champlin, F.R. and Buddington, R.K. (1993) Postnatal Changes in Selected Bacterial Groups of the Pig Colonic Microflora. *Biology of the Neonate*, **63**, 191-200.

Tan, S. and Hooi, S.C. (2000) Syncollin is differentially expressed in rat proximal small intestine and regulated by feeding behaviour. *American Journal of Physiology - Gastrointestinal and Liver Physiology*, **278**, G308-G320.

Tremel, H., Kienle, B., Weilemann, L.S., Stehle, P. and Fürst, P. (1994) Glutamine dipeptide-supplemented parenteral nutrition maintains intestinal function in the critically III. *Gastroenterology*, **107**, 1595-1601.

Vagianos, C., Karatzas, T., Scopa, C.D., Panagopoulos, C., Tsoni, I., Spiliopoulou, I. and Kalfarentzos, F. (1992) Neurotensin Reduces Microbial Translocaiton and Improves Intestinal Mucosa Integrity after Abdominal Radiation. *European Surgical Research*, **24**, 77-83.

Watford, M., Lund, P. and Krebs, H.A. (1979) Isolation and Metabolic Characteristics of Rat and Chicken Enterocytes. *Biochemical Journal*, **178**, 589-596.

Watford, M. (1994) Glutamine metabolism in rat small intestine: synthesis of three products in isolated enterocytes. *Biochemical Biophysical Acta*, **1200**, 73-78.

Windmueller, H.G. and Spaeth, A.E. (1975) Intestinal Metabolism of Glutamine and Glutamate from the Lumen as Compared to Glutamine from Blood. *Archives of Biochemistry and Biophysics*, **171**, 662-672.

Windmueller, H.G. and Spaeth, A.E. (1980) Respiratory Fuels and Nitrogen Metabolism *in vivo* in Small Intestine of Fed Rats – Quantative Importance of Glutamine, Glutamate and Aspartate. *The Journal of Biological Chemistry*, **255**, 1, 107-112.

Worsaae, H. and Schmidt, M. (1980) Plasma Cortisol and Behaviour in Early Weaned Piglets. *Acta Veterinaria Scandinavica*, **21**, 640-657.

Wu, G., Knabe, D.A. and Flynn, N.E. (1994) Synthesis of citrulline from glutamine in pig enterocytes. *Biochemical Journal*, **299**, 115-121.

Wu, G., Knabe, D.A., Yan, W. and Flynn, N.E. (1995) Glutamine and glucose metabolism in enterocytes of the neonatal pig. *American Journal of Physiology -Regulatory Integrative and Comparative Physiology*, **268**, R334-R342.

Wu, G. (1996) Effects of Concanavalin A and Phorbol Myristate Acetate on Glutamine Metabolism and Proliferation of Porcine Intestinal Intraepithelial Lymphocytes. *Comparative Biochemistry and Physiology*, **114A**, 363-368.

Wu, G., Meier, S.A. and Knabe, D.A. (1996) Dietary Glutamine Supplementation Prevents Jejunal Atrophy in Weaned Pigs. *Journal of Nutrition*, **126**, 2578-2584.

Yang, D., Hazey, J.W., David, F., Singh, J., Rivchum, R., Streem, J.M., Halperin, M.L. and Brunengraber, H. (2000) Integrative physiology of splanchic glutamine and ammonium metabolism. *American Journal of Physiology – Endocrinology and Metabolism*, **278**, E469-E476.

Ziegler, TR., Estívariz, C.F., Jonas, C.R., Gu, L.H., Jones, D.P. and Leader, L.M. (1999) Interactions between nutrients and peptide growth factors in intestinal growth, repair, and function. *Journal of Parenteral and Enteral Nutrition,* 6, S174-83.

**4**

# THE INFLUENCE OF FEED COMPOSITION ON PROTEIN METABOLISM IN THE GUT

Ortwin Simon
*Institute of Animal Nutrition, Veterinary Faculty, Free University - Berlin, Germany*

## Summary

The tissues of the gastrointestinal tract are metabolically highly active and contribute to total body protein synthesis 20 to 40 % although the proportion of protein in these organs is much lower. The actual knowledge about quantitative aspects of protein turnover rates of intestinal tissues is limited due to methodical difficulties in measuring synthesis and breakdown rates and due to the continuous loss of mucosa cell and secretion of proteins. The protein turnover of the gut is highly sensitive to luminal nutrient supply and follows postprandial modifications. These are controlled by both protein synthesis and breakdown. Nutritional factors like non starch polysaccharides or lectins may induce changes in relative weights of tissues and protein contents of the gastrointestinal tract resulting in increased body protein synthesis rates and heat production. In addition, fractional protein synthesis rates and mucin secretion were shown to be increased. Feed constituents may influence protein turnover of the gut via modifications of the intestinal flora. These effects are mediated by formation of short chain fatty acids and probably by affecting the adhering bacteria to enterocytes.

## Introduction[2]

The gastrointestinal tract is one of the most metabolically active organs of the body. The gut and the small intestine mucosa in particular, have the highest rates of protein synthesis among the various body tissues. It seems to be generally valid for all animal species that tissues of the gastrointestinal tract, which contribute only 3 to 6 % of total body protein content contribute to whole body protein synthesis at far higher proportions between 20 and 40 % (Table 1). Since a considerable part of heat production is associated to protein turnover (Bergner and Hoffmann,

1996), factors which modify protein turnover rates in tissues of the gastrointestinal tract or the mass of these tissues may influence also energy expenditure of the whole organism.

Table 1. Proportional distribution of tissue protein synthesis (as percentage of whole body protein synthesis)

| | Pigs[a] | Heifers[b] | Rats | Rainbow trout[e] |
|---|---|---|---|---|
| Muscle | 29.7 – 30.3 | 19.9 – 13.8 | 25[c] | 22 |
| Digestive tract | 19.3 – 20.3 | 32.4 – 41.5 | 28[d] | 39 |
| Liver | 7.1 – 8.3 | 4.7 – 7.5 | 15[c] | 14 |
| Skin | 5.8 – 6.5 | 16.8 – 18.6 | 18[c] | n.d. |

a) Simon, 1989; based on 11 growing pigs, 50 kg body weight, applying the continuous infusion method; calculated from minimum and upper values of fractional protein synthesis rates
b) Lobley, Milne, Lovie, Reeds and Pennie, 1980a; mean of 2 animals; calculated from minimum and upper values of fractional protein synthesis rates
c) Preedy, McNurlan and Garlick, 1983; large dose technique
d) Mc Nurlan and Garlick, 1980; large dose technique
e) Fauconneau and Arnal, 1985; pulse injection technique

A high protein turnover rate is a precondition for short term adaptional response of a tissue to various factors. Due to fractional protein synthesis rates ($k_s$) of e.g. small intestinal tissue of piglets of nearly 100 % per day (Nyachoti, de Lange, McBride, Leeson and Gabert, 2000) this tissue is highly adaptable. A $k_s$ of 100 % per day means that the amount of synthesised and degraded protein per day equals the amount present in the tissue. On this basis, such metabolically active tissues have the ability of reacting noticeably to feed intake or other diurnal acting factors. On the other hand, the intensive protein turnover and the responsiveness of intestinal tissues are part of the reasons for difficulties in quantitative measurements of protein turnover data. Other factors complicating measurements of this kind in the intestine are the continual loss of mucosa cells in addition to the internal protein turnover within cells (Lobley, Connell, Milne, Newman and Ewing, 1994) and active secretion of digestive enzymes, glycoproteins, immune proteins and apolipoproteins (Alpers, 1986; McBurney, 1994; Reeds, Burrin, Davis and Fiorotto, 1993). According to Reeds, Burrin, Stoll and van Goudoever (1999), mucin secretion is probably quantitatively the most significant secretory component, but this remains a speculation as long as quantitative in vivo measurements of mucin synthesis are not available. Finally in contrast to other tissues, tissues of the digestive tract are influenced not only by arterial factors but also by luminal factors. Luminal factors are of course primarily feed constituents, however, microorganisms associated with or adhering to mucosal surfaces or microbial metabolism may affect protein turnover of intestinal tissues as well (Muramatsu, Coates, Hewitt, Salter and Garlick, 1983; Salminen, Bouley, Bourton-Ruault, Cummings, Franck, Gibson, Isolauri, Moreau, Roberfroid and Rowland, 1998).

Therefore, all quantitative data on protein turnover especially of intestinal tissues should be interpreted with caution taking into account the aspects mentioned above, including the method which was applied.

Since the number of publications on the subject is rather limited for pigs, estimates on other species will be included in this paper.

## Methodical aspects on measurements of tissue protein turnover

Protein turnover was defined by Zilversmit (1960) and Garlick and Millward (1972) as the dynamic balance between protein synthesis and protein breakdown. Because quantitative estimates of protein breakdown rates *in vivo* present particular difficulties (for review see Simon, 1989), practically all protein turnover measurements in tissues are based on measurements of protein synthesis rates. Protein breakdown rates in distinct tissues may be calculated indirectly if both protein synthesis rate and net protein gain rate are measured. However, in organs with intensive protein secretion like intestinal tissue this procedure is rather inadequate. Therefore, for tissues of the gastrointestinal tract our knowledge on quantitative turnover data is based on measurements of protein synthesis rates.

The prevalent factor for measurements of protein synthesis is the estimation of the incorporation rate of a labelled amino acid into tissue proteins. Radioactive isotopes can be used for labelling of amino acids, e.g. $^{14}C$ or $^{3}H$ or stable isotopes like $^{15}N$ or $^{13}C$. In both cases the estimation of synthesis rates requires the measurement of the specific radioactivity or isotope enrichment, respectively, of the particular amino acid in both the precursor pool and the protein pool. Due to the higher sensitivity of measurements of radioactivity, early studies were made using radioactive isotopes. However, because of the developments in gas chromatography-mass spectrometry and in isotope ratio mass spectrometry, measurements of enrichments of stable isotopes are highly sensitive as well and the use of stable isotope techniques for this type of studies is well established (e.g. Biolo, Zhang and Wolfe, 1995; Metges and Petzke, 1996). Furthermore, due to the non radioactive nature of stable isotopes they can also be used in human studies (Bouteloup-Demange, Boirie, Déchelotte, Gachon and Beaufrère, 1998; Nakshabendi, Obeidat, Russel, Downie, Smith and Rennie, 1995).

The most reliable calculations of synthesis rates are possible if the specific labelling of the amino acid in the precursor pool remains constant during the incorporation period. One way to maintain this constant is the continuous intravenous infusion of tracer doses of a labelled amino acid for a period of several hours (usually 6 h or more). Under these conditions, the specific labelling of the free amino acid in blood plasma and in intracellular pools increases towards a plateau, which can be described by a single exponential equation (Zilversmit, 1960). This technique was applied for measurements of tissue protein synthesis in pigs by e.g. Garlick, Burk and Swick (1976) and Simon, Münchmeyer, Bergner, Zebrowska and Buraczewska (1979). The main problem with the continuous infusion technique of tracer doses of amino acids is that also plateaus in specific labelling of the free amino acid in all tissues are reached, the plateau values are lower for tissue free amino acids compared to plasma due to the release of unlabelled amino acid by intracellular proteolysis and differ also between tissues (Table 2). These differences are the reason for uncertainties of calculated protein synthesis rates, as supposing a specific labelling of the amino acid in the precursor pool equal to the extracted free amino acid from the tissue will give a considerably higher synthesis rate than supposing the specific labelling in the precursor pool like in the free extracellular amino acid pool measured in blood plasma. The problem of large differences of labelling the free amino acid pools can be solved partially by applying the so called flooding or large dose technique, where the labelled amino acid is injected or infused with a large amount of the same amino acid. In this way all possible precursor pools are flooded and become nearly similar labelled and maintained constant for the period of incorporation which is usually only 10 to 15 minutes (McNurlan, Tomkins and Garlick, 1979). This method was for technical reasons mainly used in small animals, however, there is an increasing application for studies in larger species like piglets (e.g. Burrin, Shulman, Reeds, Davis and Gravitt, 1992; Nyachoti *et al.*, 2000) or sheep (e.g. Lobley *et al.*, 1994). An example for relative specific labelling of free tissue amino acids compared to plasma is given in Table 2. Under this condition the calculated protein synthesis rates of a tissue differ only little irrespective of the supposed precursor pool. The flooding (or large dose) technique is especially suitable for measurements of protein synthesis in organs with high protein turnover rates and organs with high secretory activities. Because of the short incorporation period, recycling of labelled amino acids from intracellular degradation is negligible and newly formed secretory proteins are also measured using this technique. Therefore, in organs like liver, pancreas and intestinal tissues the flooding technique gives higher values for protein synthesis rates than continuous infusion techniques (McNurlan *et al.*, 1979).

Particularly in ruminants combined techniques of veno-arterial difference measurements and stable isotope infusion were applied for studies on amino acid and protein metabolism in splanchnic tissues (e.g. Lapierre, Bernier, Dubreuil, Reynolds, Farmer, Oellet and Lobley, 1999). This technique estimates also both synthesis of constitutive and export proteins.

**Table 2.** Relative specific radioactivity of free amino acids in tissues (expressed relative to the amino acid in plasma) after 6 hours continuous infusion or 12 min infusion with a flooding dose

| | *Relative specific radioactivity of free amino acid* | |
| | *Continuous infusion technique*[1] | *Flooding technique*[2] |
| --- | --- | --- |
| Liver | 0.39 | 0.84 |
| Pancreas | 0.39 | 0.68 |
| Duodenum | 0.45 | 0.81 |
| Jejunum | 0.39 | 0.77 |
| Ileum | 0.37 | 0.80 |
| Colon | 0.42 | 0.72 |
| Muscle | 0.55 | 0.78 |

1) Simon, Berger, Münchmeyer and Zebrowska (1982); values for free leucine after 6 h infusion of $^{14}$C leucine in pigs of 42 kg body weight receiving a barley-soy bean meal based diet.
2) Nyachoti *et al.* (2000); values for free phenylalanine after flooding dose of $^{3}$H-phenylalanine for 10 min in piglets of approximately 25 kg body weight receiving a barley-canola based diet.

Finally, a further inherent problem comes from possible utilisation of amino acids that originated from both the luminal and the vascular side (Alpers, 1972). However, as pointed out recently in a review paper (Reeds *et al.*, 1999) there is evidence that for duodenal and jejunal protein synthesis, arterial amino acids are preferentially used, at least in a fed state. The proportion of these two sources of amino acids for protein synthesis may, however, be shifted along the small intestine such that the distal segments probably rely more on arterial amino acids.

Concluding the methodical aspects, it should be stressed once again that absolute data on protein turnover rates are only comparable, if identical conditions are applied. Due to the specific problems in quantifying protein turnover parameters, our knowledge in this field is rather incomplete.

## Effects of luminal nutrient supply

These effects can be studied by varying the oral nutrient supply or by comparing the effects of enteral and parenteral nutrient administration. In a study on neonatal miniature piglets protein turnover data of visceral tissues were recorded, when water, mature milk or colostrum were fed for 6 hours before suckling by large dose administration of $^{3}$H-phenylalanine in combination with other analytical procedures (Burrin *et al.*, 1992). In this study the phenylalanine incorporation into proteins of the jejunum and ileum was not significantly different from milk and colostrum feeding, but in both treatments the incorporation was approximately three times higher compared to water feeding. However, protein accretion in small intestinal tissue in colostrum fed piglets was 10 times higher than in the milk fed group and exceeded the calculated absolute protein synthesis three to four times in colostrum fed animals. This leads to the conclusion that protein accretion in the small intestine of newborn piglets is controlled by additional factors other than synthesis and degradation rates of proteins. Additional protein accretion is most probably a consequence of endocytosis of colostral immunoglobulins, particularly of IgG. The findings reported on neonatal piglets are consistent with those made for lambs (Patureau-Mirand, Mosoni, Levieux, Attaix and Bonnet, 1990).

Fasting of animals profoundly decreases the protein mass of gastrointestinal tissues and losses from the small intestine are greater than from the rest of the body. These modifications are accompanied by decreased fractional and absolute rates of protein synthesis in the stomach but to a lesser extent in the small intestine and colon according to estimates in adult rats (Samuels, Taillandier, Aurousseau, Cherel, le Maho, Arnal and Attaix, 1996). As indicated by increased mRNA levels of critical components of lysosomal, $Ca^{2+}$-activated and ubiquitin-dependent proteolytic pathways, losses in protein mass in small intestinal tissues seem to be caused primarily by stimulated protein degradation. This agrees well with measurements made for small intestinal mucosa in 36 hours fasted humans (Bouteloup-Demange *et al.*, 1998).

Parenteral administration of an elemental diet to neonatal piglets during a period of approximately one week in comparison to oral milk fed or sow-suckled piglets (Adeola, Wykes, Ball and Penchart, 1995) or to enteral administration of the same elemental diet (Dudley, Wykes, Dudley, Burrin, Nichols, Rosenberger, Jahoor, Heird and Reeds, 1998) resulted in a pronounced reduction in intestinal mass, but the protein content of mucosa was not changed while the route of administration of the same elemental diet did not influence body weight gain. It was clearly shown, that parenteral administration of nutrients reduced fractional and absolute synthesis rates of total mucosal proteins by approximately 40%. However, not all mucosal proteins seem to be controlled in the same way, since lactase phlorizin hydrolase synthesis (a specific intestinal brush border protein responsible for terminal stages of digestion) was less susceptible to the route of nutrient administration than the mucosal protein synthesis in general.

These results imply that luminal nutrient supply is an important factor in affecting protein turnover in small intestinal tissues. The modifications are selective and contribute to adaptation.

## Postprandial response

Due to the discontinuous luminal nutrient supply and the very high protein turnover rates, intestinal tissues are suggested to be nutritionally highly sensitive and postprandial responses are most probable. Due to technical difficulties in this type of studies particularly with farm animals, quantitative data for pigs are scarce and vague. Additionally, the interest on postprandial reactions of tissue protein turnover in rats was mostly focused on muscles and liver (Garlick, Millward and James, 1973; Garlick, Fern and Preedy, 1983). In minipigs variations in protein synthesis of muscles measured at various periods after intake of a meal were reported by Danfaer (1980).

In an experiment on rats which were trained for fast feed intake twice a day, protein synthesis in liver and small intestine was measured by the large dose technique before feeding (12 hours feed withdrawal), and one to 6 hours after intake of a meal (Simon and Bergner, 1983, Table 3).

**Table 3.** Postprandial changes of nitrogen content (mg N/100 g body weight) and fractional protein synthesis rates[1] (%/day) in liver and small intestine of rats

| Time after feed intake (hours) | Nitrogen content | | Protein synthesis rate | |
|---|---|---|---|---|
| | Liver | Small intestine | Liver | Small intestine |
| 0 | 127 | 78[a] | 67[bc] | 109 |
| 1 | 137 | 88[ab] | 92[abc] | 103 |
| 2 | 129 | 82[ab] | 110[ab] | 106 |
| 4 | 126 | 84[ab] | 126[a] | 128 |
| 6 | 142 | 90[b] | 86[c] | 116 |

1) Calculated by using the specific radioactivity of the tissue free amino acid as the precursor labelling

Protein synthesis rate using this technique included both synthesis of fixed and secretory proteins. Since the amount of protein in liver was not changed, the postprandial increase of protein synthesis in liver was probably accompanied by a stimulated intracellular protein degradation and/or protein secretion. The response of protein synthesis rates in intestinal tissues was not so clear, but the nitrogen content in these tissues was increased up to 15 %. This indicates that protein degradation is involved in the regulation process. Deutz and Soeters (1998) came to the same conclusion in experiments with piglets using combined measurements of portal drained viscera amino acid flux measurements and a primed constant infusion technique with labelled amino acids. During the absorptive metabolism in their study, increased protein accretion in the gut was not paralleled by increased protein synthesis rates. Therefore, decreased protein breakdown rates were made responsible for this effect. It was shown for the large intestine of restricted fed rats that both protein content and protein synthesis rates decreased progressively with increasing time interval after the last meal (Merry, Goldspink and Lewis, 1991).

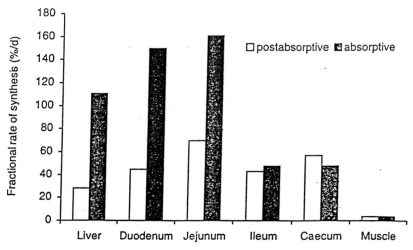

**Figure 1.** Fractional rates of tissue protein synthesis[1] (%/day) in pigs of ~ 40 kg body weight estimated at different time after intake of a meal (6 to 12 hours after feed intake = postabsorptive; 3 to 9 hours after feed intake = absorptive)[2]
1) Fractional synthesis rates calculates taking free amino acids as the precursor labelling
2) Calculated from Simon *et al.*, 1982, 1983

Protein synthesis of various tissues was measured with the large dose technique in 7- and 26-days-old piglets after a 24 hours fast and refeeding of porcine mature milk (Davis, Burrin, Fiorotto and Nguyen, 1996). As in other visceral tissues fractional protein synthesis in the jejunum was highly significantly increased of fed animals (measured 15 minutes after three meals in 60 minutes intervals). Measurements of tissue protein synthesis rates in pigs using the continuous infusion technique 6 to 12 hours (postabsorptive phase) or 3 to 9 hours (including absorptive phase) after feed intake indicates that protein synthesis in the absorptive phase is especially stimulated in the liver and in the upper small intestine (Figure 1). However, it should be remembered that continuous infusion techniques do only partially consider synthesis of secretory proteins. The interpretation of the data suffers therefore of this methodical inadequacy. And it is also an assumption that, since the main fate of free amino acids is incorporation into proteins or oxidation, mechanisms may exist in the organism by which amino acids are temporarily incorporated into proteins during the absorptive phase, thus preventing extensive oxidation of absorbed amino acids. This would be controlled by circadian modulation of protein synthesis or protein degradation or both. Postprandial stimulated secretion of proteins into the digestive tract may additionally act as a trapping mechanism for amino acids since endogenous proteins are largely reabsorbed (Fuller and Reeds, 1998) but with delay in time.

## Protein intake

In general protein synthesis of the whole body and of individual tissues in pigs correlates positively with feeding level and with protein intake at a given feeding level (Krawielitzki, 1980; Reeds, Cadenhead, Fuller, Lobley and Mc Donald, 1980; Reeds, Fuller, Cadenhead, Lobley and McDonald, 1981b; Simon, 1989). However, low protein diets affect protein turnover rates of the tissues of the digestive tract to a lesser extent than in other tissues. Reduction of protein content in feed of piglets to half of the control level (day 10 to 17 of life) resulted in decreased fractional rates of protein synthesis in muscle, liver and bone by 24, 16, and 19 %, respectively, while in tissues of the digestive tract the synthesis rate and protein deposition remained constant (Séve, Reeds, Fuller, Cadenhead and Hay, 1986). The same tendency towards maintaining constant protein synthesis rates in the liver and also in intestinal tissues was observed in pigs of 40 to 50 kg body weight, when rations containing 40 g of protein per kg instead of 160 g were fed (Simon, 1989).

## Effects of non starch polysaccharides

Non starch polysaccharides (NSP) may influence protein turnover of intestinal tissues in various ways, i.e. modifications of tissue mass, secretion of proteins into the lumen of the intestine, life span of mucosa cells and internal protein turnover. Again, technical difficulties in quantitative measurements of most of these processes limit our actual knowledge in this field.

It was shown for several animal species that increasing inclusion rates of NSP in diets induce an increase of relative and absolute weights of tissues of intestinal tract. When various NSP model substrates were included in diets for rats increases of the relative weight of small intestine from 2.4 up to 5.0 g per 100 g body weight were observed (Ikegami, Tsuchihashi, Harada, Tsuchihashi, Nishide and Innami, 1990). Furthermore it was considered, that this effect was most pronounced for NSP, which produced the highest viscosities in the intestinal digesta. The results were confirmed by experiments in broiler chickens. Inclusion of the viscosity producing model substrate carboxymethyl cellulose (CMC) into a semisynthetic diet resulted in enlargements of length of small intestine of 38 days old chickens from 139 to 181 cm (van der Klis and Van Voorst, 1993), and replacement of low viscosity CMC by high viscosity CMC caused in animals of the same age increases in relative weights of both small intestine and colon by 40 % (Smits, Veldman, Verstegen and Beynen, 1997). Even small reductions of digesta viscosity by enzyme addition to wheat based broiler chicken diets led to decreases in relative weights of small intestine between 5 to 18 % (Veldman and Vahl, 1994). In pigs receiving low (59 g/kg) or high (268 g/kg) dietary fibre diets the relative weight of the total digestive tract was 32.7 vs. 43.6 g per kg empty body weight and was significantly different (Jørgensen, Zhao and Eggum, 1996). However in contrast to rats and chickens the modifications were more pronounced for the colon than for the small intestine. Fermentable carbohydrate sources are known to increase cell turnover in the large intestine and to have trophic effects on the mucosa. The main reason for this effect is as a result of intensified formation of butyrate under these conditions (reviewed by Salminen *et al.*, 1998). One of the contributions in this workshop will especially focus on the role of butyrate for epithelial cell proliferation.

A hypertrophy of gut tissue seems therefore to be a general effect of dietary NSP constituents. The main factors for these effects are increased digesta viscosities in the content of the small intestine and intensified formation of short chain fatty acids (SCFA) in the large intestine.

Due to the very high protein turnover rate of these tissues, one may conclude, that total body protein turnover rates and resting heat production of animals will be increased in animals having elevated proportions of gastrointestinal tissues. Indeed it was shown that fasting heat production of pigs but also other species is highly related to variations in weight of metabolically active organs with high protein turnover rates as the most important influencing factor (Koong, Ferrell and Nienaber, 1985; Koong and Ferrell, 1990; Reeds *et al.*, 1999).

In experiments at our institute on broiler chickens, digesta viscosity was modulated over a wide range (between 4 and 900 mPas in jejunal digesta) by replacing crystalline cellulose with CMC, guar gum and xylans, respectively, or by replacing maize by rye. In such an experimental mode the relative intestinal weight can be almost doubled and the increases in relative weight correlated highly significantly with digesta viscosity independent of the source of viscosity producing substance (Figure 2). Under practical feeding conditions those high viscosities and changes in weights of intestines will not occur. However, increases of weights of the GIT tissues in the range of 30 % seems realistic. On this basis a model calculation was made in order to estimate the effect of an assumed increase in the amount of protein in the gastrointestinal tract on the energy metabolism (Simon, 1998; Table 4). According to these model calculations, the increase in protein content in the GIT by 30 % would mean an additional daily protein synthesis of 2.4 g associated with a heat increment of 30 kJ. This would mean an increase of heat production of 5 %. That agrees well with the measurements of Jørgensen *et al.*

(1996) who measured heat productions of 791 and 855 kJ/d and per kg empty metabolic body weight (difference 8.1 %) in pigs receiving low and high fibre diets, respectively, while total relative GIT weights differed by 37 %.

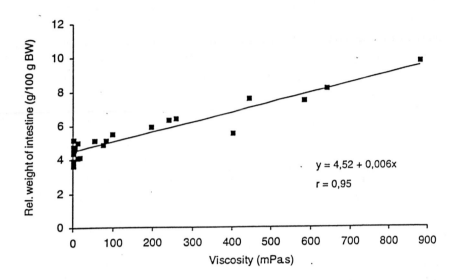

**Figure 2.** Relationship between viscosity in jejunal lumen and the relative weight of intestinal tissues in broilers (21 days of life)

**Table 4.** Model calculation for the effect of an increase of the amount of protein in the GIT by 30% on energy metabolism (calculated for 1 kg BW)[1]

|  | *Amount of protein* g | *Fractional synthesis rate* %/day | *Amount of synthesized protein* g/day | *GIT* 130 % |
|---|---|---|---|---|
| Total body | 160 | 23 | 36.8 | 39.2 |
| Skeletal muscles | 88 | 10 | 8.8 | 8.8 |
| GIT | 11.2 | 70 | 7.8 | 10.2 |
| Heat production, kJ × d⁻¹ | 625 + 30 kJ (GIT 130%) = ca. + 5% | | | |

1) based on various references

Up to this point the discussion on the effects of NSP on total protein turnover of the intestinal tissues assumes constant fractional synthesis and secretion rates of proteins. However, there are data from studies on rats showing that both crypt cell production rates as well as mucosal fractional protein synthesis rates in jejunum and ileum are significantly increased in animals receiving a diet with 75 g/kg noncellulosic NSP compared to a semisynthetic diet with 40 g/kg cellulose (Southon, Livesey, Gee and Johnson, 1985). This implies that non starch polysaccharides *per se* or viscosity producing constituents of a diet may act in a similar manner in other species too. Furthermore, again from studies on rats there is some evidence that dietary fibre components induce mucin secretion in the small intestine. In rats fed a diet containing 20 % wheat bran (compared to a fibre free diet) the relative number of mucin producing goblet cells in the epithelium of the small intestine was found to be significantly increased (Schneeman, Richter and Jacobs, 1982). Addition of guar gum or citrus fibre to a fibre free diet resulted in elevated luminal mucin contents in the small intestine of rats, as estimated by using of a quantitative enzyme-linked immunosorbent assay (Satchithanandam, Vargofcak-Apker, Calvert, Leeds and Cassidy, 1990). The significance of a stimulated secretion of mucins is only speculative, because quantitative production rates are not known. But mucins contain 20 to 30 % proteins with an amino acid composition particularly high in cystine and threonine and measurable influences on the requirements of animals for these two amino acids due to modifications in mucin secretion seem possible (Reeds *et al.*, 1999).

In order to see whether or not similar responses as in rats can be measured in farm animals more recently studies on broiler chickens were performed under the conditions of low (1.7 mPas) and high (approx. 100 mPas) viscosity of jejunal digesta (our group, not published). When the high viscosity was produced with CMC the ratio of proliferating to total epithelial cells in the crypt region was increased significantly, but similar changes were observed only as a trend when high viscosity was produced by rye inclusion. Furthermore, attempts have been made to measure protein synthesis rates in tissues of broilers when fed diets producing different digesta viscosities (Dänicke, Böttcher, Jeroch, Thielebein and Simon, 2000). The diets where based on rye, two fat sources were used and viscosity was modulated by addition of a xylanase preparation. Protein synthesis rates were measured applying the flooding technique using $^{15}$N phenylalanine. The results for jejunal tissue are presented in Table 5.

At the highest digesta viscosity (rye-tallow without xylanase addition) fractional and absolute protein synthesis rates were increased significantly in this tissue. Similar results were found for the duodenum and the ileum. The absolute protein synthesis rates of the whole small intestine were 4.80, 4.82, 7.94 and 4.47 g per day and kg body weight in treatments one to four, respectively. In a previous study (Dänicke, Jeroch and Simon, 2000) using the same diets, it was shown that animals which received rye-tallow diets without xylanase addition (treatment 3) had also the highest faecal excretion of endogenous nitrogen which was nearly three times that of animal of the other treatments. In contrast to these observations on broiler chickens, Nyachoti *et al.* (2000) failed to find any changes in protein synthesis rates in small intestines of piglets that received diets which are known to induce high losses of endogenous nitrogen.

**Table 5.** Effects of type of diet[1] on digesta viscosity and jejunal protein synthesis in broilers (after Dänicke *et al.*, 2000)

| Treat-ment | Fat type | Xyla-nase[2] | Viscosity in jejunal digesta (mPas) | Fractional protein synthesis rate (%/d) | | Absolute protein synthesis of jejunum (g/d per kg BW) |
|---|---|---|---|---|---|---|
| | | | | Jejunum | Jejunal mucosa | |
| 1 | Soya oil | - | 106[a] | 51.3[a] | 66.3[a] | 2.01[a] |
| 2 | Soya oil | + | 44[a] | 51.7[a] | 67.1[a] | 1.93[a] |
| 3 | Beef tallow | - | 206[b] | 74.8[b] | 105.1[b] | 3.28[b] |
| 4 | Beef tallow | + | 91[a] | 57.5[a] | 67.9[a] | 1.98[a] |

1) rye based diet (560 g/kg); soya oil and beef tallow inclusions 100 g/kg, respectively
2) without (-) or with (+) addition of xylanase (2700 IU/kg)

Based on the data shown above it can be concluded that non starch polysaccharides have a considerable influence on protein turnover of intestinal tissues in various ways including modifications of relative organ mass, protein synthesis rates and probably proliferation rate of enterocytes as well as mucin secretion.

As reviewed by Low and Zebrowska (1989) and more recently by Fuller and Reeds (1999) the largest part of secretion of nitrogen into the digestive tract in pigs is contributed by the small intestine. Due to a simultaneous occurrence of secretion and absorption processes, it is difficult to measure the amount and composition of protein or N secretion. In pigs of 50 to 70 kg body weight, it was approximated that 15 g of nitrogen is secreted by the whole small intestine within 24 hours (Buraczewska, 1979). The measurements were made using a perfusion technique of intestinal loops. With the same technique it was shown, that viscosity producing NSP such as guar gum may stimulate the amount of endogenous N secretion considerably from approximately 15 to 27 g per day (Low and Rainbird, 1984). Since absorption of endogenous N within the small intestine ranges between 50 and 75 % and absorption rather than secretion of endogenous nitrogen along the small intestine is influenced by nutritional factors (Grala, Buraczewska, Wasilewko, Verstegen, Tamminga, Jansman, Huisman and Korczyński, 1998), all quantitative data have the character of approximations. For further interpretations of the significance of endogenous protein secretions more information is required about the proportional contributions from the various sources e.g. pancreatic juice, mucosa cells and mucins.

## Effects of lectins

Lectins are classified as antinutritional factors which may reduce utilisation of nutrients and cause negative effects on growth and health of animals. Lectins are contained in legume seeds, but also in other feedstuffs of plant origin. The importance for practical animal feeding is not clear at present, because the degree of lectin toxicity is very much dependent on the plant species. As reviewed by Jansman and Huisman (1995) lectins from common beans (*Phaseolus vulgaris*) are very toxic and most studies are based on the effects of *Phaseolus* lectins, while lectins from pea were found to be non-toxic in piglets, but toxic in rats. Soya bean lectins were described to have low toxicity. A further problem is that most experiments on the effects of lectins are made with rats, however, it was shown that rats, piglets and chickens react in a different way when adapted to the same diets containing *Phaseolus* beans (Huisman, van der Poel, Mouwen and van Weerden, 1990a) or peas (Huisman, van der Poel, Kik and Mouwen, 1990b).

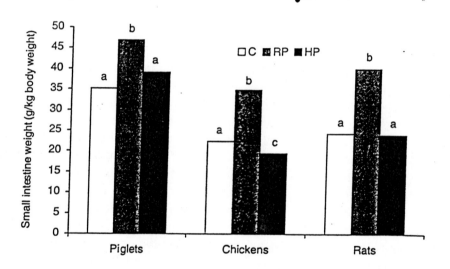

**Figure 3.** Effects of diets containing raw (RP) or heat treated (HP) *Phaseolus vulgaris* beans (200 g/kg) in comparison to a control diet (C = casein) on relative weights of small intestine of piglets, chickens and rats (after Huisman *et al.*, 1990a)
Values with different superscript letters were significantly different (P < 0.05).

The basic mechanism of the toxic effects of lectins is their ability to bind to sugar components of the luminal surface of epithelial cells in the intestine (Grant, 1991). A further probably essential event is an endocytotic uptake of lectins by epithelial cells (Pusztai, 1989) followed by an increase in protein synthesis of the mucosa cells (Oliveira, Pusztai and Grant, 1988; Palmer, Pusztai, Bain and Grant, 1987). These modifications are accompanied by drastic increases in weight, protein and DNA content of small intestine as well as increased mucin secretion (Greer, Brewer, and Pusztai, 1985). A stimulated uptake of polyamine seems to be a mechanism involved in stimulated small intestinal growth (Bardosz, Grant, Brown, Ewen, Nevions and Pusztai, 1990). Figure 3 gives an example for the effects of *phaseolus* bean inclusion in diets on small intestinal growth of piglets, chickens and rats. The relative weights were increased by 35 to 70 %. On the other hand data of Figure 3 demonstrate, that due to the protein nature of lectins these antinutritive factors can be effectively inactivated by heat treatment. Lectins from other plant species than legumes were shown to have also polyamine-dependent hyperplastic and hypertrophic growth effects on the small intestine by increasing protein, RNA and DNA contents (Pusztai, Ewen, Grant, Brown, Stewart, Peumans, van Damme and Bardocz, 1993).

It may be concluded, that lectins affect the protein turnover of the intestinal tissue in three different ways: by increasing the total organ weight (and amount of protein of the organ), by increasing cell proliferation rates and protein synthesis rates and by stimulating secretion of endogenous proteins into the gut lumen. A general consequence of the described modification is the increased cost for energy and substrates to maintain that elevated synthesis rate of protein and nucleic acids.

## Effects of other factors that influence intestinal microbial population

Interactions between feed composition and intestinal microflora with impact on protein metabolism of the gut tissue are frequently discussed. As reviewed by Salminen *et al.* (1998) carbohydrates not absorbed in the upper digestive tract are the major energy substrates for intestinal bacteria in monogastric animals resulting in SCFA as end products of bacterial fermentation. Since the most important property of SCFA in the digestive tract is their trophic effect on the intestinal epithelium, intestinal bacteria act as mediators between feed composition and gut metabolism.

Another aspect is that feed additives designed for modifying the intestinal microflora may also influence the intestinal protein metabolism. It was shown for antibiotics in pigs to have a reducing effect on the mass of intestinal tract (Yen, Nienaber, Pond and Varel, 1985) or to decrease cell proliferation rates in chickens (Krinke and Jamroz, 1996). Flavomycin treatment of sheep resulted in lowered leucine sequestration and oxidation rates in the digestive tract and an increased amino acid supply to the portal vein of 25 % (McRae *et al.*, 1999, cited by Nieto and Lobley, 1999). On the other hand, probiotics were found to stimulate epithelial cell proliferation (Ichicawa, Kuroiwa, Inagaki, Shineha, Nishihira, Satomi and Sakata, 1999). However, probiotics may influence the metabolism of the gut in a different way, i.e. by inhibition of adherence of enteropathogenic *E. coli* to enterocytes (Mack, Michail, Wie, McDougall and Holligsworth, 1999; Spencer and Chesson, 1994) which would reduce inflammation reactions. It is not reliable to draw conclusions on the significance of these modifications on the protein metabolism of the gut as the actual basis of experimental data is inadequate.

## References

Adeola, O., Wykes, L.J., Ball, R.O. and Pencharz, P.B. (1995) Comparison of oral milk feeding and total parenteral nutrition in neonatal pigs. *Nutrition Research*, **15**, 245-265.

Alpers, D.H. (1986) Uptake and fate of absorbed amino acids and peptides in the mammalian intestine. *Federation Proceedings*, **45**, 2261-2267.

Alpers, D.H. (1972) Protein synthesis in intestinal mucosa: the effect of route of administration of precursor amino acids. *Journal of Clinical Investigations*, **51**, 167-173.

Bardocz, S., Grant, G., Brown, D.S. Ewen, S.W.B., Nevison, I. and Pussztai, A. (1990) Polyamine metabolism and uptake during *Phaseolus vulgaris* lectin, PHA-induced growth of rat small intestine. *Digestion*, **46**, S2, 360-366.

Bergner, H. and Hoffmann, L. (1996) Bioenergetik und Stoffproduktion landwirtschaftlicher Nutztiere. Harwood Academic Publishers, pp. 166-176.

Biolo, G., Zhang, X.-J. and Wolfe, R.R. (1995) Role of membrane transport in interorgan amino acid flow between muscle and small intestine. *Metabolism*, **44**, 719-724.

Bouteloup-Demange, C., Boirie, Y., Déchelotte, P., Gachon, P. and Beaufrère, B. (1998) Gut mucosal protein synthesis in fed and fasted humans. *American Journal of Physiology*, **274**, *(Endocrinology and Metabolism*, **37***)*, E541-E546.

Buraczewska, L. (1979) Secretion of nitrogenous compounds in the small intestine of pigs. *Acta Physiologica Polonica*, **30**, 319-326.

Burrin, D.G., Shulman, R.J., Reeds, P.J., Davis, T.A. and Gravitt, K.R. (1992) Porcine colostrum and milk stimulate visceral organ and skeletal muscle protein synthesis in neonatal piglets. *Journal of Nutrition*, **122**, 1205-1213.

Dänicke, S., Böttcher, W., Jeroch, H., Thielebein, J. and Simon, O. (2000) Replacement of soya oil with tallow in a rye based diet increases protein synthesis in the small intestinal tissues, an effect which is eliminated if diets are supplemented with an exogenous xylanase. *Journal of Nutrition*, submitted.

Dänicke, S., Jeroch, H. and Simon, O. (2000) Endogenous N-losses in broilers estimated by a [$^{15}$N]-isotope dilution technique: effect of dietary fat type and xylanase addition. *Archives of Animal Nutrition*, **53**, 75-97.

Danfaer, A. (1980) Cited in *Dynamic Biochemistry of Animal Production* (ed. P.M. Riis), *World Animal Science. A. Basic Information*, **3** (1983), 97, Elsevier, Amsterdam-Oxford-New York-Tokyo.

Davis, T.A., Burrin, D.G., Fiorotto, M.L. and Nguyen, H.V. (1996) Protein synthesis in skeletal muscle and jejunum is more responsive to feeding in 7- than in 26-day-old pigs. *American Journal of Physiology*, **270**, (*Endocrinology and Metabolism*, **33**), E802-E809.

Deutz, N.E.P. and Soeters, P.B. (1998) The biological effects of soy and casein protein meals in interorgan amino acid metabolism in the pig as a model for man. *Bulletin of the International Dairy Federation*, **336**, 56-58.

Dudley, M.A., Wykes, L.J., Dudley, A.W., Burrin, D.G., Nichols, B.L., Rosenberger, J., Jahoor, F., Heird, W.C. and Reeds, P.J. (1998) Parenteral nutrition selectively decreases protein synthesis in the small intestine. *American Journal of Physiology*, **274**, (*Gastrointestinal Liver Physiology*, **37**), G131-G137.

Fauconneau, B. and Arnal, M. (1985) *In vivo* protein synthesis in different tissues and the whole body of rainbow trout (*Salmo Gairdnerii R.*) Influence of environmental temperature. *Comparative Biochemistry and Physiology*, **82A**, 179-187.

Fuller, M.F. and Reeds, P.J. (1998) Nitrogen cycling in the gut. *Annual Review of Nutrition*, **18**, 385-411.

Garlick, P.J., Burk, T.L. and Swick, R.W. (1976) Protein synthesis and RNA in tissues of the pig. *American Journal of Physiology*, **230**, 1108-1112.

Garlick, P.J., Fern, M. and Preedy, V.R. (1983) The effect of insulin infusion and food intake on muscle protein synthesis in post absorptive rats. *Biochemical Journal*, **210**, 669-676.

Garlick, P.J. and Millward, D.J. (1972) An appraisal of techniques for the determination of protein turnover in vivo. *Proceedings of the Nutrition Society*, **31**, 249-255.

Garlick, P.J., Millward, D.J. and James, W.P.T. (1973) The diurnal response of muscle and liver protein synthesis *in vivo* in meal-fed rats. *Biochemical Journal*, **136**, 935-945.

Grala, W., Buraczewska, L., Wasilewko, J., Verstegen, M.W.A., Tamminga, S., Jansman, A.J.M., Huisman, J. and Korczyñski, W. (1998) Flow of endogenous and exogenous nitrogen in different segments of the small intestine in pigs fed diets with soyabean concentrate, soyabean meal or rapeseed cake. *Journal of Animal and Feed Sciences*, **7**, 1-20.

Grant, G. (1991) Lectin. In *Toxic Substances in Crop Plants – 1991*, pp. 49-67. Edited by J.P.F. D'Mello, C.M. Duffus and J.H. Duffus. Royal Society of Chemistry, Cambridge.

Greer, F., Brewer, A.C. and Pusztai, A. (1985) Effect of kidney bean (*Phaseolus vulgaris*) toxin on tissue weight and composition and some metabolic functions of rats. *British Journal of Nutrition*, **54**, 95-103.

Huisman, J., van der Poel, A.F.B., Mouwen, J.M.V.M. and van Weerden, E.J. (1990a) Effect of variable protein contents in diets containing *Phaseolus vulgaris* beans on performance, organ weights and blood variables in piglets, rats and chickens. *British Journal of Nutrition*, **64**, 755-764.

Huisman, J., van der Poel, A.F.B., Kik, M.J.L. and Mouwen, J.M.V.M. (1990b) Performance and organ weights of piglets, rats and chickens fed diets containing *Pisum sativum*. *Journal of Animal Physiology and Animal Nutrition*, **63**, 273-279.

Ichicawa, H., Kuroiwa, T., Inagaki, A., Shineha, R., Nishihira, T., Satomi, S. and Sakata, R. (1999) Probiotics bacteria stimulate gut epithelial cell proliferation in rat. *Digestive Diseases and Sciences*, **44**, 2119-2123.

Ikegami, S., Tsuchihashi, F., Harada, H., Tsuchihashi, N., Nishide, E. and Innami, S. (1990) Effect of viscous indigestible polysaccharides on pancreatic-biliary secretion and digestive organs in rats. *Journal of Nutrition*, **120**, 353-360.

Jansman, A.J.M. and Huisman, J. (1995) Some antinutritional factors in feeds and feedstuffs. In *World's Poultry Science Association Proceedings, 10th European Symposium on Poultry Nutrition – Antalya-Turkey, October 15-19th, 1995.*

Jørgensen, H., Zhao, X.-Q. and Eggum, B.O. (1996) The influence of dietary fibre and environmental temperature on the development of the gastrointestinal tract, digestibility, degree of fermentation in the hind-gut and energy metabolism in pigs. *British Journal of Nutrition*, **75**, 365-378.

Koong, L.J. and Ferrell, C.L. (1990) Effects of short term nutritional manipulation on organ size and fasting heat production. *European Journal of Clinical Nutrition*, **44**, Supplement 1, 73-77.

Koong, L.J., Ferrell, C.L. and Nienaber, J.A. (1985) Assessment of interrelationship among levels of intake and production, organ size and fasting heat production in growing animals. *Journal of Nutrition*, **115**, 1383-1390.

Krawielitzki, K. (1980) Studies on growing pigs. In *Role and extent of the amino acid pool in pigs and poultry during growth*, pp 38-48. Edited by H.D. Bock. Akademie der Landwirtschaften der DDR, Berlin [in German].

Krinke, A.L. and Jamroz, D. (1996) Effects of feed antibiotic avoparcine on organ morphology in broiler chickens. *Poultry Science*, **75**, 705-710.

Lapierre, H, Bernier, J.F., Dubreuil, P., Reynolds, C.K., Farmer, Ouellet, D.R. and Lobley, G.E. (1999) The effect of intake on protein metabolism across splanchnic tissues in growing beef steers. *British Journal of Nutrition*, **81**, 457-466.

Lobley, G.E., Connell, A., Milne, E., Newman, A.M. and Ewing, T.A. (1994) Protein synthesis in splanchnic tissues of sheep offered two levels of intake. *British Journal of Nutrition*, **71**, 3-12.

Lobley, G.E., Milne, V., Lovie, J.M., Reeds, P.J. and Pennie, K. (1980a) Whole body and tissue protein synthesis in cattle. *British Journal of Nutrition*, **43**, 491-502.

Low, A.G. and Rainbird, A.L. (1984) Effect of guar gum on nitrogen secretion into isolated loops of jejunum in conscious pigs. *British Journal of Nutrition*, **52**, 499-505.

Low, A.G. and Zebrowska, T. (1989) Digestion in pigs. *In Protein Metabolism in Farm Animals – 1989*, pp 53-121. Edited by H.-D. Bock, B.O. Eggum, A.G. Low, O. Simon and T. Zebrowska. Oxford Science Publications, Deutscher Landwirtschaftsverlag, Berlin.

Mack, D.R., Michail, S., Wie, S., McDougall, L. and Holligsworth, M.A. (1999) Probiotics inhibits enteropathogenic *E. coli* adherence *in vitro* by inducing intestinal mucin gene expression. *American Journal of Physiology*, **276**, G941-G950.

McBurney, M.I. (1994) The gut: central organ in nutrient requirements and metabolism. *Canadian Journal of Physiology and Pharmacology*, **72**, 260-265.

McNurlan, M.A. and Garlick, P.J. (1980) Contribution of rat liver and gastrointestinal tract to whole body protein synthesis in the rat. *Biochemical Journal*, **186**, 381-383.

McNurlan, M.A., Tomkins, A.M. and Garlick, P.J. (1979) The effect of starvation on rate of protein synthesis in rat liver. *Biochemical Journal*, **178**, 373-379.

Merry, B.J., Goldspink, D.F. and Lewis, S.E.M. (1991) The effects of age and chronic restricted feeding on protein synthesis and growth of the large intestine of the rat. *Comparative Biochemistry and Physiology*, **98A**, No.3/4, 559-562

Metges, C.C. and Petzke, K.-J. (1996) Gas chromatography/combustion/isotope ratio mass spectrometric comparison of *N*-acetyl- and *N*-pivaloyl amino acid esters to measure $^{15}N$ isotopic abundances in physiological samples: A pilot study on amino acid synthesis in the upper gastro-intestinal tract of minipigs. *Journal of Mass Spectrometry*, **31**, 367-376.

Muramatsu, T., Coates, M.E., Hewitt, D., Salter, D.N. and Garlick, P.J. (1983) The influence of the gut microflora on protein synthesis in liver and jejunal mucosa in chicks. *British Journal of Nutrition*, **49**, 453.

Nakshabendi, I.M., Obeidat, W., Russell, R.I., Downie, S., Smith, K. and Rennie, M.J. (1995) Gut mucosal protein synthesis measured using intravenous and intragastric delivery of stable tracer amino acids. *American Journal of Physiology*, **269**, *(Endocrinology and Metabolism*, **32**), E996-E999.

Nieto, R., and Lobley, G.E. (1999) Integration of protein metabolism within the whole body and between organs. *In Protein Metabolism and Nutrition, Proceedings of the VIII$^{th}$ International Symposium on Protein Metabolism and Nutrition – Aberdeen, UK, 1.-4. September 1999*, pp

127-153. Edited by G.E. Lobley, A. White and J.C. MacRae. EAAP Publication No. 96, Wageningen Pers, 1999.

Nyachoti, C.M., De Lange, C.F.M., McBride, B.W., Leeson, S. and Gabert, V.M. (2000) Endogenous gut nitrogen losses in growing pigs are not caused by increased protein synthesis rates in the small intestine. *Journal of Nutrition*, 130, 566-572.

Oliveira, J.T.A. de, Pusztai, A. and Grant, G. (1988) Changes in organs and tissues induced by feeding of purified kidney bean (*Phaseolus vulgaris*) lectins. *Nutrition Research*, 8, 943-947.

Palmer, R.M., Pusztai, A., Bain, P. and Grant, G. (1987) Changes in rates of tissue protein synthesis in rats induced *in vivo* by consumption of kidney bean (*Phaseolus vulgaris*) lectins. *Comparative Biochemistry and Physiology*, 88C, 179-183.

Patureau-Mirand, P., Mosoni, L., Levieux, D., Attaix, D. and Bonnet, Y. (1990) Effect of colostrum feeding on protein metabolism in the small intestine of newborn lambs. *Biology of the Neonate*, 57, 30-36.

Pusztai, A. (1989) Biological effects of dietary lectins. *In Recent Advances of Research in Antinutritional Factors in Legume Seeds – 1989*, pp. 17-29. Edited by J. Huisman, A.F.B. van der Poel and I.E. Liener. Pudoc. Wageningen, Netherlands.

Pusztai, A., Ewen, S.W.B., Grant, G., Brown, D.S., Stewart, J.C., Peumans, W.J., van Damme, E.J.M. and Bardocz, S. (1993) Antinutritive effects of wheat-germ agglutinin and other N-acetylglucosamine-specific lectins. *British Journal of Nutrition*, 70, 313-321.

Preedy, V.R., McNurlan, M.A. and Garlick, P.J. (1983) Protein synthesis in skin and bone of the young rat. *British Journal of Nutrition*, 49, 517-523.

Reeds, P.J., Burrin, D.G., Davis, T.A. and Fiorotto, M.L. (1993) Postnatal growth of gut and muscle: competitors or collaborators. *Proceedings of the Nutrition Society*, 52, 57-67.

Reeds, P.J., Burrin, D.G., Stoll, B. and van Goudoever, J.B. (1999) Consequences and regulation of gut metabolism. *In Protein Metabolism and Nutrition, Proceedings of the VIII[th] International Symposium on Protein Metabolism and Nutrition – Aberdeen, UK, 1.-4. September 1999*, pp. 127-153. Edited by G.E. Lobley, A. White and J.C. MacRae. EAAP Publication No. 96, Wageningen Pers, 1999.

Reeds, P.J., Cadenhead, A., Fuller, M.F., Lobley, G.E. and McDonald, J.D. (1980) Protein turnover in growing pigs. Effects of age and food intake. *British Journal of Nutrition*, 43, 445-455.

Reeds, P.J., Fuller, M.F., Cadenhead, A., Lobley, G.E. and McDonald, J.D. (1981b) Effect of changes in the intakes of protein and non-protein energy on whole-body protein turnover in growing pigs. *British Journal of Nutrition*, 45, 539-546.

Salminen, S., Bouley, C., Boutron-Ruault, M.-C., Cummings, J.H., Franck, A., Gibson, G.R., Isolauri, E., Moreau, M.-C., Roberfroid, M. and Rowland, I. (1998) Functional food science and gastrointestinal physiology and function. *British Journal of Nutrition*, **80**, Supplement 1, 147-171.

Samuels, S.E., Taillandier, D., Aurousseau, E., Cherel, Y., Le Maho, Y., Arnal, M. and Attaix, D. (1996) Gastrointestinal tract protein synthesis and mRNA levels for proteolytic systems in adult fasted rats. *American Journal of Physiology*, **271**, (*Endocrinology and Metabolism*, **34**), E232-E238.

Satchithanandam, S., Vargofcak-Apker, M., Calvert, R.J., Leeds, A.R. and Cassidy, M.M. (1990) Alteration of gastrointestinal mucin by fiber feeding in rats. *Journal of Nutrition*, **120**, 1179-1184.

Schneeman, B.O., Richter, B.D. and Jacobs, L.R. (1982) Response of dietary wheat bran in the exocrine pancreas and intestine of rats. *Journal of Nutrition*, **112**, 283-286.

Séve, B., Reeds, P.J., Fuller, M.F., Cadenhead, A. and Hay, S.M. (1986) Protein synthesis and retention in some tissues of the young pig as influenced by dietary protein intake after early weaning. Possible connection to the energy metabolism. *Reproduction, Nutrition, Développement*, **26**, 849-861.

Simon, O. (1989) Metabolism of proteins and amino acids. *In Protein Metabolism in Farm Animals – 1989*, pp 273-366. Edited by H.-D. Bock, B.O. Eggum, A.G. Low, O. Simon and T. Zebrowska. Oxford Science Publications, Deutscher Landwirtschaftsverlag, Berlin.

Simon, O. (1998) The mode of action of NSP hydrolyzing enzymes in the gastrointestinal tract. *Journal of Animal and Feed Sciences*, **7**, 115-123.

Simon, O. and Berger, H. (1983) Veränderungen der Proteinsynthese in Leber und Dünndarm von Ratten nach Futteraufnahme. *Biomedica Biochimica Acta*, **42**, 1299-1388.

Simon, O., Berger, H., Münchmeyer, R. and Zebrowska, T. (1982) Studies on the range of tissue protein syntheses in pigs: the effect of thyroid hormones. *British Journal of Nutrition*, **48**, 571-581.

Simon, O., Münchmeyer, R., Berger, H., Zebrowska, T. and Buraczewska, L. (1978) Estimation of rate of protein synthesis by constant infusion of labelled amino acids in pigs. *British Journal of Nutrition*, **40**, 243-252.

Smits, C.H.M., Veldman, A., Verstegen, M.W.A. and Beynen, A.C. (1997) Dietary carboxymethylcellulose with high instead of low viscosity reduces macronutrient digestion in broiler chickens. *Journal of Nutrition*, **127**, 483-487.

Southon, S., Livesey, G., Gee, J.M. and Johnson, I.T. (1985) Differences in intestinal protein synthesis and cellular proliferation in well-nourished rats consuming conventional laboratory diets. *British Journal of Nutrition*, **53**, 87-95.

Spencer, R.J. and Chesson, A. (1994) The effect of *Lactobacillus spp.* on the attachment of enterotoxigenic *Escherichia coli* to isolated porcine enterocytes. *Journal of Applied Bacteriology*, **77**, 215-220.

Van der Klis, J.D. and Van Voorst, A. (1993) The effect of carboxymethylcellulose (a soluble polysaccharide) on the rate of marker excretion from the gastrointestinal tract of broilers. *Poultry Science*, **72**, 503-512.

Veldman, A. and Vahl, H.A. (1994) Xylanase in broiler diets with differences in characteristics and content of wheat. *British Poultry Science*, **35**, 537-550.

Yen, J.T., Nienaber, J.A., Pond, W.G. and Varel, V.H. (1985) Effects of carbadox on growth, fasting metabolism, thyroid function and gastrointestinal tract in pigs. *Journal of Nutrition*, **115**, 970-979.

Zilversmit, D.B. (1960) The design and analysis of isotope experiments. *American Journal of Medicine*, **29**, 832-848.

5

# ORGANIC ACID PRODUCTION IN THE LARGE INTESTINE: IMPLICATION FOR EPITHELIAL CELL PROLIFERATION AND CELL DEATH

Takashi Sakata and Akiko Inagaki
*Ishinomaki Senshu University, School of Science and Engineering, Ishinomaki 986-8580, Japan*

## Summary

Organic acids produced by large bowel bacteria are relatively well known examples of lumen factors that affect gut functions. This chapter summarises the effects of different organic acids produced in the large intestine on epithelial cell proliferation and epithelial cell loss of the intestine and discusses factors to regulate microbial organic acid production.

## Background

Germ-free rats that lack gut microbes and their production of short chain fatty acids (SCFA) have enlarged, however, lighter colon (Yajima and Sakata, 1987; Pell, Johnson and Goodlad, 1995). Epithelial cell proliferation is less active in the small and large intestine of germ-free rats than in conventional animals (Komai, Takehisa and Kimura, 1982; Sakata, 1987). The lack of fermentable fibre in the diet or total parenteral nutrition depresses epithelial cell proliferation of rat colon (Jane, Carpentier and Willems, 1977). Crypt cell production rate is lower in rats with their caecum and colon bypassed than in their intact counterparts (Sakata, 1988).

Thus, conditions that avoid the presence of hindgut bacteria (germ-free animals), substrates for these bacteria or substrate entrance into the bacterial habitat (bypass surgery) all reduce the proliferative activity of intestinal epithelial cells, suggesting the role of bacterial metabolites such as organic acids in maintaining normal tissue mass and epithelial cell proliferation of the intestine. It is also to note that the effects of bacterial metabolism in the large intestine are not restricted to the large intestine but also affect the small intestine. Accordingly, the present paper focuses on influences of SCFA and other organic acids on the tissue mass of the intestine and on epithelial cell kinetics of the intestinal tract.

## Influence of SCFA on gut tissue mass

Infusion of a physiologic mixture of SCFA for 2 weeks increases the wet tissue mass relative to empty body weight of the caecum of rats fed an elemental diet (Sakata, 1988). Further, intracaecal infusion of a mixture of SCFA for 36 days increased the caecal tissue mass, but not that of the distal colon, in the rat but pH or co-existing succinic acid had no effect on the tissue mass (Hoshi, 1994). The instillation of butyrate to defunctioned distal colon also increased the mass of the segment (Kissmeyer-Nielsen, Mortensen, Laurberg and Hessov, 1995).

## Influence of SCFA on the mucosa

SCFA stimulate mucosal growth. Kripke, Fox, Berman, Settle and Rombeau (1989) showed that intracolonic infusion of butyric acid stimulated mucosal growth of atrophied colon. They also found that intracaecal or intracolonic infusion of SCFA stimulated mucosal growth in the ileum and increased mucosal DNA in the jejunum and ileum. Thus, SCFA in the hindgut increase the mucosal tissue mass of the large intestine as well as that of the small intestine. It is likely that the effect of SCFA on the distant mucosa (small intestine) is mediated by a systemic mediatory mechanism.

## Effect of SCFA on non-mucosal tissue

Tropic effect of SCFA is not restricted to the mucosa. Intracolonic infusion of SCFA enhanced the healing of a colonic anastomosis and increased the bursting strength of the anastomosis (Rollandelli, Koruda, Settle and Rombeau, 1986), suggesting the effect of SCFA on submucosal tissue and collagen synthesis. Further, daily instillation of a mixture of sodium acetate, sodium propionate and sodium n-butyrate into isolated and defunctioned rat distal colon for 14 days increases the tissue mass of not only the mucosa but also the submucosa and muscularis externa of the distal colon (Kissmeyer-Nielsen *et al.*, 1995). The mechanism for such a tropic action of SCFA on non-mucosal tissue has not been clarified.

## Influence of organic acids on epithelial cell proliferation

Organic acids influences on epithelial cell proliferation of the small and large intestine, however, differ among different experimental settings.

# INFLUENCE OF SCFA ON CRYPT FISSION

Epithelial cell division is confined to the crypt in normal mammalian intestinal epithelia. Thus, intestinal crypt is a proliferative unit for the epithelium. Accordingly, there are two ways to regulate the rate of epithelial cell supply for an intestinal segment. One is to change the number of proliferative unit, the crypt. Another way is to change the cell production rate per crypt.

Study on the influence of SCFA on crypt fission is scarce. The percentage of dividing crypts reaches the peak (25% in the small intestine, and 52% in the colon) at 21 days after birth in rats (Clair and Osborne, 1985). This is the time when the mass of the small and large intestine increases 3 times faster than that of the whole body mass growth (Sakata and Setoyama, 1997). Crypt fission should be responsible for the very rapid growth of the small and large intestine during the suckling period.

As the crypt fission is a relatively slow process that takes 5-6 days in rats (Park, Goodlad and Wright, 1995), it is not easy to detect changes in crypt fission rate in short-term studies.

We have not detect any changes in percentage of crypts in fission when we incubated isolated pig colonic mucosa for 24 hours (Sakata and Sato, unpublished results). However, crypt fission rate and crypt cell production rate (CCPR) negatively correlated in this study. This may indicate the existence of an overall regulatory mechanism to integrate the total epithelial cell production rate per segment both by crypt fission and cell production in the crypt.

# INFLUENCE OF SCFA ON THE PROLIFERATION OF ISOLATED CELLS

SCFA inhibit the proliferation of isolated cells including colorectal cancer cell lines in a dose-dependent manner (Ginsburg, Salamon, Sreevalsan and Freese, 1973; Kruh, Defer and Tichonicky, 1995). This effect is reversible at lower doses and becomes irreversible at higher doses (Ginsburg *et al.*, 1973). The effect varies among acids: n-butyrate > propionate > acetate (Ginsburg *et al.*, 1973). Histone hyperacetylation seems to be responsible for this inhibitory effect (Kruh *et al.*, 1995). However, recent studies suggest that SCFA may stimulate normal (not transformed) gut epithelial cells in vitro (Young and Gibson, 1995).

# EFFECT OF ORGANIC ACIDS ON EPITHELIAL CELL PROLIFERATION OF ISOLATED MUCOSA OF LARGE INTESTINE

SCFA stimulate epithelial cell proliferation of human caecal or colonic biopsy specimens within 3 hours (Scheppach, Bartram, Richter, Richter, Liepold, Dusel, Hofstetter, Ruthlein and Kasper, 1992). On the other hand, SCFA inhibit epithelial cell proliferation of normal rat mucosa in vitro (Sakata, 1987). The effect varies among acids: n-butyrate > propionate > acetate (Sakata, 1987).

On the contrary, n-butyric or succinic acid inhibits epithelial cell proliferation of isolated pig caecal mucosa in short-term culture (Inagaki and Sakata, poster at this symposium). The inhibitory effect of these acids is stronger when only the lumenal side of the mucosa is exposed to the acid than when both lumenal and serosal sides are exposed. The effects of these acids are dose-dependent with different time-courses. The inhibitory effect of n-butyric acid appears within a few hours of exposure, while that of succinic acid takes more than 15 hours to appear. It is interesting that low pH itself (pH 5 vs. 7) inhibits the epithelial cell proliferation of pig caecal mucosa in short-term organ culture. This clearly shows that it is not the acidity but the chemical structure of SCFA or succinic acid that is responsible for the inhibitory effect of these acids.

We have no explanation for the contradiction between studies.

## EFFECTS OF ORGANIC ACIDS ON EPITHELIAL CELL PROLIFERATION IN VIVO

Daily intermittent or continuous administration of SCFA into the caecum or colon stimulates epithelial cell proliferation of the small and large intestine (Sakata, 1995; Sakata, 1997). Non-fermentable dietary bulk (kaolin) neither stimulates epithelial cell proliferation nor modifies the effect of SCFA (Sakata, 1986). Therefore, it is not likely that physical abrasion by solid dietary fibre stimulates epithelial cell proliferation. Considering the nature of highly viscous caecal or colonic contents (Takahashi and Sakata, unpublished results), the flow rate of contents at the very surface of the mucosa should be so slow that there may not be enough abrasive force even when a coarse particles are in direct contact with the mucosal surface.

The effect of SCFA is dose-dependent and varies among acids (acetic < propionic < n-butyric) (Sakata, 1987). The effect appears within 1 to 2 days and lasts at least for 2 weeks (Sakata, 1986; Sakata, 1987; Ichikawa and Sakata, 1997). It should be protonized SCFA or SCFA-anions that have the stimulatory effect, but not protons. Because, SCFA have the stimulatory effect at neutral pH (Sakata, 1986; Sakata, 1987) and the stimulatory effect is abolished by lowering the pH (Ichikawa and Sakata, 1997).

Continuous infusion of lactic acid into the caecum increases the crypt cell production rate (Ichikawa and Sakata, 1997). This stimulatory effect is stronger at pH 5 than at pH 7 (Ichikawa and Sakata, 1997).

The above effect of daily SCFA administration is mediated by a systemic mediatory mechanism (Sakata, 1995). The afferent transmission involves neural transmission, very likely a cholinergic mechanism (Frankel, Zhang, Singh, Klurfeld, Sakata, Modlin and Rombeau, 1992; Reilly, Frankel, Klurfeld, D and Rombeau, 1993; Frankel, Zhang, Singh, Klurfeld, Don, Sakata, Modlin and Rombeau, 1994). Efferent transmission to the gut does not require mesenteric neural transmission, suggesting either humoral or cellular transmission (Sakata, 1989). Gastrin is a possible stimulator for the tropic effect of hindgut SCFA on jejunal epithelium (Frankel *et al.*, 1994; Reilly, Frankel, Bain and Rombeau, 1995). The systemic stimulatory effect should be stronger than the local inhibitory effect of SCFA. The mechanism for the stimulatory effect of lactic acid is unknown.

Continuous infusion of succinic acid into the colon inhibits the epithelial cell production in this segment (Sakata, Ichikawa and Inagaki, 1999). The mechanism for this effect is unknown.

## Effect of organic acids on cell death of colonic epithelium

Epithelial tissue mass is the result of a dynamic balance between the cell production and cell loss. There are two routes of cell loss for intestinal epithelial cells, desquamation and apoptosis. Butyric acid stimulates apoptosis of transformed cells (Hague, Manning, Hanlon, Hutschtscha, Hart and Paraskeva, 1993; Hague and Paraskeva, 1995; Hague, Butt and Paraskeva, 1996). On the other hand, loss of mucosal n-butyric acid increases the apoptosis of colonic mucosa in vitro (Luciano, Hass, Busche, Vonengelhardt and Reale, 1996). However, the latter results may be due to the lack of energy substrate or growth factor in the serosal medium (Hague, Singh and Paraskeva, 1997).

## Among acid variance in kinetic effects of organic acids

As stated above, SCFA increases the mucosal and submucosal tissue mass and crypt cell number, however lactic acid does not. This reflects that SCFA stimulates epithelial cell proliferation to exceed the rate of epithelial cell loss, while lactic acid stimulates both epithelial cell proliferation and cell loss to a similar extent. Thus, SCFA might be important physiologic stimuli to maintain the normal tissue mass, but lactic acid may not. The inhibitory effect of low pH (Ichikawa and Sakata, 1997) and succinic acid (Inagaki, Ichikawa and Sakata, unpublished results) on cell proliferation indicate that neither proton nor carboxyl residue contributes to the tropic effect of SCFA or lactic acid.

It is also to note that effects of organic acids on epithelial cell proliferation vary among acids and are affected by pH. Both succinic and lactic acids, but not SCFA, are major determinants of the pH in large intestinal contents (Hoshi, Sakata, Mikuni, Hashimoto and Kimura, 1994). Therefore, the shift of bacterial metabolism from SCFA to the production of lactic or succinic acid can modify the epithelial cell kinetics considerably due to the different effects among acids and additional modification of low pH due to the accumulation of these poorly absorbable acids (Umesaki, Yajima, Yokokura and Mutai, 1978). Since the net bacterial production of succinic acid and lactic acid is greatly enhanced by low pH (Ushida and Sakata, 1998), it should be important to keep the lumen pH of the large intestine above 6.0 to maintain normal epithelial cell number.

In this regard, it is of prime importance to regulate the hindgut fermentation toward the direction to produce SCFA mainly and to avoid the accumulation of lactic or succinic acid.

## Regulation of organic acid production by large intestinal bacteria

There are many factors that regulate bacterial organic acid production in the large intestine.

Type of substrate is one of the major factors that affect fermentation profile and organic acid composition in the lumen. For instance, meal feeding of xylosylfrucoside results in the accumulation of succinic acid in the rat caecum, while SCFA are the major anions in the caecum when rats are meal-fed with galactosylsucrose (Hoshi *et al.*, 1994).

The lumen pH is another major factor. Studies using batch cultures of mixed pig caecal bacterial showed that pH below 6.0 leads to the shift from SCFA production to lactic acid production and pH below 5.0 results in the accumulation of succinic acid beside lactic acid in place of SCFA (Ushida and Sakata, 1998). The effect of pH is far larger than the difference among different substrate oligosaccharides. Our recent study showed that changes in both production and consumption of lactic and succinic acid are involved in the pH-dependent accumulation of these acids (Inagaki, Sato and Sakata, unpublished results). Production of these acids seems to increase when the pH of the culture is below 5 and the consumption of these acids are depressed at pH below 5 and abolished when the pH is below 4.

Considering the above mentioned effect of pH, it is likely that both the particle size and the rate of entry into the large intestine of substrates affect the fermentation profile. The smaller particle size means larger surface area of substrate particles available for bacterial attack. Thus, the small particles should favour the production of lactic and succinic acids when the rate of bacterial breakdown exceeds the capacity of the large intestine to absorb produced organic acids. The entrance rate of substrates into the large intestine should affect the fermentation profile as well. In other words, processing of feeds/diets or way of intake (e.g. drinking vs.

nibbling) can affect the gut fermentation often more than chemical composition of the diet. One unstudied area in this regard is the secretion of bicarbonate from digestive organs. Because, bicarbonate can neutralize and buffer the acidity. Usually bicarbonate secretion via salivary, gastric, biliary, pancreatic and intestinal secretion is under the control of autonomic nerve system. Accordingly, the hindgut fermentation can be modulated by modulating the effect of autonomic nerve system, e.g. by beta-blockers.

One thing we should keep in mind is the danger of employing the organic acid concentration in the bulk phase of caecal or colonic contents as the measure of either organic acid production or the concentration of organic acids at the very surface of mucosa. Since more than 95% of SCFA produced in the large intestine is absorbed, what we measure in these samples might represent only at most 5% left unabsorbed. Further, the viscosity of the lumen contents in the caecum or colon of pigs is so high (Takahashi and Sakata, unpublished observation) that the rate of absorption of SCFA exceeds the rate of diffusion of these acids. The higher concentration of SCFA in the core of caecal or caecal contents than in peripheral contents in rats (Yajima and Sakata, 1992) and the positive correlation between caecal SCFA concentration and the size of the caecum (Sakata, 1987) indirectly indicate the very slow diffusion of SCFA across the caecal or colonic contents. Thus, the actual SCFA concentration at the mucosal surface or around the crypt bottom (proliferative zone) should be far lower than their concentration in the bulk phase.

We should also be careful for the time-dependent change in the organic acid composition in the caecal or colonic contents. We recently found that lactic acid dominated in the caecal contents of rats just after the meal feeding of a purified diet containing 7.5% fructooligosaccharide but the proportion of this acid dramatically decreases at 15 hours after the end of feeding (Inagaki, Ichikawa and Sakata, unpublished results). This warns us that a single-point measurement of organic acid concentration in the lumen does not always represent the lumen condition at other time point.

## References

Clair, W.S. and Osborne, J. (1985) Crypt fission and crypt number in the small and large bowel of postnatal rats. *Cell Tissue Kinet*, **18**, 255-262.

Frankel, W., Zhang, W., Singh, A., Klurfeld, D., Don, S., Sakata, T., Modlin, I. and Rombeau, J. (1994) Mediation of the trophic effects of short-chain fatty acids on the rat jejunum and colon. *Gastroenterology*, **106**, 375-380.

Frankel, W., Zhang, W., Singh, A., Klurfeld, D., Sakata, T., Modlin, I. and Rombeau, J. (1992) Stimulation of the autonomic nervous system (ANS) mediates short-chain fatty acid (SCFA) induced jejunal trophism. *Surgical Forum,* **43**, 24-25.

Ginsburg, E., Salamon, D., Sreevalsan, T. and Freese, E. (1973) Growth inhibition and morphological changes caused by lipophilic acids in mammalian cells. *Proc Nat Acad Sci USA,* **70**, 2457-61.

Hague, A., Butt, A. and Paraskeva, C. (1996) The role of butyrate in human colonic epithelial cells: an energy source or inducer of differentiation and apoptosis? *Proc Nutr Soc,* **55**, 937-43.

Hague, A., Manning, A., Hanlon, K., Hutschtscha, L., Hart, D. and Paraskeva, C. (1993) Sodium butyrate induces apotosis in human colonic tumour cell lines in a p53-independent pathway: implications for the possible role of dietary fiber in the prevention of large-bowel cancer. *Int J Cancer,* **55**, 498-505.

Hague, A. and Paraskeva, C. (1995) The short-chain fatty acid butyrate induces apoptosis in colorectal tumour cell lines. *Eur J Cancer Prev,* **4**, 359-364.

Hague, A., Singh, B. and Paraskeva, C. (1997) Butyrate acts as a survival factor for colonic epithelial cells: Further fuel for the in vivo versus in vitro debate. *Gastroenterology,* **112**, 1036-1040.

Hoshi, S. (1994) Nutritional and physiological influences of indigestible saccharides on the digestible tract. PhD Thesis, School of Agricultural Sciences.Tohoku University, Sendai.

Hoshi, S., Sakata, T., Mikuni, K., Hashimoto, H. and Kimura, S. (1994) Galactosylsucrose and xylosylfructoside alter digestive tract size and concentrations of cecal organic acids in rats fed diets containing cholesterol and cholic acid. *J Nutr,* **124**, 52-60.

Ichikawa, H. and Sakata, T. (1997) Effect of L-lactic acid, short-chain fatty acids, and pH in cecal infusate on morphometric and cell kinetic parameters of rat cecum. *Dig Dis Sci,* **42**, 1598-1610.

Jane, P., Carpentier, Y. and Willems, G. (1977) Colonic mucosal atrophy induced by a liquid elemental diet in rats. *American Journal of Digestive Diseases,* **22**, 808-812.

Kissmeyer-Nielsen, P., Mortensen, F., Laurberg, S. and Hessov, I. (1995) Transmural trophic effect of short chain fatty acid infusions on atrophic, defunctioned rat colon. *Dis Colon Rectum,* **38**, 946-951.

Komai, M., Takehisa, F. and Kimura, S. (1982) Effect of dietary fiber on intestinal epithelial cell kinetics of germfree and conventional mice. *Nutritional Report International,* **26**, 255-261.

Kripke, S.A., Fox, A.D., Berman, J.M., Settle, R.G. and Rombeau, J.L. (1989) Stimulation of intestinal mucosal growth with intracolonic infusion of short-chain fatty acids. *JPEN,* **13**, 109-16.

Kruh, J., Defer, N. and Tichonicky, L. (1995) Physiological and clinical aspects of short-chain fatty acids, pp. 275-288. Edited by Cummings, J., Rombeau, J. and Sakata, T. Cambridge University Press, Cambridge.

Luciano, L., Hass, R., Busche, R., Vonengelhardt, W. and Reale, E. (1996) Withdrawal of butyrate from the colonic mucosa triggers "mass apoptosis" primarily in the G(0)/G(1), phase of the cell cycle. *Cell Tissue Res*, **286**, 81-92.

Park, H., Goodlad, R. and Wright, N. (1995) Crypt fission in the small intestine and colon: A mechanism for the emergence of G6PD locus-mutated crypts after treatment with mutagens. *American Journal of Pathology*, **147**, 1416-1427.

Pell, J.D., Johnson, I.T. and Goodlad, R.A. (1995) The effects of and interactions between fermentable dietary fiber and lipid in germfree and conventional mice. *Gastroenterology*, **108**, 1745-1752.

Reilly, K., Frankel, W., Bain, A. and Rombeau, J. (1995) Colonic short chain fatty acids mediates jejunal growth by increasing gastrin. *Gut*, **37**, 81-86.

Reilly, K., Frankel, W., Klurfeld, D., D, D.C. and Rombeau, J. (1993) The parasympathetic (PSNS) and sympathetic (SNS) nervous system mediate the systemic effects of short chain fatty acids (SCFA) on jejunal structure and function. *Surgical Forum* XLIV, 20-22.

Rollandelli, R., Koruda, M., Settle, R. and Rombeau, J. (1986) Effects of intraluminal infusion of short chain fatty accids on the healing of colonic anastomosis in the rat. *Surgery*, **100**, 198-203.

Sakata, T. (1986) Effects of indigestible dietary bulk and short chain fatty acids on the tissue weight and epithelial cell proliferation rate of the digestive tract in rats. *J Nutr Sci Vitaminol*, **32**, 355-362.

Sakata, T. (1987) Short-chain fatty acids and water in the hindgut contents and feces of rats after hindgut bypass surgery. *Scand J Gastroenterol*, **22**, 961-968.

Sakata, T. (1987) Stimulatory effect of short-chain fatty acids on epithelial cell. proliferation in the rat intestine: a possible explanation for trophic effects of fermentable fibre, gut microbes and luminal tropic factors. *Br J Nutr*, **58**, 96-103.

Sakata, T. (1988) Depression of intestinal epithelial cell production rate by hindgut bypass in rats. *Scand J Gastroenterol*, **23**, 1200-1202.

Sakata, T. (1989) Stimulatory effect of short-chain fatty acids on epithelial cell proliferation of isolated and denervated jejunal segment of the rat. *Scand J Gastroenterol*, **24**, 886-890.

Sakata, T. (1995) Dietary fibre: mechanisms of action in human physiology, pp. 61-68. Edited by Cherbut, C. and Barry, J.L. John Libbey Eurotext, Paris.

Sakata, T. (1995) Physiological and clinical aspects of short chain fatty acids, pp. 289-305. Edited by Cummings, J.H., Rombeau, J.L. and Sakata, T., Cambridge University Press, Cambridge.

Sakata, T. (1997) Dietary Fiber in Health and Disease, pp. 191-199. Edited by

Kritchevsky, D. and Bonfield, C. Plenum Press, New York.

Sakata, T., Ichikawa, H. and Inagaki, A. (1999) Influences of lactic acid, succinic acid and ammonia on epithelial cell proliferation and motility of the large bowel. APJCN 8.

Sakata, T. and Setoyama, H. (1997) Bi-phasic allometric growth of the small intestine, cecum and the proximal, middle, and distal colon of rats (Rattus norvegicus Berkenhout, 1764) before and after weaning. *Comp Biochem Physiol [A]*, **118**, 897-902.

Scheppach, W., Bartram, P., Richter, A., Richter, F., Liepold, H., Dusel, G., Hofstetter, G., Ruthlein, J. and Kasper, H. (1992) Effect of short-chain fatty acids on the human colonic mucosa in vitro. *JPEN*, **16**, 43-48.

Umesaki, Y., Yajima, T., Yokokura, T. and Mutai, M. (1978) Effect of organic acid absorption on bicarbonate transport in rat colon. *Pflügers Arch*, **379**, 43-47.

Ushida, K. and Sakata, T. (1998) Effect of pH on Oligosaccharide fermentation by porcine cecal digesta. *Anim. Sci. Technol.*, **69**, 100-107.

Yajima, T. and Sakata, T. (1987) Influences of short-chain fatty acids on the digestive organs. *Bifidobacteria Microflora*, **6**, 13-20.

Yajima, T. and Sakata, T. (1992) Core- and periphery-concentrations of short-chain fatty acids in luminal contents of the rat colon. *Comp Biochem Physiol*, **103A**, 353-355.

Young, G. and Gibson, P. (1995) *Physiological and clinical aspects of short-chain fatty acids*, pp. 319-335. Edited by Cummings, J., Rombeau, J. and Sakata, T. Cambridge University Press, Cambridge.

6

# ACTION OF N-BUTYRATE AT THE LEVEL OF GENE EXPRESSION IN THE COLONIC MUCOSA : LESSONS FROM PIG AND RAT EXPERIMENTS

Claire Cherbuy[1], Claude Andrieux[2], Pierre-Henri Duée[1], Béatrice Darcy-Vrillon[1]
[1] *Laboratoire de Nutrition et Sécurité Alimentaire,* [2] *Unité d'Ecologie et Physiologie du Système Digestif, Institut National de la Recherche Agronomique, 78350 Jouy-en-Josas, France*

## Summary

n-butyrate produced by bacterial fermentation, and circulating glutamine are the main oxidative substrates of the colonic epithelium. In the presently reported studies, we have used various colonic preparations from pigs and rats, and investigated : 1/ whether changes of the luminal environment related to fermentation could modulate the capacities of the colonic epithelial cells to metabolise these substrates; 2/ if n-butyrate could be a factor in these changes; and 3/ which mechanisms were involved, including possible effects on gene expression. We show that the capacities of colonic cells to metabolize nutrients adapt to changes of the luminal milieu, such as changes in SCFA (mainly n-butyrate) or ammonia levels, or changes in the bacterial status. We present evidence that, through n-butyrate production, the intestinal flora can control the expression of target genes involved in substrate metabolism in epithelial colonic cells.

## Introduction

Due to their hydrolysis and transport functions and to their high turn-over rate, epithelial intestinal cells have high metabolic requirements (Duée, Darcy-Vrillon, Blachier and Morel, 1995). Glutamine and glucose, originating both from luminal environment and circulating blood, are important metabolic substrates for small intestinal cells. Colonic cells are differently fuelled : glucose and glutamine are also available at their basolateral surface; however, they are exposed to differentiated substrates at their apical surface. Among these, are short chain fatty acids (SCFA), mainly acetate, propionate and n-butyrate, derived from carbohydrate fermentation.

Colonic cells display metabolic adaptation to their local nutritional environment. *In vivo* experiments in rats (Demigné and Rémésy, 1985) and pigs (Rérat, Fizlewicz, Giusi and Vaugelade, 1987) have shown that most of the n-butyrate absorbed is efficiently metabolized in the colonic mucosa. A high capacity for n-butyrate utilisation for energetic purposes has been demonstrated in colonocytes isolated from rats and humans (Roediger, 1980 and 1982, Ardawi and Newsholme, 1985). Moreover, there is increasing evidence that some pathological conditions such as ulcerative colitis correlate with impaired n-butyrate metabolism, due to a lack of substrate or a defective metabolic pathway (Roediger and Nance, 1990; Roediger, Duncan, Kapaniris, and Millard, 1993).

In the presently reported studies, our objectives were to investigate 1/ whether changes of the luminal environment related to the fermentation process could modulate the capacities of the colonic epithelial cells to metabolise n-butyrate, glutamine, or glucose; 2/ if n-butyrate could be a factor in these changes; and 3/ which mechanisms were involved, including possible effects on gene expression.

## Materials and methods

Various experimental strategies have been used to induce or mimic changes in the amounts of SCFA or other bacterial products present in the colonic milieu : dietary manipulation in the pig, bacterial manipulation in the rat, or addition of nutrients or bacterial metabolites in acute conditions.

### ANIMAL MODELS

The pig is a convenient animal model, in which bacterial fermentation, and thus SCFA production, can be significantly enhanced by feeding an increased amount of highly fermentable carbohydrates such as soluble fibres (Bergman, 1990; Fleming and Arce, 1986). Changes in the colonic environment can be easily monitored, and its effect on specific portions of the colonic mucosa (proximal, distal) assessed. Pigs (30-45 kg) were either adapted to a high fibre (12 % sugar beet fibre added) *vs* a low fibre diet, or to a standard pig diet, for at least 4-5 weeks (Darcy-Vrillon, Morel, Cherbuy, Bernard, Posho, Blachier, Meslin, and Duée, 1993; Darcy-Vrillon, Cherbuy, Morel, Durand and Duée, 1996).

The rat allows manipulation of the bacterial status. Several groups of 3 month-old rats (Cherbuy, Darcy-Vrillon, Morel, Pégorier and Duée, 1995) were used : germ-free rats, raised in sterile conditions and harbouring no intestinal flora (GF); conventional rats (CV); initially germ-free rats used 2, 14, or 30 d after inoculation of the fecal flora coming from CV rats fed the same diet; initially germ-free rats used 30 d after inoculation of a bacterial strain which produces (*Clostridium paraputrificum*, CP) or does not produce (*Bifidobacterium breve*, BB) n-butyrate.

## CELLULAR TOOLS

Absorbing colonic cells have been successfully isolated from pig (Darcy-Vrillon et al., 1993, Darcy-Vrillon et al., 1996) or rat (Cherbuy et al., 1995) colon, using a combination of previously reported methods (Roediger and Truelove, 1979; Vidal, Comte, Beylot, and Riou, 1988). Colonocytes isolated by this method have been shown to display metabolic characteristics which can respond to nutritional factors (Duée et al., 1995).

Metabolic fluxes were compared on cell populations (comprising more than 85 % absorbing cells) of similar histological origin and viability (85-90 % at the onset of incubation). The cell suspensions were incubated (30 min, 37 °C, 100 rpm) in the presence of $^{14}[C]$ labelled substrates. Net substrate disappearance and/or metabolite production was measured. Maximum activities of key-enzymes could also be measured on these cell preparations.

## MOLECULAR TOOLS

Messenger RNAs were analysed by northern blotting, after extraction of total RNA (Chomczynski and Sacchi, 1987) from mucosal scrapings of the colon. Immunoreactive proteins were analysed by western blotting, following isolation of mitochondria from the colonic mucosa (Herbin, Pégorier, Duée, Kohl, Girard, 1987) when appropriate.

## Results and Discussion

### N-BUTYRATE, GLUCOSE AND GLUTAMINE METABOLISM IN PIG COLONOCYTES

In pigs, as in rats and humans, n-butyrate and glutamine are major cell substrates (Darcy-Vrillon et al., 1993). Despite differences in n-butyrate utilisation capacities according to species (2-5μmol/min/g cell dry weight), n-butyrate metabolic fate is similar: it is extensively oxidized, with $CO_2$ production accounting for around 40 % of total metabolism, the remainder consisting of total ketone body (acetoacetate and ß-OH-butyrate) production (Fig. 1).

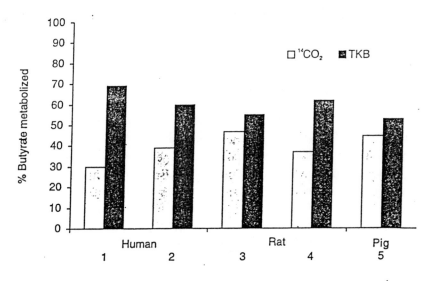

**Figure 1.** Metabolic fate of n-butyrate in isolated colonic epithelial cells

    1: human ascending colon (Roediger, 1980)
    2: human descending colon (Roediger, 1980)
    3: rat colon (Roediger, 1982)
    4: rat colon (Clausen and Mortensen, 1994)
    5: pig proximal colon (Darcy-Vrillon et al., 1993)
    TKB : Total ketone bodies

Pig colonocytes also use glutamine and glucose (Darcy-Vrillon et al., 1993), essentially for non oxidative purposes, as oxidation accounts for about 5 % of substrate disappearance, as in rats and humans.

## EFFECT OF LUMINAL ENVIRONMENT ON NUTRIENT METABOLISM IN COLONOCYTES

Though n-butyrate production must have been enhanced in the colon of pigs receiving highly fermentable fibre in the diet, n-butyrate metabolism in their colonic cells was not substantially affected (Darcy-Vrillon et al., 1993). The main effect observed with the latter diet was a substantial decrease in the capacity of the cells to utilize glucose (5 mM), due to a lower capacity for glycolysis (Fig. 2A). This long term effect was paralleled by a short term effect of n-butyrate (10 mM) added during incubation, which strongly reduced both glycolysis and glucose oxidation (Fig. 2B). Ammonia, another bacterial product, was found to be a strong modulator of both glucose (5 mM) and n-butyrate (10 mM) metabolism (Fig. 3) in pig colonocytes

(Darcy-Vrillon et al., 1996). Interestingly, n-butyrate and ammonia had adverse effects on glucose metabolism.

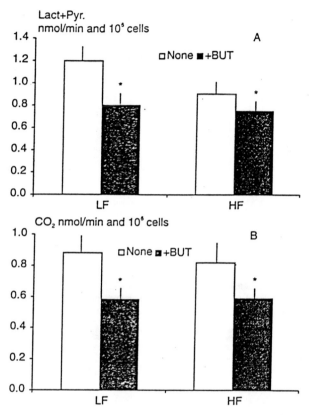

**Figure 2.** Effect of n-butyrate on glucose metabolism in colonocytes isolated from pigs adapted to a low (LF) *vs* high (HF) fiber diet (courtesy of *Journal of Nutrition*)

A: net production of lactate and pyruvate
B: net production of ¹⁴CO₂
* : significant effect of n-butyrate (p<0.05; paired Student's t test)

Possible changes in n-butyrate and glutamine metabolism have also been investigated in germ-free rats which do not have SCFA production in their colon (Cherbuy et al., 1995). Specific alterations have been observed : although the capacity to use n-butyrate is preserved in germ-free rats, the capacity for ketogenesis is significantly lower than that of conventional rats. In parallel, the capacity for glutamine utilisation is higher than in the conventional situation (Fig. 4). These changes take place at the level of two enzymatic steps, respectively the mitochondrial 3-hydroxy 3-methyl glutaryl CoA (HMGCoA) synthase, controlling

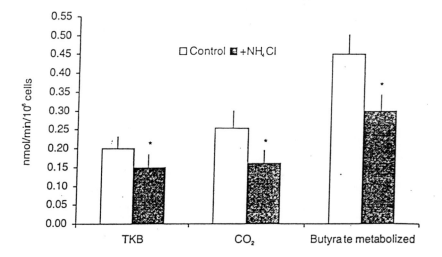

**Figure 3.** Effect of ammonia on n-butyrate metabolism in isolated pig colonocytes (courtesy of *Molecular and Cellular Biochemistry*)

TKB : net production of total ketone bodies
$^{14}$ $CO_2$ : net conversion of 1-[ $^{14}$C] n-butyrate into $^{14}CO_2$
n-butyrate metabolized : estimated as the sum of TKB + $^{14}$ $CO_2$
* : significant effect of $NH_4Cl$ (10 mM); $p<0.05$, paired Student's t test

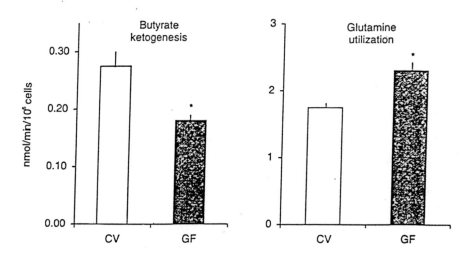

**Figure 4.** Effect of the bacterial status on the metabolic capacities of rat colonocytes

CV : conventional, GF : germfree
* : statistically different from CV rats ($p<0.05$, Student's t test)

ketone body production from n-butyrate, and the glutaminase, responsible for the first step of glutamine utilisation in these cells.

## ROLE OF INTESTINAL FLORA AND n-BUTYRATE IN CONTROLLING THE EXPRESSION OF TARGET METABOLIC GENES

The mitochondrial HMGCoA synthase, responsible for ketone body production in the liver, is also expressed in the colonic mucosa (Cherbuy et al., 1995). In the latter tissue, n-butyrate derived from colonic fermentation is the main precursor for ketone body production. In accordance with data on ketone body production flux (Fig. 4), the level of the HMGCoA synthase protein and mRNA was found to be much lower in the mucosa of germ-free rats (Fig. 5). Thirty days after having inoculated the flora obtained from control conventional rats, the differences in mRNA and protein were abolished. This effect was observed as soon as SCFA production was established in the colon, i.e. 2 days after inoculation.

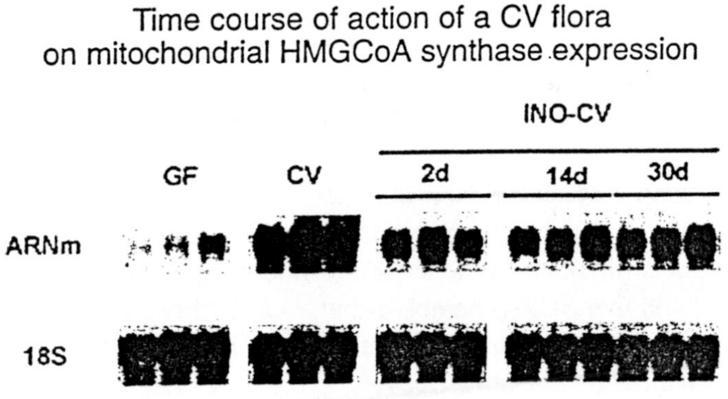

Time course of action of a CV flora
on mitochondrial HMGCoA synthase expression

**Figure 5.** Northern blot analysis of mitochondrial HMGCoA synthase mRNA

Total RNA deposit of 20 µg; 18 S RNA used as an internal standard
CV : conventional, GF : germfree, INO-CV : initially germfree rats inoculated with the flora of CV rats, for 2, 14 or 30 d.

Moreover, mRNA levels were similar between germ-free rats and rats inoculated by a bacterial strain (*B. breve*) which does not produce n-butyrate, whereas it was restored to the control level (3-4 fold higher) when rats were inoculated by a flora (*C. paraputrificum*) which produces n-butyrate at a concentration of 10 mM, which is in the physiological range (Fig. 6). Taken together, these data strongly suggest that SCFA, and specifically n-butyrate, are responsible for these changes.

## Mitochondrial HMGCoA synthase expression after inoculation by strains producing butyrate or not

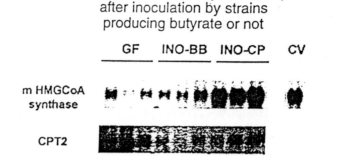

Figure 6. Northern blot analysis of mitochondrial HMGCoA synthase mRNA

Total RNA deposit of 20 µg; CPT2 mRNA used as a control
CV : conventional, GF : germfree, INO-BB : initially germfree rats inoculated with a *Bifido -
bacterium breve* strain (producing no n-butyrate) for 30 d, INO-CP : initially germfree rats
inoculated with a *Clostridium paraputrificum* strain (producing n-butyrate) for 30 d.

However, HMGCoA synthase expression could not be induced in the same rat model (*B. breve* strain) receiving n-butyrate by rectal administration as a bioadhesive thermogel (Tuleu et al., 1999). In the latter case, differences in the dose and time-course of supply of additional n-butyrate, as compared to production by the flora *in situ*, could possibly explain the lack of effect.

The results obtained in the same rat models for glutaminase activity support the conclusion that SCFA, namely n-butyrate are involved : as soon as two days after inoculation, the glutaminase activity was similar to the conventional value, i.e. half that measured in germ-free rats; in the *B. Breve* group, glutaminase activity was similar to that measured in colonocytes of the germ-free group, whereas it was restored to the conventional value when rats were inoculated with *C. paraputrificum*. Preliminary data indicate that this effect takes place at the level of the glutaminase gene expression.

## Conclusions and perspectives

Taken together, these data indicate that n-butyrate controls the expression of two enzymes, one involved in the metabolic pathway of its own utilization, and one involved in the metabolism of glutamine, a key-substrate for intestinal cells. It raises an important issue: what are the respective roles of n-butyrate and glutamine, as nutrients for colonocytes? Our data suggest that, in the absence or lack of n-butyrate, glutamine may represent an alternative substrate. In this regard, the enzymes studied, i.e. HMGCoA synthase and glutaminase, can be used as metabolic biomarkers of the colonic mucosa. Finally, it must be emphasized that, through n-butyrate production, the intestinal flora can control the expression of target genes involved in the metabolism of epithelial colonic cells.

# References

Ardawi M.S., and Newsholme E.A. (1985) Fuel utilization in colonocytes of the rat. *Biochemical Journal*, **231**, 713-719.

Bergman E.N. (1990) Energy contributions of volatile fatty acids from the gastrointestinal tract in various species. *Physiological Reviews*, **70**, 567-590.

Cherbuy C., Darcy-Vrillon B., Morel M.T., Pégorier J.P., and Duée P.H. (1995) Effect of germfree state on the capacities of isolated rat colonocytes to metabolise n-butyrate, glucose and glutamine. *Gastroenterology*, **109**, 1890-1899.

Chomczynski P., and Sacchi N. (1987) Single-step method of RNA isolation by acid guanidinium thiocyanate-phenol-chloroform extraction. *Analytical Biochemistry*, **162**, 156-159.

Clausen M.R. and Mortensen P.B. (1994) Kinetic studies on the metabolism of short-chain fatty acids and glucose by isolated rat colonocytes. *Gastroenterology*, **106**, 423-432.

Darcy-Vrillon B., Cherbuy C., Morel M.T., Durand M. and Duée P.H. (1996) Short chain fatty acid and glucose metabolism in isolated pig colonocytes : modulation by NH4+. *Molecular and Cellular Biochemistry*, **156**, 145-151.

Darcy-Vrillon B., Morel M.T., Cherbuy C., Bernard F., Posho L., Blachier F., Meslin J.C., and Duée P.H. (1993) Metabolic characteristics of pig colonocytes after adaptation to a high fiber diet. *Journal of Nutrition*, **123**, 234-243.

Demigné C., and Rémésy C. (1985) Stimulation of absorption of volatile fatty acids and minerals in the cecum of rats adapted to a very high fiber diet. *Journal of Nutrition*, **115**, 53-60.

Duée P.H. Darcy-Vrillon B. Blachier F., and Morel M.T. (1995) Fuel selection in intestinal cells. *Proceedings of the Nutrition Society*, **54**, 83-94.

Fleming S.E., and Arce D.S. (1986) Using the pig to study digestion and fermentation in the gut *in* Swine in Biomedical Research (Tumbleson M., ed.), 123-134. Plenum Press, New York, N.Y.

Herbin C. Pégorier J.P., Duée P.H., Kohl C., and Girard J. (1987) Regulation of fatty acid oxidation in isolated hepatocytes and liver mitochondria from newborn rabbits. *European Journal of Biochemistry*, **165**, 201-207.

Rérat A. Fizlewicz M. Giusi A., and Vaugelade P. (1987) Influence of meal frequency on post prandial variations in the production and absorption of volatile fatty acids in the digestive tract of conscious pigs. *Journal of Animal Science*, **64**, 448-456.

Roediger W.E.W. (1980) Role of anaerobic bacteria in the metabolic welfare of the colonic mucosa in man. *Gut*, **21**, 793-798.

Roediger W.E.W. (1982) Utilization of nutrients by isolated epithelial cells of the rat colon. *Gastroenterology*, **83**, 424-429.

Roediger W.E.W., Duncan A., Kapaniris O., and Millard S. (1993) Reducing sulfur compounds of the colon impair colonocyte nutrition : implications for ulcerative colitis. *Gastroenterology*, **104**, 802-809.

Roediger W.E.W, and Nance S. (1990) Selective reduction of fatty acid oxidation in colonocytes : correlation with ulcerative colitis. *Lipids*, **25**, 646-652.

Roediger W.E.W, and Truelove S.C. (1979) Method of preparing isolated colonic epithelial cells (colonocytes) for metabolic studies. *Gut*, **20**, 484-488.

Tuleu C., Andrieux C.,Cherbuy C., Meslin J.C., Darcy-Vrillon B., Duée P.H., Charrueau C., and Chaumeil J.C. (1999) Optimisation de la supplémentation colique en n-butyrate de sodium par voie rectale. *Nutrition Clinique et Métabolique*, **13 suppl.1**, 72.

Vidal H., Comte B., Beylot M., and Riou J.P. (1988) Inhibition of glucose oxidation by VIP in isolated rat enterocytes. *Journal of Biological Chemistry*, **263**, 9206-9211.

7

# MICROORGANISMS EXERT BIOACTIVE AND PROTECTIVE EFFECTS THROUGH THE INNATE IMMUNE SYSTEM

Bror Morein and Ke-Fei Hu
*Department of Veterinary microbiology, Swedish University of Agricultural Sciences, Box 585, S-751 23 Uppsala, Sweden*

## Summary

The gut is entry for many pathogens but also the natural residence for many commensal bacteria. The protection against pathogens in the gut is in part provided by the microenvironment, in part by the innate immune system and a part of the protection is due to specific acquired immunity. To provoke and activate the innate immunity against an invader, e.g. a bacteria, the invader has to be recognised. The marker for recognition can be any molecular structure deviating from such structures of the host including prokaryotic peptides, lipids, DNA motifs e.g. CpG and above all carbohydrate structures. LPS is a well known bacterial molecule stimulating the innate immunity. The recognition of LPS leads to an effector phase with activation of the complement system, production of a number of chemokines and cytokines including IL-1, IL-6, IFN-$\gamma$, TNF-$\alpha$, production of reactive oxygen intermediates (ROI) all indirectly or directly exerting antimicrobial effects. Several bacteria in the natural gut flora or non-pathogenic bacteria which can colonise the gut have been shown to have preventive or even therapeutic effects on pathogens. Most commonly used and studied are lactic acid bacteria (LAB) and they have been shown to stimulate the innate immune system to produce cytokines and products mentioned above. Another mechanism so far unique for Lactobacillus planetarum is to use mannose specific adhesions thereby likely to compete against Gram-negative pathogens. An interesting prospect is the use of probiotic in the management of food allergy supposingly by stimulation of local regulatory cytokines.

## Recognition of the first signal

Probiotic activities are based on host reactions against microbes and mostly bacteria are studied. The first signal of a host to react is based on *recognition* of molecular structures on the invader, which differ from those of the host. In hosts with eucaryotic cells a long evolution time has past since divergence from prokaryotes and therefore many molecular structures have evolved suitable for recognition Almost all kinds of bacterial molecules can be targets for recognition but most common are carbohydrate structures in the form of glycolipids in the outer membrane, microbial cell wall carbohydrates and DNA CpG motifs. Anatomically carbohydrates are covering the bacterial surfaces presenting a wide range of molecular structures and patterns serving as finger prints for recognition by targeting matching receptors. In the host the soluble mannose binding protein (MBP) can serve as an example as well as the cell surface mannose binding receptor (not limited to mannose), which are able to recognize these patterns of prokaryotes discerning self from non-self and thereby motivated to activate the innate immunity. MBP is produced in the liver and has a carboxy terminal carbohydrate recognition domain (CRD) and is highly flexible due to a helix region broadening the freedom for ligand binding to carbohydrates of microorganisms. MBP can activate the complement cascade in more than one way and enhances the antibody response and promotes antigen uptake by antigen presenting cells (APC). The binding of MBP to bacterial carbohydrates is nicely explained by Frazer, Koziel and Ezekowitz (1998). Carbohydrate structures in O-linked polysaccharides of Gram-negative bacteria and in lipoteichoic acid of Gram-positive bacteria are important for activation of the innate immune response. Co-crystallisation of the carbohydrate domain of rat MBP with a defined oligomannose ligand binding site shows that an equatorial orientation of the C3 and C4-OH groups of the hexoses is required for the binding. This orientation of hydroxyl groups is found not only in mannose, but also in glucose, N-acetylglucosamine and fucose (Weis, Drickamer and Hendrickson, 1992) in the cell walls of Gram-positive and Gram-negative bacteria, yeasts, and certain parasites. These structures in O-linked polysaccharides of Gram-negative bacteria, in lipoteichoic acid of Gram-positive bacteria are certainly important for activation of the innate immune response. The analyses of defining the key amino acids in the rat MBP binding region clarifies also the requirements for the galactose binding to the C type lectin binding domains. In contrast the ultimate and penultimate sialic acid and galactose sugars of mammalian cells, probably constituting a marker of self for the innate immune system are not bound to the MBP binding site. Thus, the MBP is a target for the innate immune system with its recognition and opsonin functions. Also viral carbohydrates are bound to MBP as exemplified by herpes viruses and HIV-1. Conceptionally, recognition of adjuvant e.g. for vaccine use by the innate immunity is similar to that of the innate immune system recognizing microorganisms, which initiate the danger signal (Matzinger, 1998) or mimic pathogen-associated molecular pattern (PAMP) to target the corresponding pattern recognition receptors (PRR) and provoke a cascade of events in the good cases stimulate protective reactions in the innate system and eventually leading to protective specific immunity. The endocytic and phagocytic activities mediated by mannose receptor are independently regulated. IFN-γ enhances mannose receptor-mediated phagocytic activity connected with Th1 response while the IL-4 induced endocytosis leads to Th2 response (Lefkowitz, Lincoln, Lefkowitz, Bollen and Moguilevsky, 1997; Shepherd, Lane and Abdolrasulnia, 1997). In vivo the expression of the mannose receptors is regulated by immunoglobulins, corticosteroids and prostaglandins (Fraser et al., 1998).

## Effector mechanisms

Recognition leads to an *effector phase*. Microbial carbohydrate structures activate complement in the host through the classical pathway by binding to collectin or through an alternative pathway by interacting with sialic free carbohydrates. Both ways mediate killing of microbes. Lipopolysaccharids or endotoxins (LPS) of Gram-negative bacteria (for review see Ulevitch and Tobias, 1999) has since long been known to stimulate the innate immune system resulting in positive and negative effects. Considerable understanding has been gained in the molecular mechanisms controlling the cellular responses. The biological active endotoxic structure within this complex glycolipid is the lipid A moiety which is a phosphorylated glucosamine, with multiple fatty acids anchoring the structure in the outer membrane of the Gram-negative bacteria. LPS binds to soluble LPS-binding serum proteins (LBP) (Lamping, *et al.* 1996) or the homologous bacterial/permeability-increasing protein (BPI) (Tobias, Soldau, Iovine, Elsbach and Weiss, 1997). The LBP-binding promotes delivery of LPS to the CD14 receptor of monocytes constituting a LBP/CD14 pathways leading to cellular activation and TNF-α production. No other serum proteins are able to replace LBP as an opsonin for LPS that promotes transfer to CD14 and phagocytosis. However, CD14 only increases the sensitivity of macrophages to LPS because it does not have a cytoplasmic signalling domain. The evidence suggests that CD14 recruits LPS to Toll like receptor (TLR) proteins, thereby facilitating signal transduction, leading to the release of cytokines and expression of costimulatory molecules from macrophages, and also the recruitment of interleukin-1 receptor-associated kinase 2 and tumour necrosis factor receptor-associated factor 6, activation of nuclear factor-kB, and subsequent gene transcription (Muzio, Natoli, Saccani, Levrero and Mantovani, 1998; Kirschning, Wesche, Merrill Ayres and Rothe, 1998). Apparently, agonists of TLRs in the form of probiotic microorganisms like vaccine adjuvants could prove useful to stimulate innate immunity and thereby enhance adaptive immune responses (Modlin, Brightbill and Godowski, 1999). This pathway is down-regulated by the BPI-LPS complex and may control LPS aggregation and delivery to monocytes. The inflammatory reaction follows the recognition as seen with Gram-negative bacteria resulting in production of chemokines, proinflammatory cytokines like IL-1, IL-6, IL-8 GM-CSF and TNF-$\alpha$. Subsequent to inflammation regulatory cytokines are produced with IL-12 (in synergism with IL-15 and IL-18) and IL-4 and IL-10 as main actors for Th1 and Th2 responses respectively. Besides carbohydrate structures of microorganisms the innate immune system recognizes lipids e.g. in LPS, and prokaryote peptides or their derivatives (e.g. MDP, GMDP and MTP), bacterial cell walls components e.g. trehalose dimycolate (TDM) from mycobacterium tuberculosis and prokaryotic DNA (e.g. non-methylated DNA) giving signals for activation of the innate system. These products are also found in various adjuvant delivery systems and formulations, provoke also other cells than DCs and macrophages in the innate immune system, such as, NK cells and neutrophils (Fearon DTal, 1996). Cellular elements that evoke Th2 response include "natural" T cells producing IL-4 (Fearon DTal, 1996). Also mast cells and basophils produce IL-4 and have, therefore, a regulative role to push a type 2 response. In Freunds complete adjuvant, which contains whole cell mycobacteria, a Th1 type of response is promoted, while the incomplete Freunds adjuvant favours a Th2 type response. A peptide derived from this mycobacteria is MDP from which various derivatives have been made. In general lipophilic derivatives MDP, MTP, GMDP induce a type 1 like response and the hydrophilic a type 2 response and DNA CpG motifs induce Th1 type of response, all being used as adjuvants and in adjuvant formulations. Effector cells of the innate immune system being recruited by activated Th1 cells are above all macrophages and neutrophils producing a number of inflammatory products and respiratory burst.

## Effector mechanisms in the enteric flora

The CD1 pathway of antigen presentation, which functions similar to that of MHC class II molecules, opens a new channel for the presentation of a novel chemical universe of lipids. Studies suggest that CD1 may not be primarily involved with presenting foreign ligand, but rather would function in triggering regulating cells to respond to danger signals, such as stress or damage, by exerting or recruiting appropriate protective responses (for review see Park, Chiu, Jayawardena, Roark, Kavita and Bendelac, 1998). It is also well established that mycolic acids and ceramides, which can be presented by CD1, are strong adjuvants of adaptive immune responses (Bendelac, 1995; Sallusto, Nicolo, De Maria, Corinti and Testi, 1996), implicating its importance in glycolipid vaccine formulation e.g. vaccine against Mycobacterium tuberculosis. These activities are likely probiotic functions.

The enteric flora comprise more than 90% of the total number of cells in the body with a vast number of foreign antigens and therefore able to activate the innate immune system and subsequently evoke acquired immune response. How these effects of a "natural" gut flora interfere with invading pathogens is empirical and not yet rationally explained. However, the few examples above are likely or even proven mechanisms by which the probiotic flora of the gut work. The innate immunity lacking antigenic specificity but being triggered by molecular patterns is an effector system active at primary infections as well as being required by the acquired immune reaction. Lactic acid bacteria (LAB) are the most studied organisms exhibiting beneficial probiotic effects e.g. in chronic conditions such us inflammatory bowel disease (IBD) (for ref see Dunne, *et al.*, 1999). These bacteria exhibit bile tolerance, acid resistance, adherence to host epithelial tissue and in vitro antagonism of pathogens. Probiotic combinations of Lactobacillus salivarius and Bifidobacterium longum infantis showed beneficial effects in prevention of illness-related weight loss. Selected strains of LAB have been shown to have preventive and therapeutic effects on viral- and bacterial-induced intestinal infections positively influencing immunological parameters (Kasper, 1998). Lactobacillus planetarum seems to be unique among the lactobacilli to use mannose-specific adhesions, uncommon among Gram-positive but common among Gram-negative bacteria, which makes it possible to compete with the Gram-negative pathogens for receptors (Bengmark, 1998). Concrete mechanisms by which LAB exert their probio-active effects has been reviewed by Naidu, Bidlack and Clemens (1999) and include prevention of adherence and establishment of mucosal pathogens. LAB also release enzymes having a synergetic effects on digestion and alleviate symptoms of intestinal malabsorption. Cellular components of LAB strains exert adjuvant effects by stimulation of cell-mediated immune responses, activation of the reticuloendothelial system, promoting production of cytokines including TNF-$\alpha$ and IL-8. Bifidobacterium breve has been shown to activate antibody and cell mediated immune systems. Also IgE production was inhibited (Yasui, Shida, Matsuzaki and Yokokura, 1999). Recently it has also been suggested that selected probiotics may used in the management of food allergy supposedly by stimulation of local regulatory cytokines (Kirjavainen, Apostolou, Salminen and Isolauri, 1999).

This review has attempted to give examples of how the innate immune system is triggered by microorganisms and tie such knowledge to known and prospective mechanisms of probiotic microorganisms.

# References

Bendelac, A. (1995) CD1: presenting unusual antigens to unusual T lymphocytes [comment]. *Science* **269** (5221), 185-186.

Bengmark, S. (1998) Immunonutrition: role of biosurfactants, fiber, and probiotic bacteria. *Nutrition,* **14,** 585-94.

Dunne, C., Murphy, L., Flynn, S., O'Mahony, L., O'Halloran, S., Feeney, M, et al. (1999) Probiotics: from myth to reality. Demonstration of functionality in animal models of disease and in human clinical trials. *Antonie Van Leeuwenhoek*, **76**, 279-92.

Fearon DTaL, R. M. (1996) The instructive role of innate immunity in the acquired immune response. *Science*, **272**, 50-54.

Fraser, I. P., Koziel, H. and Ezekowitz, R. A. (1998) The serum mannose-binding protein and the macrophage mannose receptor are pattern recognition molecules that link innate and adaptive immunity. *Seminars in Immunolog*, **10** (5), 363-372.

Kasper, H. (1998) Protection against gastrointestinal diseases-present facts and future developments. *International Journal of Food Microbiology*, **41**, 127-31.

Kirjavainen, P. V., Apostolou, E., Salminen, S. J. and Isolauri, E. (1999) New aspects of probiotics-a novel approach in the management of food allergy. *Allergy*, **54**, 909-15.

Kirschning, C. J., Wesche, H., Merrill Ayres, T. and Rothe, M. (1998) Human toll-like receptor 2 confers responsiveness to bacterial lipopolysaccharide. *Journal of Experimental Medicine*, **188** (11), 2091-2097.

Lamping, N., Hoess, A., Yu, B., Park, T. C., Kirschning, C. J., Pfeil, D., et al. (1996) Effects of site-directed mutagenesis of basic residues (Arg 94, Lys 95, Lys 99) of lipopolysaccharide (LPS)-binding protein on binding and transfer of LPS and subsequent immune cell activation. *Journal of Immunology*, **157** (10), 4648-4656.

Lefkowitz, D. L., Lincoln, J. A., Lefkowitz, S.S., Bollen, A. and Moguilevsky, N. (1997) Enhancement of macrophage-mediated bactericidal activity by macrophage- mannose receptor-ligand interaction. *Immunology and Cell Biology*, **75** (2), 136-141.

Matzinger, P. (1998) An innate sense of danger. *Seminars in Immunology*, **10** (5), 399-415.

Modlin, R. L., Brightbill, H. D. and Godowski, P. J. (1999) The toll of innate immunity on microbial pathogens. *New England Journal of Medicine*, **340** (23), 1834-1835.

Muzio, M., Natoli, G., Saccani, S., Levrero, M. and Mantovani, A. (1998) The human toll signaling pathway: divergence of nuclear factor kappaB and JNK/SAPK activation upstream of tumor necrosis factor receptor- associated factor 6 (TRAF6). *Journal of Experimental Medicine*, **187** (12), 2097-2101.

Naidu, A. S., Bidlack, W. R. and Clemens, R. A. (1999) Probiotic spectra of lactic acid bacteria (LAB). *Critical Reviews in Food Science and Nutrition*, **39** (1), 13-126.

Park, S. H., Chiu, Y. H., Jayawardena, J., Roark, J., Kavita, U. and Bendelac, A. (1998) Innate and adaptive functions of the CD1 pathway of antigen presentation. *Seminars in Immunology,* **10** (5), 391-398.

Sallusto, F., Nicolo, C., De Maria, R., Corinti, S. and Testi, R. (1996) Ceramide inhibits antigen uptake and presentation by dendritic cells. *Journal of Experimental Medicine,* **184** (6), 2411-2416.

Shepherd, V.L., Lane, K.B. and Abdolrasulnia, R. (1997) Ingestion of Candida albicans down-regulates mannose receptor expression on rat macrophages. *Archives of Biochemistry and Biophysics,* **344** (2), 350-356.

Tobias, P. S., Soldau, K., Iovine, N. M., Elsbach, P. and Weiss, J. (1997) Lipopolysaccharide (LPS)-binding proteins BPI and LBP form different types of complexes with LPS. *Journal of Biological Chemistry,* **272** (30), 18682-18685.

Ulevitch, R. J. and Tobias, P. S. (1999) Recognition of gram-negative bacteria and endotoxin by the innate immune system. *Current Opinion in Immunology,* **11** (1), 19-22.

Weis, W.I., Drickamer, K. and Hendrickson, W. A. (1992) Structure of a C-type mannose-binding protein complexed with an oligosaccharide. *Nature,* **360** (6400), 127-134.

Yasui, H., Shida, K., Matsuzaki, T. and Yokokura, T. (1999) Immunomodulatory function of lactic acid bacteria. *Antonie Van Leeuwenhoek,* **76**, 383-9.

**8**

# LUMINAL BACTERIA: REGULATION OF GUT FU[...]
# IMMUNITY

Kelly, D. and King, T.P.
*Gut Immunology Group, Rowett Research Institute, Greenburn Road, Bucksburn, Aberdeen, Scotland. AB21 9SB.*

## Summary

The normal or indigenous microbiota inhabit body sites whose surfaces are easily accessible from the environment. Thus the skin surface, oral cavity, respiratory tract and gastrointestinal tract are all sites of microbial colonization. Microbial colonization is a complex process and is influenced by a number of regulatory factors of both bacterial and host origin. The intestinal microflora comprise an estimated 400 different bacterial species that colonize the entire tract and reach their highest numbers in the terminal ileum and colon. Variables that contribute to regional compositional diversity include immune reactivity, the presence of gut receptors, nutrient availability and composition, the flow of digesta, pH and Eh (oxidation/reduction potential) and molecular oxygen.

Bacteria play an important role in molding the structure and the biochemistry of the gut. This feature is well illustrated in comparative studies on the intestine of germ-free and conventional animals. Bacteria can influence directly the genetic programming of the gut and are critical to the induction of certain differentiation-related genes. This process appears to require bacterial recognition through association with intestinal cell surface domains such as oligosaccharides or toll-like proteins and/or secretion of bacterial proteins that activate host signalling pathways. Exposure to bacterial antigen is also a prerequisite for promoting the expansion and function of immune organs and the establishment of regulatory networks that profoundly influence the effectiveness of immune defence mechanisms. This relationship is thought to be dependent on continuous bacterial antigen sampling and presentation to the underlying lymphoid tissues. Bacteria can also communicate directly with mucosal epithelial cells and differentially modulate cytokine profiles. Epithelial cytokines are thought to direct the activities of underlying lymphoid cells in the gut and to influence immunological outcome. In addition to regulating acquired immunity, cytokines also exert important effects on

...nate mechanisms of defence. Important intrinsic features of the gut that ...ovide first line defence and protect underlying tissues against pathogen invasion include tight junctions, mucins and epithelial defensins.

## Introduction *muito bem!*

The intestinal mucosa represents a dynamic interface where the processes of digestion, nutrient transport, antigen and bacterial recognition, uptake or exclusion occur. Optimal mucosal function is essential to intestinal health and protection and is determined by the concerted actions of specific immunological and non-immunological defence mechanisms. Non-specific defence mechanisms including innate immune reactivity, the indigenous microbiota, the mucin and mucous barriers, gastric acidity and bile salts contribute to the 'front line' defence. The indigenous flora is recognized to play a critical role in stimulating mucosal protection, primarily by interfering with colonization of the intestinal tract by exogenous microorganisms, including opportunistic pathogens. This feature, variably referred to as colonization resistance, competitive exclusion and bacterial interference (Rolfe, 1996), is achieved by active competition for nutrients, competition for mucosal receptor sites and production of protein and /non-protein bacterial inhibitors including bacteriocins, organic acids and amines. The commensal flora also stimulates gut function and primes the gut immune system. The precise mechanisms whereby bacteria potentiate and modulate the function and immune reactivity of the gut have not been fully elucidated.

## BACTERIAL COLONIZATION AND FORMATION OF MICRO-NICHES IN THE GUT

Several hundred microbial species have been documented as components of the indigenous microflora and their origin appears to be maternal and environmental (Finegold, Sutter and Mathiesen, 1983; Conway, 1996). The pattern of colonization is similar for humans and most animals, with lactic acid bacteria, enterobacteria and streptococci appearing first, followed by obligate anaerobes (Conway, 1996). Microbial colonization is a complex process of natural selection and ecological succession (Rolfe, 1996) and is influenced by numerous regulatory factors of both bacterial and host origin including bacterial antagonisms, animal genotype and physiology, and importantly, nutrition (Kelly, Begbie and King., 1994; Conway, 1996). Several microhabitats exist within the intestine that exert a selective influence on the local composition and metabolic activity of the microflora. These microniches are found in the proximal and distal intestine associated with the villus surface, crypts, epithelial associated mucins and luminal mucus. Variables that contribute to the regional compositional diversity include immune reactivity, the presence of gut receptors, nutrient availability and composition, the flow of digesta, pH and Eh (oxidation/reduction potential) and available molecular oxygen (Stewart, Hillman, Maxwell, Kelly and King, 1993).

## BACTERIAL DIVERSITY AND SUBSTRATE SUPPLY

For growth bacteria require energy sources and nutrients, derived either exogenously from the host diet or endogenously from sloughed-off epithelial cells, and cell secretions from the mucus blanket that coats much of the inner surface of the gut (Stewart *et al.*, 1993).

Competition for substrates is a major determining factor in the composition of the intestinal microbial population. Dietary residues influence the composition and metabolic activities of gut microorganisms (Gibson and McCartney, 1998). During both animal and human development, alterations in diet are believed to induce a succession of related changes in the gut microbial ecosystem (Conway, 1996). Through the process of fermentation, hind gut bacteria are able to produce a wide range of compounds that have both positive and negative effects on gut physiology as well as other systemic influences (Gibson and Roberfroid, 1995). Short chain fatty acids (SCFAs; acetate, propionate and butyrate) are major anions of the colonic lumen, produced as a result of fermentation of dietary fibre by the microflora in the lumen of the large intestine. SCFAs, in particular butyrate, are believed to have a pivotal role in maintaining homeostasis in the colon (Ritzhaupt, Ellis, Hosie and Shirazi-Beechey, 1998). However, although butyrate promotes the growth and proliferation of the normal colon, a specific therapeutic role for SCFAs in the colon remains to be defined (Cook and Sellin, 1998). In recent years there have been attempts to introduce so-called functional foods to selectively enhance hindgut fermentation processes by improving the 'balance' of the microflora (Gibson and Fuller, 2000). Gibson and Roberfroid (1995) defined prebiotics as nondigestible food ingredients that beneficially affect the host by selectively stimulating the growth and/or activity of one or a limited number of bacteria in the colon, thus improving health. The prebiotic properties of non-digestible oligosaccharides such as inulin and fructo-oligosaccharides have been analysed in several recent reports but the only confirmed benefit is an increase in the population of bifidobacteria and lactic-acid bacteria in the hind gut (German, Schiffrin, Reniero, Moilet, Pfeier and Nesser, 1999). Increased numbers of these bacterial species is believed to be associated with health-promoting functions such as the production of SCFAs, immunostimulation and inhibitory effects on the growth of harmful bacteria (Gibson and Roberfroid, 1995).

Non-dietary or endogenous nutrient sources are recognized as important regulators of gut microbial populations (Stewart *et al.*, 1993). The oligosaccharide chains (glycans) attached to intestinal cell surface and secreted proteins and lipids mediate in many important biological roles. It has been suggested that a large part of the observed intra- and inter-species glycan diversity on mucosal surfaces is driven by exogenous selection pressures mediated by enteric organisms (Gagneux and Varki, 1999). Recent evidence suggests that during evolution microbial pressure has led to the diverse expression of enteric glycans as essential nutrient sources for selected commensal bacterial populations. Studies of a gut commensal, *Bacteroides thetaiotaomicron*, have revealed a novel signalling pathway that allows the microbe and host to actively collaborate to produce a nutrient foundation that can be used by this bacterium (Hooper, Xu, Falk, Midvedt and Gordon, 1999; Hooper, Falk and Gordon, 2000). *B thetaiotaomicron* uses a repressor, FucR, as a molecular sensor of L-fucose availability. FucR coordinates expression of an operon encoding enzymes in the L-fucose metabolic pathway with expression of another locus that regulates production of fucosylated glycans in intestinal enterocytes. Coordinating the immediate nutritional requirements of this commensal with production of a host-derived energy source is consistent with its need to enter and persist within a competitive ecosystem (Hooper *et al.*, 1999). It remains to be determined whether other components of the commensal microflora similarly utilise other outer chain sequences on intestinal glycans.

## COLONIZATION RESISTANCE AND COMPETITIVE EXCLUSION

The resident microflora exists in a symbiotic relationship with the host and receives a rich and continuous nutrient supply and complements this by improving nutrient bioavailability and augmenting disease resistance mechanisms of the host. The protection afforded by the indigenous flora is thought to be related to direct suppression of pathogens by microbial by-products mainly acid, organic acids and bacteriocins, through direct stimulation of the immune system, and by competitive exclusion and interference with attachment to mucosal surfaces. Many indigenous and pathogenic bacteria specifically adhere to complex oligosaccharides associated with proteins and/or lipids of intestinal membranes and secreted mucin glycoconjugates. The inter- and intra-species diversity of intestinal glycosylation patterns/ carbohydrate epitopes is well established (Kelly and King, 1991; King, 1995). This significantly influences bacterial colonization and composition and can, at critical points in development such as weaning, result in deleterious alterations in the microbial balance (Kelly *et al.*, 1994). The interaction of bacteria with binding sites may involve direct recognition or recognition of cryptic receptors following the action of secreted exoglycosidase enzymes.

# BACTERIAL INTERACTIONS IN THE GUT

*Fimbrial and non-fimbrial mediated interactions*

The chemistry and distribution of bacterial binding sites on gut mucosal surfaces play important roles in determining host and tissue susceptibility and in triggering host responses. This is particularly noticeable in neonates where both beneficial and harmful swings in microbial balance can accompany epithelial differentiation (Kelly, Begbie and King, 1992, Stewart *et al.*, 1993). Enteric bacterial strains that cause diarrhoea in animals have been partially classified according to the nature of their fimbrial adhesins or lectins. These lectins are constituents of proteinaceous appendages that protrude from surfaces of bacteria and recognize sugar moieties of glycoproteins and/or glycolipids on intestinal surfaces. The synthesis of these appendages and the production of enterotoxins are essential virulence factors that enable pathogens to compete successfully with commensals in the intestine.

The structural diversity of oligosaccharides found on intestinal membranes and mucins is theoretically enormous. Monosaccharides can be combined with each other in a variety of ways that differ not only in sequence and chain length, but also in anomery (a and b), position of links and branching points (Lis and Sharon, 1993). In reality, regions of structural variation are often restricted and the assembly of oligosaccharide chains is at least partially based upon sets of structural rules. Membrane and secretory glycoconjugates are not themselves primary gene products, but are constructed in a stepwise manner as monosaccharides are added to precursor oligosaccharides via several glycosyltransferases coded for by different genes (for review see Roth, 1997). Most glycoproteins carry oligosaccharide side chains N-glycosidically linked to the amide nitrogen of asparagine and/or O-glycosidically linked to the hydroxyl groups of the amino acids serine/threonine. A diverse group of bioactive oligosaccharides is also linked to lipids.

The affinity of bacterial lectins for particular oligosaccharides is relative rather than absolute. In some instances, binding to intestinal glycoconjugates involves precise matching of the tertiary structures of both fimbrial lectin and receptor molecules, so resulting in highly species- or tissue-specific interactions. Other lectin, receptor interactions are less precise in nature or the minimal binding epitopes for the lectins may be sufficiently small to be recognized as constituents of diverse groups of glycoconjugates. This results in a wider tissue and host range for some bacteria.

The Red Queen effect (named after the enigmatic character, whom Alice met in *Through the Looking Glass*) suggests that large multicellular organisms with long life cycles must constantly change to survive the onslaught of lethal microorganisms that have much shorter life cycles and hence evolve faster (Varki,

1997). For any enteropathogens (or their toxins), binding to host target cells via recognition of specific oligosaccharide sequences is a key virulence feature. A large part of the intra- and inter-species variation in glycosylation in the intestine may be a consequence of such ongoing host-pathogen interactions during evolution (Gagneux and Varki, 1999).

Many of the intestinal glycosylation patterns associated with microbial attachment have their basis in only small changes in oligosaccharide chain termination by a-linked sialic acid, galactose, N-acetylgalactosamine or fucose (King, 1995). These relatively simple glycosylation changes may be sufficient to create or mask binding epitopes for bacterial fimbriae. Variations in glycosylation within populations means that individual animals may be more or less susceptible to infection by selected organisms. In the wild, there are advantages to animal herds if some individuals survive epidemics. Similar arguments may hold true in agricultural units, where variations in host susceptibility to pathogens, and faecal shedding of commensal and pathogen strains strongly influence the spread of enteric infections.

Other non-fimbrial interactions can occur between bacteria and host cells but perhaps some of the more intriguing are those that arise as a result of insertion of bacterial receptors into host cells. The adhesion of enteropathogenic and enterohemorrhagic *E coli* (EPEC and EHEC) strains to intestinal cell surfaces is a multistage process that begins with a loose attachment mediated by so-called bundle forming type IV pili. Intimin, a 94-kDa outer membrane protein expressed by EPEC and EHEC, is required for intimate attachment to the host cell. The bacteria inserts its own receptor (translocated intimin receptor or Tir) into the host cell surface, to which it then adheres to trigger additional host signaling events, actin nucleation, cytoskeletal reorganization and the formation of so-called 'attaching and effacing' lesions (Kenny, Devinney, Stein, Reinscheid, Frey and Finlay, 1997; DeVinney, Stein, Reinscheid, Abe, Ruschkowski and Finlay, 1999). The ability to insert receptors into host cells is a mechanism that has been described for pathogenic bacteria and as yet has not been documented amongst commensal species.

### Other receptor-mediated interactions

An important family of receptors have recently been described that appear to play a critical role in bacterial recognition (Janeway and Medzhitov, 1999). Toll receptors are integral transmembrane proteins that possess an extracellular leucine-rich repeat domain and a cytoplasmic domain homologous to the cytoplasmic domain of the interleukin (IL)-1 receptor. Toll receptors have been shown to bind bacterial components including lipopolysaccharides and lipotechoic acids (Takeuchi, Hoshino,

Kawai, Sanjo, Takada, Ogawa, Takeda and Akira, 1999). Using targeted disruption of toll-receptor genes, it has recently been shown that the toll-like receptors display differential recognition of bacterial cell wall components (Takeuchi *et al.*, 1999). Toll-like receptor 2 has been shown to recognize gram-positive bacterial cell wall components whereas toll-like receptor 4 recognises gram-negative lipopolysaccharides. Toll receptors have been found on antigen presenting cells such as macrophages but, more recently, they have also been shown to be expressed on intestinal epithelial cells (Cario, Rosenberg, Brandwein, Beck, Reinecker and Podolsky, 2000). Epithelial cells are also able to respond to molecules such as bacterial LPS by activating cell signalling pathways (Cario *et al.*, 2000). Such data suggests that intestinal cells may play a pivotal role in detecting the presence of luminal bacteria and in communicating their presence to the underlying lymphoid tissues. The intestinal epithelial cell may thus play an important role in modulating or directing the immune response to colonizing and invading bacteria.

### Bacterial/receptor mediated signalling in the gut

Apart from establishing an organism on the host surface, attachment can permit communication between host and bacterium. For example, attachment of pathogenic organisms such as *Salmonella typhimurium* or enteroaggregative *Escherichia coli* (EAEC) to epithelial cells, stimulates the release of the chemokine IL8 and other proinflammatory mediators (Gewirtz, Rao, Simon, Merlin, Carnes, Madara and Neish, 2000; Steiner, Nataro, Poteet-Smith, Smith, J.A. and Guerrant, 2000). Cytokines can exert dramatic effects on both lymphoid and non-lymphoid cells via paracrine and autocrine mechanisms. For example, IL8 release from epithelial cells triggers a rapid recruitment of polymorphonuclear leukocytes through the lamina propria to the subepithelial space and, in part, is responsible for the inflammatory infiltrate associated with many enteric infections. The IL8 releasing activity of EAEC has been ascribed to synthesis of a flagellar protein that interacts with epithelial cells to stimulate cytokine production (Steiner *et al.*, 2000). The production of inflammatory cytokines by epithelial cells is thought to be mediated by the activation of the transcription factor, nuclear factor kappa B (NFκB). Other bacterial strains have been found to secrete immuno-suppressive factors (Schesser *et al.*, 1998; Sangari *et al.*, 1999). The enteropathogen *Yersinia pseudo-tuberculosis* is able to deliver a plasmid-encoded protein into the cytoplasm of eukaryotic cells that inhibits the activation of NF-κB and impairs proinflammatory cytokine release. In this way this pathogen is able to evade immune recognition. Bacteria can also directly influence the function of the epithelial cell by altering specific gene expression. For example, intestinal barrier function is determined by the assembly of tight junctional proteins, such as the occludins and claudins, that collectively regulate the permeability or the 'leakiness' of the intestinal epithelium (Madara, 1998). Bacteria and bacterial products have been shown to influence the level of expression of both the mRNA and protein of junctional constituents (McClane, 2000). This effect can dramatically alter intestinal barrier integrity and is likely to be driven by bacterial-induced cytokine activation (Madara and Stafford, 1989; Schmitz, *et al.*, 1999).

Much of the work to date has focused on enteric pathogens, mainly because the effects driven by pathogens are more easily detected. However, recent work has shown that commensal bacteria also possess mechanisms that permit communication with the host and that the net outcome can be to augment non-immune and immune mechanisms of defence (Mack, Michail, Wei, McDougall and Hollingsworth, 1999; Hooper *et al.*, 1999; Lopez-Boado, Wilson, Hooper, Gordon, Hultgren and Parks, 2000). For example, colonization of the germ-free mouse with *Bacteroides thetaiotaomicron* has been shown to induce matrilysin expression, a matrix metalloproteinase, required to active gut defensins (Lopez-Boada *et al.*, 2000).

There is now an emerging view that intestinal bacteria, commensals and pathogens, have evolved a diverse range of mechanisms that promote their survival within the gut ecosystem. Bacteria can produce a vast array of cytokine-inducing or cytokine-modulating molecules that will regulate or direct the host response. Certain of these factors may promote the virulence and pathogenic potential of bacteria but others, paradoxically, may facilitate the maintenance of the indigenous microflora by beneficially regulating the immuno-inflammatory status of the gut.

## BACTERIAL MODULATION OF GUT FUNCTION

### Germ-free intestine

Very little antigen exposure occurs *in utero*. Hence, at birth the gut of a healthy newborn is sterile and the immune system is immunologically naïve. During early postnatal life, exposure to dietary and bacterial antigens is a prerequisite for the normal development of the intestinal tract and to drive the expansion of immune organs. Bacterial antigens play a very significant role in the proliferation and development of the gut associated lymphoid tissues (GALT) (Helgeland *et al.*, 1996; Umesaki, Setoyama, Matsumoto, Imaokaq and Itok, 1999). The importance of bacterial exposure to the function of gut and its associated immune system is highlighted by investigations on germfree animals. These animals are exposed exclusively to dietary antigens but not bacterial antigens and as a consequence possess an immature gut and are highly susceptible to infection.

*Bacteria and gut differentiation*

In the intestine, membrane glycoconjugates have attracted extensive interest as digestive enzymes, transporter proteins and growth factor receptors. The carbohydrate moieties of these intestinal components may be implicated in their physiological function but in addition they are often targets for wide range of biologically active proteins of both dietary and microbial origin.

Postnatal intestinal development involves extensive epithelial cell proliferation and cytodifferentiation, including changes in the expression of enzymes, receptors and transport systems. Age-related intestinal glycosylation changes play an important role in modifying the properties of intestinal receptors for dietary constituents as well as commensal and pathogenic bacteria (Kelly *et al.*, 1992, Stewart *et al.*, 1993). Increased levels of glycoprotein fucosylation have been observed in the intestines of several species at the time of weaning (King, 1995). Bry, Falk, Midvedt and Gordon (1996) compared genetically identical germ-free mice with mice raised with a functional microbiota and determined that the production of fucosylated glycoconjugates, appearing in the intestine and colon after the age of weaning, requires components of the microbiota. Fucoconjugates were largely absent from weaned germfree mice; inoculation with the commensal bacterium *Bacteroides thetaiotaomicron* restored the same fucosylation pattern as in conventional mice and induced the accumulation of mRNA encoding for $\alpha 1,2$ fucosyltransferase (Bry *et al.*, 1996). Molecular studies on *B. thetaiotaomicron* have identified a transcriptional repressor that serves as molecular sensor of fucose availability that coordinates bacterial fucose metabolism and host fucosylated glycan production (Hooper *et al.*, 2000). The identity and mode of action of the fucosylation-inducing signal produced by the commensal has not been determined (Hooper *et al.*, 2000). The signals may be polyamines. In the weaned rats *B. thetaiotaomicron* contributes high amounts of putrescine and spermidine in the caecum and ileum of pectin-fed gnotobiotic rats (Noack, Dongowski, Hartmann and Blaut, 2000). Polyamines have recently been shown to be potent maturation factors implicated in the expression of increased $\alpha 1,2$ fucosylation in the rat gut at the time of weaning (Greco, Hugueny, Louisot and Biol, 1999; Greco, Hugueny, George, Perrin and Biol, 2000).

Epithelial mucins are major glycoprotein components of the mucus that coats the mucosal surfaces of the gastrointestinal tract. They are believed to function to protect epithelial cells from infection, dehydration and physical or chemical injury, as well as to aid the passage of materials through the tract (Perez-Villar and Hill, 1999). Mucin production may therefore be considered a key innate defence mechanism of intestinal epithelial cells. Intestinal mucins are an extremely diverse group of structural glycoproteins. Some mucin species are small molecules whereas others are contain several thousands of residues and are among the largest known proteins. All mucins exhibit domains of tandemly repeated peptides rich in threonine and/or serine whose hydroxyl groups are in O-glycosidic linkage with N-acetyllactosamine. These moieties form the core structures for carbohydrate chains that may account for as much as 90% of the weight of the mucin glycoproteins.

The dietary composition, microbial flora, as well as interactions between the dietary constituents and the flora, influence the composition and functional characteristics of intestinal mucins (Sharma, Schumacher, Ronaasen and Coates, 1995) Many enteric bacteria produce mucolytic or glycosidic enzymes that alter the chemical characteristics of mucins (Sharma and Schumacher, 1995; Meslin, Fontaine and Andrieux, 1999). Bacterial/mucosal crosstalk may lead to changes in gene expression for mucin peptides. For example, the ability of selected probiotic strains of *Lactobacillus* to inhibit the adherence of attaching and effacing bacteria is mediated through their ability to increase expression of MUC2 and MUC3 intestinal mucins (Mack *et al.*, 1999).

Several commensal species of bacteria colonize the mucus layer overlying the intestinal epithelial cells. In chronic inflammatory bowel disease (IBD), an altered protective efficacy of intestinal mucus results in an increased association of luminal bacteria with the mucus layer (Schultsz, van den Berg, Ten Kate, Tytgat and Dankert, 1999). Such an increased association may enhance or sustain the inflammatory process by exposing the epithelial cells and the mucosal immune system to bacterial antigens. Factors leading to bacterial penetration of the mucus layer are uncertain but are believed to include genetically determined changes in the glycosylation of mucin glycoproteins that result in weakening of the mucus barrier structure (Rhodes, 1996).

## BACTERIAL COLONIZATION AND INTESTINAL IMMUNITY

The primary function of the immune system is to eliminate infectious agents and to minimise the damage they cause. Immune defence relies on the two arms of the immune system, the innate and the acquired. The immune system consists of organs and several cell types that recognize foreign antigen. The primary immunological organs consist of the bone marrow and the thymus and the secondary organs include spleen, mesenteric lymph nodes and Peyer's patches. The immune cells can be grouped into two major categories, lymphocytes and phagocytes. The latter group includes monocytes, macrophages and neutrophils. The lymphocytes are exclusively involved in the specific immune recognition of foreign antigens (acquired immunity) whereas phagocytes function in the production of innate immune responses. Intestinal transport of antigen is vital to drive the expansion and maturation of lymphoid organs.

The mechanisms by which microbes influence the phenotype and function of lymphoid cells associated with the gut associated lymphoid tissue (GALT) are largely unknown but are likely to involve complex events that are probably triggered following the 'normal' route of antigen uptake and processing. This refers to uptake of bacterial antigens by specialized microfold cells (M cells) overlying the follicle-associated epithelium called Peyer's patches. Commensal bacteria and pathogens can also directly influence immune function by modulating intestinal cytokine profiles. These signalling molecules can have very dramatic effects on immune parameters such as the polarisation of the immune response and T cell subset development (Delespesse *et al.*,1998).

*Innate immunity*

The innate immune system is the first line defence of the gut and is believed to predate the acquired or adaptive immune system as it is found in all multicellular organisms whereas, the adaptive is found only in vertebrates (Medzhitov and Janeway, 1997; Dyrynda and Ratcliffe, 1998). The major immune cell types involved in mediating innate responses are macrophages, neutrophils and natural killer cells. These cells recognize bacterial antigens, such as lipopolysaccharides or techoic acids via specific cell surface pattern recognition receptors expressed on activated macrophages. Cellular recognition and signalling induces killing mechanisms including phagocytosis and opsonisation. Other important intrinsic features of the gut that provide first line defence, protecting underlying tissues against pathogen invasion, include tight junctions, mucins and associated epithelial defensins. The influence of enteric bacteria on the innate mechanisms of defence are not well defined. However, recent studies clearly indicate that bacteria exist in a dynamic cross-talk with the host. Commensal bacteria can differentially regulate the gut cytokine response (Haller, 2000). Potentially these cytokines can target immune and non-immune cells and generate a wide range of effects that could influence significantly the innate mechanisms of defence. The precedent that bacteria can regulate intestinal factors that influence the immune barrier function of the gut has already been established (Mack et al., 1999; Lopez-Boado et al., 2000).

## ADAPTIVE IMMUNITY

Resistance to infection relies on a balance between the innate and acquired (antigen driven) immunity. The acquired immune responses are initiated following antigen uptake and presentation to T and B cells. The major route of antigen uptake has long been considered to be via M cells. Antigens are transported into the GALT and are presented to T and B cells by antigen presenting cells (APC), a process, which involves antigen recognition and has inherent fine molecular specificity. Antigen primed T and B lymphocytes migrate through the lymph and reach the peripheral blood for homing to mucosal effector sites, including the mammary gland. In this way the maternal experience of environmental antigens, or protective immunity, is passed to the sucking neonate. The possibility that enterocytes in the gut also transport and present antigen (Kaiserlian and Etchart, 1999) remains contentious.

Segmented filamentous bacteria (SFB) are one of the single most potent nonspecific microbial stimuli of the mucosal immune system. SFB are a group of autochthonous, strictly anaerobic, spore-forming, gram-positive bacteria that occur in the intestines of many vertebrate species (Klaasen, Koopman, Poelma and Beynen, 1992). The epithelium overlying the Peyer's patches is frequently colonised by SFBs. Initial attachment of the bacteria to the intestinal epithelium occurs via specialised holdfast segments. An accumulation of actin-rich filamentous material occurs in the intestinal cytoplasm adjacent to the protruding appendage of attached holdfasts (Jepson, Clark, Simmons and Hirst, 1993). Several investigations have shown that SFBs contribute to host resistance to enteropathogens. Snel, Vandenbrink, Bakker, Poelma and Heidt (1996) noted that SFB stimulate small intestine transit, leading to increased clearance of some bacterial species. Colonization with SFB has been shown to correlate with upregulation of class II histocompatibility antigens and a transient increase in fucosyl asialo GM1 glycolipid expression by intestinal epithelial cells (Umesaki, Okada, Matsumoto, Imaoka and Setoyma, 1995). Talham, Jiang, Bos and Cebra (1999) found that SFB stimulate a large increase in total IgA; with only a small fraction being specific for SFB. As with innate immunity, the nature or mechanisms whereby SFB and other enteric bacteria contribute to the maintenance of the gut lymphoid tissues or, beneficially enhance protective immune function are not clearly established.

## Bacteria and education of intestinal immunity

Analogous to the brain, the immune system requires stimulation and input in order to function properly. Exposure to bacterial antigen is now recognized to be of immense importance, both in early life, in order to prime the immune system in the correct way and throughout life, to maintain a functional immune system. The idea of an 'optimum' functional immune system has now crept into the equation, and with this, the challenge to identify bacteria and bacterial antigens that can be employed to provide appropriate and optimal stimulation of the immune system. Recent evidence in humans suggests that preoccupation with hygiene has drastically reduced our contact with bacteria, both beneficial commensals and pathogens, and is having a detrimental influence on the protective function of the gut immune system (Rook and Stanford, 1998). This is also likely to be the case with animals maintained on antibiotics and with those housed in high health status environments. Hence knowledge of the gut bacteria that provide the correct signals to the gut immune system to optimize function is now recognized to be of major importance. In addition to stimulation of protective immunity, the immunomodulatory potential of bacteria or bacterial antigens may be used to adjust or correct immune dysfunction or hyperfunction. Such an application may be particularly relevant for the treatment of autoimmune and inflammatory diseases in humans.

## PRACTICAL ALTERNATIVES TO CHEMOTHERAPEUTICS

Since their introduction in the late 1940's, there has been an extensive worldwide exploitation of antibiotics in human medicine, animal care and agriculture. As a direct consequence of over-use, transmissible antibiotic resistance genes are present in pathogenic and commensal bacteria. Public health concern about the risks associated with excessive use of antibiotics has resulted in new EU legislation that will curtail their future use in veterinary and agricultural practices. Research directed towards establishing alternative strategies to combat widespread endemic diseases normally controlled by antibiotics and other chemotherapeutics is now recognised as a high priority.

Many important bacterial pathogens are transmitted via the gut. The gut immune system can respond selectively and specifically to pathogenic challenge and is generally activated after the mucosal barrier has been breached. As discussed earlier, the ability of pathogenic bacteria to colonise and invade intestinal surfaces is related to the expression of virulence factors including adhesins and enterotoxins that facilitate entry across the gut. One potential strategy to reduce or prevent bacterial entry is to interfere with the attachment process using specific competing receptor analogues. This strategy however, is limited by the very nature of its specificity, requiring unique blocking analogues for each pathogen. A potentially more effective anti-microbial strategy could be achieved by augmenting the natural defence mechanisms of the gut thereby providing protection against a diverse range of pathogens. Development and exploitation of this approach requires a basic understanding of how the innate and adaptive immune responses of the gut are regulated upon exposure to bacteria.

## Summary and conclusion

Clearly, members of the commensal flora exert differential effects on gut function and on intestinal immune responses. These effects can be triggered by luminal bacteria, following secretion of metabolites or by the adherent flora, through direct contact and activation of host receptor systems. The mechanisms by which the gut immune system recognizes, processes and responds to diverse bacterial antigens is of immense importance to animal and human health. Identification of those bacteria that improve gut function and upregulate host immunity could lead to the development of novel disease therapies based on the manipulation of bacterial colonization or the administration of efficacious bacterial antigens.

## Acknowledgement

This work was supported by grants from the Scottish Executive Rural Affairs Department.

## References

Cario, E., Rosenberg, I.M., Brandwein, S.L., Beck, P.L., Reinecker, H.C. and Podolsky, D.K. (2000) Lipopolysaccharide activates distinct signaling pathways in intestinal epithelial cell lines expressing toll-like receptors. *The Journal of Immunology*, **164**, 966-972.

Conway, P.L. (1996) Development of intestinal microbiota. Gastrointestinal microbes and host interactions *In Gastrointestinal Microbiology Vol 2 - 1996*, pp3-39 . Edited by R.I. Mackie, B.A. Whyte and R.E. Isaacson. Chapman & Hall, London.

Conway, P.L., Gorbach S.L. and Goldin, B.R. (1987) Survival of lactic acid bacteria in the human stomach and adhesion to intestinal cells. *Journal of Dairy Science*, **70**, 1-12.

Cook, S.I., and Sellin, J.H. (1998) Review article: short chain fatty acids in health and disease. *Alimentary Pharmacology and Therapeutics*, **12**, 499-507.

Delespesse, G., Yang, L.P., Ohshima, Y., Demeure, C., Shu, U., Byun, D.G. and Sarfati, M. (1998) Maturation of human neonatal CD4+ and CD8+ T lymphocytes into Th1/Th2 effectors. *Vaccine*, **16**, 1415-1419.

DeVinney, R., Stein, M., Reinscheid, D., Abe, A., Ruschkowski, S. and Finlay, B.B. (1999) Enterohemorrhagic *Escherichia coli* 0157:H7 produces Tir, which is translocated to the host cell membrane but is not tyrosine phosphorylated. *Infection and Immunity*, **6**, 2389-3298.

Finegold, S.M., Sutter, V.L. and Mathisen, G.E. (1983) Normal indigenous intestinal flora. *In Human intestinal microflora in health and disease-1983*, pp 3-31. Edited by D.J. Hentges, Academic Press, New York.

Gagneux, P. and Varki, A., (1999) Evolutionary considerations in relating oligosaccharide diversity to biological function. *Glycobiology,* 9, 747-755.

German, B., Schiffrin, E.J., Reniero, R., Mollet, B., Pfeifer, A. and Neeser, J.R. (1999) The development of functional foods: lessons from the gut. *Trends in Biotechnology,* 12, 492-499.

Gewirtz, A.T., Rao, A.S., Simon, P.O., Merlin, D., Carnes, D., Madara, J.L.and Neish, A.S. (2000) Salmonella typhimurium induces epithelial IL8 expression via Ca2+-mediated activation of the NF-kB pathway. *Journal of Clinical Investigation,* 105, 79-92.

Gibson, G.R. and Fuller, R. (2000) Aspects of in vitro and in vivo research approaches directed toward identifying probiotics and prebiotics for human use. *Journal of Nutrition,* 130, (2S Suppl):391S-395S.

Gibson, G.R. and McCartney, A.L. (1998) Modification of the gut flora by dietary means. *Biochemical Society Transactions,* 26, 222-228.

Gibson, G.R. and Roberfroid, M.B. (1995) Dietary modulation of the human colonic microbiota: introducing the concept of prebiotics. *Journal of Nutrition,* 125, 1401-1412.

Greco, S., Hugueny, I., George, P., Perrin, P., Louisot, P. and Biol, M.C. (2000) Influence of spermine on intestinal maturation of the glycoproteins glycosylation process in neonatal rats. *Biochemical Journal,* 345, 69-75.

Greco, S., George, P., Hugueny, I., Louisot, P. and Biol M.C. (1999) Spermidine-induced glycoprotein fucosylation in immature rat intestine. *C R Academy of Science,* 322, 543-549.

Haller, D., Bode, C., Hammes, W.P., Pfeifer, A.M., Schiffrin, E.J. and Blum, S. (2000) Non-pathogenic bacteria elicit a differential cytokine response by intestinal epithelial/leucocyte co-cultures. *Gut,* 47, 79-87.

Helgeland, L., Vaage, J.T. and Rolstad, B. (1996) Microbial colonization influences composition and T-cell receptor V beta repertoire of intraepithelial lymphocytes in rat intestine. *Immunology,* 89, 494-501.

Hooper, L.V., Xu, J., Falk, P.G., Midvedt, T. and Gordon J.I. (1999) A molecular sensor that allows a gut commensal to control its nutrient foundation in a competitive ecosystem. *Proceedings of the National Academy of Science of the USA,* 96, 9833-9838.

Hooper LV, Falk PG, Gordon JI (2000) Analyzing the molecular foundations of commensalism in the mouse intestine. *Current Opinion in Microbiology,* 3, 79-85.

Janeway, C.A. and Medzhitov, R. (1999) Innate immunity: Lipoproteins take their toll on the host. *Current Biology,* 9, R879-R882.

Jepson, M.A., Clark, M.A., Simmons, N.L., Hirst, B.H. (1993) Actin accumulation at sites of attachment of indigenous apathogenic segmented filamentous bacteria to mouse ileal epithelial cells. *Infection and Immunity,* 61, 4001-4004.

Kaiserlian, D. and Etchart, N. (1999) Entry sites for oral vaccines and drugs: A role for M cells, enterocytes and dendritic cells? *Seminal Immunology,* **11**, 217-224.

Kinugasa, T., Sakaguchi, T., Xuibin, G. and Reinecker, H.C. (2000) ). Claudins regulate the intestinal barrier in response to immune mediators. *Gastroenterology,* **118**, 1001-1011.

Kelly, D. and King, T.P. (1991) The influence of lactation products on the temporal expression of histo-blood group antigens in the intestines of suckling pigs: lectin histochemical and immunohistochemical analysis. *Histochemical Journal,* **23**, 55-60.

Kelly, D., Begbie, R. and King, T.P. (1992) Postnatal Intestinal Development. *In Neonatal Survival and Growth, BSAP occasional publication Number 15.-1992,* pp 63-79. Edited by M.A. Varley, P.E.V. Williams and T.L.J. Lawrence, Edinburgh, British Society of Animal Production.

Kelly, D., R. Begbie and King, T.P. (1994) Nutritional influences on interactions between bacteria and the small intestinal mucosa. *Nutrition Research Reviews,* **7**, 233-257.

Kenny, B., DeVinney, R., Stein, M., Reinscheid, D.J., Frey, E.A. and Finlay, B.B. (1997) Enteropathogenic E. coli (EPEC) transfers its receptor for intimate adherence into mammalian cells. *Cell,* **14**, 511-520.

King, T. P. (1995) Lectin cytochemistry and intestinal epithelial cell biology *In Lectins : Biomedical Perspective -1995,* pp 183-210. Edited by A. Pusztai and S. Bardocz, Taylor and Francis, London and Bristol.

King, T.P., Begbie, R., Slater, D., McFadyen, M., Thom, A. and Kelly, D. (1995). Sialylation of intestinal microvillar membranes newborn, sucking and weaned pigs. *Glycobiology,* **5**, 525-534.

Klaasen H.L, Koopman J..P, Poelma F.G. and Beynen, A.C. (1992) Intestinal, segmented, filamentous bacteria. *FEMS Microbiology Reviews,* **88,**165-180

Lis, H. and Sharon, N. (1993) Protein glycosylation. Structural and functional aspects. *European Journal of Biochemistry,* **218**, 1-27.

Lopez-Boada, Y.S., Wilson, C.L., Hooper, L., Gordon, J.I., Hultgren, S.J. and Parks, W.C. (2000) Bacterial exposure induces and activates matrilysin in mucosal epithelial cells. *The Journal of Cell Biology,* **148**, 1305-1315.

Madara, J. L. (1998) Regulation of the movement of solutes across tight junctions. *Annual Reviews in Physiology,* **60**, 143-159.

Madara, J.L. and Stafford, J. (1989) Interferon gamma directly affects barrier function of cultured epithelial monolayers. *Journal of Clinical Investigation,* **83,**724-727.

Mack, D.R., Michail, S., Wei, S., McDougall, L. and Hollingsworth, M.A. (1999) Probiotics inhibit enteropathogenic *E. coli* adherence in vitro by inducing intestinal mucin gene expression. *American Journal of Physiology*, **276**, G941-G950.

Medzhitov, R. and Janeway, C.A. (1997) Innate immunity: impact on the adaptive immune response. *Current Opinions in Immunology*, **9**, 4-9.

Meslin, J.C., Fontaine, N., and Andrieux, C. (1999) Variation of mucin distribution in the rat intestine, caecum and colon: effect of the bacterial flora. *Comparative Biochemistry and Physiology. Part A Molecular and Integrative Physiology*, **123**, 235-239.

Mouricout, M., Petit, J.M., Carias, J.R. and Julien, R. (1990) Glycoprotein glycans that inhibit adhesion of *Escherichia coli* mediated by K99 fimbriae: treatment of experimental colibacillosis. *Infection and Immunity*, **58**, 98-106.

McClane, B.A.(2000) Clostridium perfringens enterotoxin and intestinal tight junctions. *Trends in Microbiology*, **8**, 145-146.

Noack, J., Dongowski, G., Hartmann, L. and Blaut, M. (2000) The human gut bacteria Bacteroides thetaiotaomicron and Fusobacterium varium produce putrescine and spermidine in cecum of pectin-fed gnotobiotic rats. *Journal of Nutrition*, **130**, 1225-1231.

Perez-Vilar, J. and Hill, R. (1999) The structure and assembly of secreted mucins. *The Journal of Biological Chemistry*, **274**, 31751-31754.

Rhodes, J.M. (1996) Unifying hypothesis for inflammatory bowel disease and associated colon cancer: sticking the pieces together with sugar. *Lancet*, **347**, 40-44.

Ritzhaupt, A., Ellis, A., Hosie, K.B. and Shirazi-Beechey, S.P. (1998) The characterization of butyrate transport across pig and human colonic luminal membrane. *Journal of Physiology (London)*, **507**, 819-30.

Rolfe, R.D. (1996) Colonisation resistance. *In Gastrointestinal Microbiology Vol 2 Gastrointestinal microbes and host interactions.- 1996*, pp501-536 Edited by R.I. Mackie, B.A. Whyte & R.E. Isaacson. Chapman & Hall, London.

Rooke, G.A.W. and Stanford, J.L. (1998) Give us our daily germs. *Immunology Today*, **19**, 113-116.

Roth, J. (1997) Topology of glycosylation in the Golgi apparatus. *In The Golgi Apparatus – 1997* pp131-161. Edited by E.G. Berger and J. Roth. Birkhauser Verlag Basel, Switzerland.

Sangari, F.J., Petrofsky, M. and Bermudez, L.E. (1999) Mycobacterium avium infection of epithelial cells results in inhibition or delay in the release of interleukin-8 and RANTES. *Infection and Immunity*, **67**, 5069-5075.

Schesser, K., Spiik, A.K., Dukuzumuremyi, J.M., Neurath, M.F., Petterson, S. and Wolf-Watz, H. (1998) The yopJ locus is required for Yersinia-mediated inhibition of NF-kappaB activation and cytokine expression: YopJ contains a eukaryotic SH2-like domain that is essential for its repressive activity.

*Molecular Microbiology*, **28**, 1067-1079.

Schmitz, H., Fromm, M., Bentzel, C. J., Scholz, P. et al. (1999) Tumor necrosis factor alpha (TNFa) regulates the epithelial barrier in the human intestinal cell line HT-29/B6. *Journal of Cell Science*, **112**, 137-146.

Schultsz, C., van den Berg, F.M., Ten Kate F.W., Tytgat, G.N. and Dankert, J. (1999) The intestinal mucus layer from patients with inflammatory bowel disease harbors high numbers of bacteria compared with controls. *Gastroenterology*, **117**,1089-1097.

Seignole, D., Mouricout, M., Duval Iflah, Y., Quintard B.and. Julien, R. (1991) Adhesion of K99 fimbriated *Escherichia coli* to pig intestinal epithelium: correlation of adhesive and non-adhesive phenotypes with the sialoglycolipid content. *Journal of General Microbiology*, **137**,1591-1601.

Sharma R, Schumacher U (1995) The influence of diets and gut microflora on lectin binding patterns of intestinal mucins in rats. *Laboratory Investigation,*73, 558-64.

Sharma, R., Schumacher, U., Ronaasen, V. and Coates, M. (1995) Rat intestinal mucosal responses to a microbial flora and different diets. *Gut*, 36, 209-214

Snel, J., VandenBrink, M.E., Bakker, M.H., Poelma, F.G.J. and Heidt, P.J. (1996) The influence of indigenous segmented filamentous bacteria on small intestinal transit time in mice. *Microbial Ecology in Health and Disease,* **9**, 207-214.

Steiner, T.S., Nataro, J.P., Poteet-Smith C.E., Smith, J.A., and Guerrant, R.L.(2000) Enteroaggregative Escherichia coli expresses a novel flagellin that causes IL8 release from intestinal epithelial cells. *Journal of Clinical Investigation*, **105**, 1769-1777.

Stewart, C., Hillman, K., Maxwell, F., Kelly, D. and King, T.P. (1993) Recent advances in probiosis in pigs: observations on the microbiology of the pig gut. *In Recent Advances in Animal Nutrition - 1993* pp197-219. Edited by P.C. Garnsworthy and D.J.A Cole Nottingham University Press, Nottingham.

Takeuchi, O., Hoshino, K., Kawai, T., Sanjo, H., Takada, H., Ogawa, T., Takeda, K. and Akira, S. (1999) Differential roles of TLR2 and TLR4 in recognition of gram-negative and gram-positive bacterial cell wall components. *Immunity*, **11**, 443-451.

Talham, G.L., Jiang, H.Q., Bos, N.A., and Cebra, J.J. (1999) Segmented filamentous bacteria are potent stimuli of a physiologically normal state of the murine gut mucosal immune system. *Infection and Immunity*, **67**,1992-2000.

Umesaki Y, Okada Y, Matsumoto S, Imaoka A, and Setoyama H (1995) Segmented filamentous bacteria are indigenous intestinal bacteria that activate intraepithelial ymphocytes and induce MHC class II molecules and fucosyl asialo GM1 glycolipids on the small intestinal epithelial cells in the ex-germ-free mouse. *Microbiology and Immunology*, **39**, 555-562.

Umesaki, Y., Setoyama, H., Matsumoto, S., Imaoka, A. and Itok, K. (1999) Differential roles of segmented filamentous bacteria and clostridia in development of the intestinal immune system. *Infection and Immunity*, **67**, 504-511.

Varki, A. (1997) Relationship of oligosaccharide diversity to biological function : how much do we owe to the red queen ? *Glycobiology*, **14**, Suppl.1. S3.

9

# THE USE OF NONDIGESTIBLE OLIGOSACCHARIDES TO MANAGE THE GASTROINTESTINAL ECOSYSTEM

Randal K. Buddington
*Department of Biological Sciences, Mississippi State University, Mississippi State, MS 39759, USA*

## Abstract

The gastrointestinal tract represents a small, complex ecosystem that has several distinct habitats. Exclusive use of parenteral nutrition has shown that dietary inputs are critical to maintain the structural components (physical, chemical, and biotic features) and functional elements (transfer of energy and materials) of the gastrointestinal ecosystem. Similar to other ecosystems, the gastrointestinal ecosystem is responsive to the types and amounts of dietary inputs. Nondigestible oligosaccharides (NDO) are recognized as a vital component of a healthy diet. Supplementing diets with NDO increases the densities of lactic acid producing bacteria and provides numerous health benefits. These include enhanced enteric and systemic immune functions, increased energy and nutrient availability, inhibition of pathogen growth, reduced risk of carcinogenesis, and improved levels and profiles of serum lipids. This review describes how the various types of NDO can be used as "management tools" to beneficially affect the bacteria resident in the gastrointestinal ecosystem and thereby enhance health during development and in healthy and diseased states. There is a need to better understand how variation among the gastrointestinal ecosystems of different species, individuals, and age groups, particularly the resident bacteria, influences the responses to different amounts and types of NDO.

## Introduction

Ecosystems consist of structural components that include the physical and chemical features and the resident biota. Interactions among the structural components influence the functional elements, which involve the transfer of energy and materials and are the critical indicators of ecosystem health and productivity. The gastrointestinal tract (GIT) also includes structural components and functional elements and, as such, the GIT can be considered as a small, but quite complex ecosystem (Bry, Falk, Midtvedt and Gordon, 1996; Buddington, 2000).

The health and productivity of ecosystems is dependent on inputs of energy and matter. This is also true for the GIT, which is dependent on dietary inputs. What is of interest is identifying the specific components of diet that can be used as management tools to improve the health and productivity of the GIT in maturity, during development, and will accelerate recovery from disturbances, such as diarrhea and other GIT diseases. Several different diet based approaches have been used to manage the GIT ecosystem (Table 1). Nutrients are of obvious importance. When luminal nutrients are absent, as during parenteral nutrition, the health and productivity of the GIT are severely compromised. Dietary supplements of enzymes, growth factors, and hormones can be used to influence the physical and chemical features of the GIT ecosystem, and by doing so, these approaches also have an impact on the resident organisms. Antibiotics, probiotics, and prebiotics directly influence the resident biota. In response to growing concern about antibiotics and restrictions on their use in diets, probiotics and prebiotics are considered to provide attractive alternative approaches to manage the GIT bacteria.

**Table 1.** Diet based approaches that can be used to manage the gastrointestinal ecosystem

Nutrients
Hormones and Growth Factors
Enzymes
Probiotics and Prebiotics
Antibiotics

A better understanding of the GIT ecosystem will enhance the ability to effectively utilize dietary inputs to enhance health and productivity. Therefore, this contribution first familiarizes readers with the concept of the GIT as an ecosystem. Subsequent sections describe how nondigestible oligosaccharides (NDO), which are prebiotics, can be used to manage the GIT ecosystem in maturity, during development, and for accelerating recovery from disturbances.

## GIT and river ecosystems

Among the various types of ecosystems that have been studied, perhaps the GIT shares the most similarities with river systems (Figure 1). Both are continua with progressive changes in the structural components and functional elements. The differences among the regions of the GIT ecosystem are evident by comparing the stomach, small intestine, and colon, each of which provides distinct habitats with different assemblages of resident organisms. The gradients that exist between, and even within, GIT regions (habitats) can be abrupt (the pyloric sphincter separating the stomach and small intestine) or gradual (the virtually indistinguishable boundary between the jejunum and ileum).

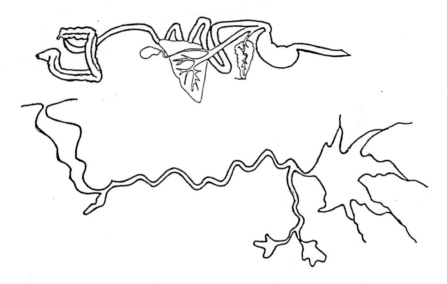

**Figure 1.** The general structure and features of the gastrointestinal tract share several obvious similarities with river ecosystems.

## PHYSICAL AND CHEMICAL FEATURES OF THE GIT ECOSYSTEM

The GIT, like many rivers, has several different habitats, each with distinct physical and chemical characteristics. The GIT begins as a reservoir (stomach) and movement of digesta into the upper region of the GIT (small intestine) is regulated by the pyloric sphincter. The digesta in the proximal small intestine is characterized by relatively faster flow and higher oxygen content, and lower densities and diversity of resident organisms. In this region the composition of the contents is determined largely by the combination of dietary inputs and secretions from the stomach, intestine, and accessory organs (e.g., gall bladder and pancreas). The composition of the digesta gradually changes as it proceeds distally due to the processes of hydrolysis and absorption and microbial metabolism. Digesta in the colon moves slower, has higher sediment levels, is lower in oxygen, and has higher species density and diversity. Movement of digesta between the small intestine and colon is regulated by the ileocolonic junction (Faussone-Pellegrini, Pantalone, and Cortesini, 1993). When it is removed, such as in ileostomy patients, there is a faster flow of digesta in the distal small intestine and the population and metabolic characteristics of the resident organisms are altered.

The mucosa of the GIT is a boundary and the epithelial cells that line the mucosa represents a semipermeable barrier that regulates the exchange of energy and materials between the lumenal contents and the organism As such, the mucosa is similar to the riparian zone of rivers that separates the water column from the underlying terrestrial ecosystem. The mucosa is a very metabolically active tissue (Cant, McBride and Coom, 1994) and has the four basic functions of digestion, osmoregulation, defense (i.e., immunity), and endocrine secretions. There are regional differences in the architecture and functions of the mucosa and these influence the resident bacteria (Kelly, Begbie and King, 1994).

## THE BIOTIC COMPONENTS

Although over 500 bacteria have been identified in the GIT, this underestimates the actual diversity. Similar to river systems, there is a "horizontal zonation" of organisms along the length of the GIT, with qualitative and quantitative differences among the various GIT regions (Simon and Gorbach, 1986; Toskes, 1993). There is also a "vertical zonation" with the population and metabolic characteristics of the bacteria present in the lumenal contents differing from those associated with the mucosa. The specific assemblages of bacteria and patterns of zonation are determined by a combination of GIT anatomy and physiology, dietary inputs, and the complex interactions among the various species (Buddington, 2000). It is not surprising that even within a species, because of subtle differences in GIT characteristics and diet, individuals have different assemblages of GIT bacteria, with differences apparent even among siblings (Hinton and Linton, 1987).

The GIT bacteria have been differentiated into different groups based on various criteria. One approach involves separating the bacteria into resident and transient species (Simon and Gorbach, 1986). The bacteria have also been grouped, based on their metabolic activities and interactions with the host, into those that are perceived as being beneficial and those that have the potential of being detrimental (Gibson and Roberfroid, 1995).

## Interactions between the resident bacteria and the GIT

Studies of other ecosystems have shown that their health and productivity are related to the densities, diversity, and functional roles of the resident organisms.

Although the linkage between the GIT bacteria and health has long been recognized, the complex interactions with the host and the implications in health and disease are still not well understood (Bry *et al.*, 1996). There is increasing awareness that the four functions of the mucosa are responsive to the assemblages of bacteria (MacFarlane and Cummings, 1991; Kinouchi, 1993; Buddington, Buddington and Sunvold, 1999). The interactions between the bacteria and the mucosa can be mediated directly by the attachment of the bacteria to the epithelial cells. Alternatively, products of bacterial metabolism can influence mucosal characteristics. Because of the high metabolic activity and numerous interactions with the host, some have considered the GIT bacteria to constitute another "organ"

The bacteria in the GIT influence mucosal architecture and the expression of genes by the epithelial cells (Bry *et al.*, 1996). By doing so the bacteria alter the physical and chemical features of the GIT environment. Historically, the majority of research has been directed at understanding the impact of pathogenic bacteria when they invade and colonize the GIT. Exemplary are the numerous studies of food borne pathogens and more recently Crohn's disease, a chronic disorder of the GIT (Favier, Neut, Mizon, Cortot, Colombel and Mizon, 1997).

Certain species of the resident bacteria are known to provide benefits to the host. Exemplary are the lactic acid producing bacteria (LAB), which include the *Lactobacilli*, *Bifidobacteria*, members of the *Streptococci*, and several other species (Gibson and Roberfroid, 1995). Increasing the densities of LAB is purported to provide several health benefits (Table 2). Of particular interest are the abilities of LAB to stimulate immune functions and reduce the densities of potential pathogens. In addition, the adherence of LAB to the mucosa limits the interactions of pathogens with enterocytes (Bernet, Brassart, Neeser and Servin, 1993), thereby diminishing the adverse impact on health. These findings have led to efforts to increase the densities of LAB and the relative proportion of the bacterial assemblages that they represent. The two most commonly used approaches are to supplement the diet with live microbes (probiotics) or with compounds that enhance the proliferation of LAB (prebiotics).

Table 2. Some of the health benefits associated with increasing the densities of lactic acid producing bacteria in the gastrointestinal tract. Assembled from several references

| |
|---|
| Inhibition of pathogen growth |
| Stimulation of enteric and systemic immune functions |
| Reduced risk of carcinogenosis |
| Treatment of intestinal disorders |
| Utilization of indigestible dietary components |
| Increased mineral absorption |
| Improved serum lipids |
| Improved stool characteristics |

# Using nondigestible oligosaccharides to manage the GIT ecosystem

The reductions in GIT structure and functions caused by total parenteral nutrition (Zaloga, Roberts, Black and Prielipp, 1993) highlight the importance of dietary inputs for maintaining the GIT. However, dietary inputs need to provide more than just energy and nutrients for the host to maintain GIT health. Exemplary of this is how nutritionally complete enteral diets devoid of fiber are associated with reduced mucosal barrier functions (Spaeth, Berg, Specian, and Deitch, 1990). Therefore a healthy d*iet al*so needs to contain compounds that are not digestible by the host, but can be metabolized by at least some representatives of the GIT bacteria, preferably the LAB.

## NONDIGESTIBLE OLIGOSACCHARIDES

Of the possible prebiotics that have been considered as diet supplements, the nondigestible oligosaccharides (NDO) have received the most attention. The NDO include a wide diversity of forms (Table 3), and more are being described regularly. The NDO are characterized by being resistant to hydrolysis by the enzymes secreted by vertebrates, but can be fermented by bacteria present in the GIT. Although considered by some to be "fiber", this designation for NDO is controversial. The various NDO vary in the specific changes they elicit in the assemblages of GIT bacteria (Buddington, 2000), the concentrations and relative proportions of short chain fatty acids that result from their fermentation (Campbell, Fahey and Wolf, 1997; Djouzi and Andrieux, 1997), and the rates of fermentation (Roberfroid, Van Loo and Gibson, 1998). Most of our knowledge about the influences of NDO are based on analysis of fecal samples. This may provide only a partial understanding since the responses to NDO are likely to be more pronounced in proximal regions compared to feces (Macfarlane and McBain, 1997).

**Table 3.** A partial listing of the different types of nondigestible oligosaccharides that can be added used as prebiotics

Fructans (inulin and oligofructose)
Transgalactosylated oligosaccharides
Soybean oligosaccharides
Xylooligosaccharides
Lactosucrose
Verbascose
Polydextrose
Lactulose
Palatinose

The mechanisms by which NDO influence the microecology of the GIT are complex and involve interactions among several factors. Fructans and other NDO are often considered to be selective substrates for the bifidobacteria, but other GIT bacteria are capable of using NDO (Hartemink, Van Laere and Rombouts, 1998). Interestingly, under certain conditions lactobacilli are able to use fructooligosaccharides even better than bifidobacteria (Sghir, Chow and Mackie, 1998). NDO are not fermented by all bacteria, notably many of the pathogenic and putrefactive bacteria have either reduced abilities or are unable to do so. As a consequence, NDO results in higher densities and relative proportions of LAB (Gibson and Roberfroid, 1995) and can therefore be considered as selective substrates.

Fermentation of NDO by the LAB yields short chain fatty acids (SCFA) and these provide several benefits, including serving as energy substrates for the host (Molis, Flourié, Ouarne, Gailing, Lartigue, Guibert, Bornet and Galmiche, 1996). Production of SCFA lowers the lumenal pH and the resulting changes in the chemical environment inhibit the growth of other bacteria. Other products of LAB metabolism inhibit the growth of many other species of bacteria (Russell and Diez-Gonzalez, 1998).

## Nondigestible oligosaccharides for managing the mature GIT

The bacterial assemblages present in the mature GIT are often mistakenly considered to be stable and to respond only to large scale changes in diet. It is now known that diet can be used to manage the microecology of the GIT (Collins and Gibson, 1999) and that relatively small amounts of NDO do elicit changes in the quantitative, qualitative, and metabolic characteristics of the GIT bacteria (Buddington, Williams, Chen and Witherly, 1996). The changes in the GIT bacteria can be accompanied by changes in the amount and functional properties of small intestinal mucosa (Buddington *et al.*, 1999). These findings are important in that they provide further information about how the resident bacteria can modify their environment and how NDO can be used to influence the specific changes. Furthermore, the higher densities of LAB that result from supplementing the diet with NDO provides basically the same benefits known to be provided by increasing the densities of LAB. NDO also increase resistance to invasion by pathogens (Bovee-Oudenhoven, Termont, Heidt and Van der Meer, 1997), reduce translocation of pathogens out of the GIT into the host (Berg, 1993), and lower the availability of some toxins and carcinogens (Zhang and Ohta, 1993).

Although geriatric issues are generally not of concern for agricultural species, there are changes in the GIT bacteria with increasing age. With relevance to health, there are decreases in bacterial groups perceived as beneficial with concomitant increases in the densities of pathogens and putrefactive bacteria (Mitsuoka, Hideka and Eida, 1987; Mitsuoka, 1992; Toskes, 1993). The changes in bacterial assemblages may be related to the higher incidence of GIT disorders suffered by elderly patients. Therefore, the elderly may especially benefit from dietary supplements of NDO.

## Nondigestible oligosaccharides for managing the developing GIT

The profound changes in the GIT ecosystem during development, including the resident bacteria, provide an opportunity to study successional ecology on a small, but complex scale (Mackie, Sghir and Gaskins, 1998). The first, and perhaps most dramatic period is at birth when neonates begin to drink milk and the GIT that was sterile *in utero* is rapidly colonized by bacteria. During suckling there are changes in the relative proportions of the different groups of fecal bacteria, notably a decline in aerobic forms and their replacement by anaerobes (Swords, Wu, Champlin and Buddington, 1993). The changes in species composition are accompanied by changes in the metabolic characteristics of the bacteria, as evident from quantitative and qualitative shifts in SCFA production (Murray, McClung, Li and Ailabouni, 1987).

Weaning, regardless of the age when it occurs, is another period with dramatic changes in dietary inputs and GIT characteristics (Buddington, 1994). The shift from a milk diet to solid food brings changes in the types and quantities of nutrients and a concurrent loss of the protective and regulatory factors that are present in milk (antibodies, growth factors, and hormones). There are concurrent changes in the amount, architecture, and functional characteristics of the mucosa. Also to be considered are the changes in the volumes and composition of secretions from the pancreas and gall bladder. Collectively, these changes influence the ability of the different resident bacteria to adhere to the mucosa and exert influences on the host, whether beneficial or detrimental (Krause, Easter, White and Mackie, 1995). When the changes in the physical and chemical features of the GIT are considered collectively, it is not surprising that weaning triggers changes in the assemblages and metabolic characteristics of the GIT bacteria. Of greatest concern are the rapid increases in the densities of some pathogens, even though they are transient. The changes in the GIT bacteria continue for weeks and even months in pigs (Swords *et al.*, 1993) and involve a series of successional stages (Conway, 1996).

The growing concerns about the use of antibiotics has increased the interest in using NDO as feed supplements to enhance GIT health of young, growing production animals. The results to date have been promising. Supplementing a milk replacer with fructooligosaccharides increases the densities of bifidobacteria in the GIT of suckling pigs (our unpublished data) and prevents the mucosal atrophy caused by the feeding of an elemental diet (Howard, Gordon, Garleb and Kerley, 1995). Including NDO into the diet of newly weaned pigs lowers lumenal pH (Bolduan, Beck and Schubert, 1993) and increases feed intake and growth (Morimoto, Horo, Ohtaki and Yamazki, 1984). These findings are not unique to pigs. Adding lactulose to the diet increases the densities of LAB and lowers the lumenal pH in the GIT of weaned rats (Nagendra and Rao, 1992). Supplementing a chick diet with fructooligosaccharides leads to competitive exclusion of *Salmonella* in a dose-response manner (Bailey, Blankenship and Cox, 1991), with the benefits more pronounced when a probiotic is included (Fukata, Sasai, Miyamoto and Baba, 1999). Interestingly, the type of diet influences the metabolism of NDO (Parrett and Edwards, 1997), and this interaction needs to be considered.

## Influence of nondigestible oligosaccharides on the disturbed GIT

Eating exposes the normal GIT to frequent, small scale increases in the volume and flow rates of digesta. These disturbances are essential for maintaining the structural components and functional elements of the GIT. In contrast, the extreme conditions of no inputs (parenteral nutrition) and extremely high volumes and flow rates (diarrhea) detrimentally influence the health and productivity of the GIT. Similarly, the most productive ecosystems with the greatest diversity of organisms are considered to be those that experience disturbances of intermediate frequency and magnitude (Buddington and Weiher, 1999).

During severe, chronic diarrhea the assemblages of GIT bacteria are disrupted (Bhan, *et al.*, 1989; Oli, Petschow and Buddington, 1998), the mucosa is damaged (Fagundes-Neto, Toccalino and Dujovney, 1997), and the immune system is overstimulated (Fink, 1994). Since pathogens generally have shorter generation times than members of the LAB, during diarrhea and the initial stages of GIT recovery there is a higher relative abundance of pathogens. Collectively, these factors increase the risk of bacterial translocation and sepsis. Even though the impact of disturbances is considered to be greater for young developing ecosystems, it is not known if this applies to the GIT. It is known that the GIT of infants is less resistant to invasion by pathogens (Shah and Sanderson, 1999). Historically, antibiotics have been used to address the pathogens. However, antibiotics also disrupt the bacterial assemblages (Jackson, Smith and Rowe, 1989; Nord, 1993) and can actually lead to the proliferation of some pathogens, such as *Clostridium difficile* (Wilson, 1993).

Fermented milks have long been known to provide health benefits to patients recovering from diarrhea and other GIT problems (Robinson and Samona, 1992). Similarly, probiotic preparations enhance recovery from diarrhea (reviewed by Buddington and Weiher, 1999). However, there has been reluctance for the routine use of fermented milks and probiotics. There are also demonstrated benefits associated with using NDO. Dietary NDO lessens the severity of enteropathies and other disturbances caused by some therapeutics, apparently by helping to maintain or restore the normal flora (Honda, Matsumoto, Kuroki, Iida, Oka and Sawatani, 1999). Supplementing the diet with NDO also accelerates the recovery of the LAB following disturbances to the GIT (Oli *et al.*, 1998), including experimental necrotizing enterocolitis (Catala, Butel, Bensaada, Popot, Tessedre, Rimbault and Szylit, 1999). The faster recovery of the LAB helps to restore and maintain mucosal structure and functions (Salminen and Salminen, 1997). NDO may also reduce the risk of chronic inflammatory bowel diseases that are mediated by interactions between the resident bacteria and the mucosa (Teramoto, Rokutan, Kawakami, Fujimura, Uchida, Oku, Oka and Yoneyama, 1996).

## Perspectives

There is a need to identify the NDO that are best at promoting GIT health and productivity. The best forms will selectively encourage the abundance of LAB, decrease the densities of pathogens and putrefactive bacteria, will enhance the structural and functional characteristics of the entire GIT, and will improve the growth and health of the host. There are compounds other than NDO that promote the growth of LAB, with several present in milk (Poch and Bezkorovainy, 1988; Petschow and Talbott, 1990). Choosing which dietary supplement, or combination, is best is similar to decisions that are routinely faced in agriculture about fertilization. Multidisciplinary studies that incorporate various fields of study, such as nutrition, microbiology, physiology, and pathology are needed to guide the choice.

There is a need to consider dosage levels and the phrase "enough, but not too much" is very appropriate. Despite being fermented by the bacteria, higher doses of NDO can cause osmotic diarrhea (Clausen, Jorgensen and Mortensen, 1998). Even lower doses can cause flatulence and in some individuals bloating and other GIT discomfort.

## References

Bailey, J.S., Blankenship, L.C. and Cox, N.A. (1991) Effect of fructooligosaccharide on Salmonella colonization of the chicken cecum. *Poultry Science* **70**, 2433-2438.

Berg, R.D. (1999) Bacterial translocation from the gastrointestinal tract. *Adv Exp Med Biol.* **473**, 11-30.

Bernet, M.-F., Brassart, D., Neeser, J.R., and Servin, A.L. (1993) Adhesion of human bifodobacterial strains to cultured human intestinal epithelial cells and inhibition of enteropathogen-cell interactions. *Applied Environmental Microbiology* **59**, 4121-4128.

Bhan, M.K., Raj, P., Khoshoo, V., Bhandari, N., Sazawal, S., Kumar, R., Srivastava, R., and Arora, N.K. (1989) Quantitation and properties of fecal and upper small intestinal aerobic microflora in infants and young children with persistent diarrhea. *Journal of Pediatric Gastroenterology and Nutrition* **9**, 40-45.

Bolduan, G., Beck, M. and Schubert, C. (1993) The effect of oligosaccharides on piglets. *Archiv fur Tierernahrung* **44**, 21-27.

Bovee-Oudenhoven, I.M.J., Termont, D.S.M.L., Heidt, P.J. and Van der Meer, R.. (1997) Increasing the intestinal resistance of rats to the invasive pathogen *Salmonella enteritidis*: additive effects of dietary lactulose and calcium. *Gut* **40**, 497-504.

Bry, L., Falk, P.G., Midtvedt, T., and Gordon, J.I. (1996) A model of host-microbial interactions in an open mammalian ecosystem. *Science* **273**, 1380-1383.

Buddington R.K. (1994) Nutrition and ontogenetic development of the intestine. *Canadian Journal of Physiology and Pharmacology* **72**, 251-259.

Buddington, R.K. (2000) The use of fermentable fibers to manage the gastrointestinal ecosystem. In: *Phytochemicals as Bioactive Agents* (Bidlack, W.R., Omaye, S.T., Meskin, M.S. and Topham, DKW., eds) Technomic Publ. Co., Lancaster, PA, pp.87-103.

Buddington, R.K., Buddington, K.K. and Sunvold, G.D. (1999) The influence of fermentable fiber on the small intestine of the dog: Intestinal dimensions and transport of glucose and proline. *American Journal of Veterinary Research* **60**, 354-358.

Buddington, R.K. and Weiher, E. (1999) The application of ecological principles and fermentable fibers to manage the gastrointestinal tract ecosystem. *Journal of Nutrition* **129**, 1446S-1450S.

Buddington, R.K., Williams, C.H., Chen, S.-C. and Witherly, S.A. (1996) Dietary supplement of neosugar alters the fecal flora and decreases activities of some reductive enzymes in human subjects. *American Journal of Clinical Nutrition* **63**, 709-716.

Campbell, J.M., Fahey Jr. G.C. and Wolf, B.W. (1997) Selected indigestible oligosaccharides affect large bowel mass, cecal and fecal short-chain fatty acids, pH and microflora in rats. *Journal of Nutrition* **127**, 130-136.

Cant, J.P., McBride, B.W. and Croom, W.J. Jr. (1996) The regulation of intestinal metabolism on whole animal energetics. *Journal of Animal Science* **74**, 2541-2553.

Catala, I., Butel, M.J., Bensaada, M., Popot, F., Tessedre, A.C., Rimbault, A. and Szylit, O. (1998) Oligofructose contributes to the protective role of bifidobacteria in experimental necrotizing enterocolitis in quails. *Journal of Medical Microbiology* **48**, 89-94.

Clausen, M.R., Jorgensen, J. and Mortensen. P.B. (1998) Comparison of diarrhea induced by ingestion of fructooligosacchare, Idolax, and disaccharide lactulose: role of osmolarity versus fermentation of malabsorbed carbohydrate. *Digestive Disease Science* **43**, 2696-2707.

Collins, M.D. and Gibson, G.R. (1998) Probiotics, prebiotics and synbiotics: approaches for modulating the microbial ecology of the gut. *American Journal of Clinical Nutrition* 69, 1052S-1057S.

Conway, P.L. (1996) Development of intestinal microbiota. In: *Gastrointestinal Microbes and Host Interactions* (Mackie, R.I., Whyte, B.A. and Isaacson, R.E., eds) Chapman and Hall, New York, pp. 3-38.

Djouzi, Z. and Andrieux, C. (1997) Compared effects of three oligosaccharides on metabolism of intestinal microflora in rats inoculated with a human faecal flora. *British Journal of Nutrition* 78, 313-324.

Fagundes-Neto, U., Toccalino, H. and Dujovney, F. (1976) Stool bacterial aerobic overgrowth in the small intestine of children with acute diarrhoea. *Acta Paediatrica Scandinavia* **65**, 609-615.

Faussone-Pellegrini, M.-S., Pantalone, D. and Cortesini, C. (1993) Morphological evidence for a cecocolonic junction in man and functional implications. *Acta Anatomica* **146**, 22-30.

Favier, C., Neut, C., Mizon, C., Cortot, A., Colombel, J.F. and Mizon, J. (1997) Fecal ß-D-galactosidase production and *Bifidobacteria* are decreased in Crohn's disease. *Digestive Disease Sciencies* **42**, 817-822.

Fink, M.P. (1994) Effect of critical illness on microbial translocation and gastrointestinal mucosa permeability. *Seminar Respiratory Infections* **9**, 256-280.

Fukata, T., K. Sasai, T. Miyamoto and E. Baba. (1999) Inhibitory effects of competitive exclusion and fructooligosaccharide, singly and in combination, on Salmonella colonization of chicks. *Journal of Food Protection* **62**, 229-233.

Gibson, G.R., Beatty, E.R., Wang, X. and Cummings, J.H. (1995) Selective stimulation of bifidobacteria in the human colon by oligofructose and inulin. *Gastroenterology* **108**, 975-982.

Gibson, G.R. and Roberfroid, M.B. (1995) Dietary modulation of the human colonic microflora: introducing the concept of prebiotics. *Journal of Nutrition* **125**, 1401-1412.

Hartemink, R., Van Laere, K.M. and Rombouts, F.M. (1997) Growth of Enterobacteria on fructooligosaccharides. *Journal of Applied Microbiology* **83**, 367-374.

Hinton, M. and Linton, A.H. (1987) The ecology of *Escherichia coli* in healthy newborn piglets. *British Veterinary Journal* **143**, 541-548.

Honda, K., Matsumoto, T., Kuroki, F., Iida, M., Oka, M. and Sawatani, I. (1999) Protective effect of lactosucrose on intracolonic indomethacin-induced small intestinal ulcers in rats. *Scandinavian Journal of Gastroenterology* **34**, 264-269.

Howard, M.D., Gordon, D.T., Garleb, K.A. and Kerley, M.S. (1995) Dietary fructooligosaccharide, xylooligosaccharide and gum arabic have variable effects on cecal and colonic microbiota and epithelial cell proliferation in mice and rats. *Journal of Nutrition* **125**, 2604-2609.

Jackson, R.J., Smith, S.D. and Rowe, M.I. (1989) The effect of cefoxitin and cefotaxime on gut flora and bacterial translocation. *Microecology Therapy.* **19**, 179-184.

Kelly, D., Begbie, R. and King, T.P. (1994) Nutritional influences on interactions between bacteria and the small intestinal mucosa. *Nutrition Research Reviews* **7**, 233-257.

Kinouchi, T., Kataoka, K., Miyanishi, K., Akimoto, S. and Ohnishi, Y. (1993) Biological activities of the intestinal microflora in mice treated with antibiotics or untreated and the effects of the microflora on absorption and metabolic activation of orally administered glutathione conjugates of K-region epoxides of 1-nitropyrene. *Carcinogenesis* **14**, 869-874.

Krause, D.O., Easter, R.A., White, B.A. and Mackie, R.I. (1995) Effect of weaning diet on the ecology of adherent lactobacilli in the gastrointestinal tract of the pig. *Journal of Animal Science* **73**, 2347-2354.

Macfarlane, G.T. and Cummings, J.H. (1991) The colonic flora, fermentation, and large bowel digestive function. In *The Large Intestine: Physiology, Pathophysiology, and Disease* (Phillips, S.F., Pemberton, J.H. and Shorter, R.G., eds) Raven Press, New York, pp.51-92.

Mackie, R.I., Sghir, A. and Gaskins, H.R. (1998) Developmental microbial ecology of the neonatal gastrointestinal tract. *American Journal of Clinial Nutrition* **69**, 1035S-1045S.

McBain, A.J. and MacFarlane, G.T. (1997) Investigations of bifidobacterial ecology and oligosaccharide metabolism in a three-stage compound continuous culture system. *Scandinavian Journal of Gastroenterology* **32**, Suppl 222: 32-40.

Mitsuoka, T. (1992) Intestinal flora and aging. *Nutrition Reviews* **50**, 438-446.

Mitsuoka T., Hideka, H. and Eida, T. (1987) Effect of fructo-oligosaccharides on intestinal microflora. *Die Nahrung* **31**, 427-436.

Molis, C., Flourié, B. Ouarne, F., Gailing, M.-F., Lartigue, S., Guibert, A., Bornet, F. and Galmiche, J.-P. (1996). Digestion, excretion, and energy value of fructooligosaccharides in healthy humans. *American Journal of Clinical Nutrition* **64**, 324-328.

Morimoto, H., Noro, H., Ohtaki, H. and Yamazaki, H. (1984) Study on feeding fructooligosaccharides (Neosugar G) in suckling pigs. *Japanese Science Feedstuffs*. Assoc. Report 59-88, 1-17.

Murray, E.D., McClung, H. J., Li, B.U.K and Ailabouni, A. (1987) Short-chain fatty acid profile in the colon of newborn piglets using fecal water analysis. *Pediatric Research* **22**, 720-724.

Nagendra, R. and Rao, S.V. (1992) Effect of incorporation of lactulose in infant formulas on the intestinal bifidobacterial flora in rats. *International Journal Food Science Nutrition* **43**, 169-173.

Nord, C.E. (1993) The effect of antimicrobial agents on the ecology of the human intestinal microflora. *Veterinary Microbiology* **35**, 193-197.

Oli, M.W., Petschow B.W. and Buddington, R.K. (1998) Evaluation of fructooligosaccharide supplementation of oral electrolyte solutions for treatment of bacteria. Recovery of the intestinal bacteria. *Digestive Disease Sciences* **43**, 138-147.

Parrett, A.M. and Edwards, C.A. (1997) In vitro fermentation of carbohydrate by breast fed and formula fed infants. *Archives Diseases Children* **76**, 249-253.

Petschow, B.W. and Talbott, R.D. (1990) Growth promotion of *Bifidobacterium* species by whey and casein fractions from human and bovine milk. *Journal of Clinical Microbiology* **28**, 287-292.

Poch. M. and Bezkorovainy, A. (1988) Growth-enhancing supplements for various species of the genus *Bifidobacterium*. *Journal Dairy Science* **71**, 3214-3221.

Roberfroid, M., Van Loo, J. and Gibson, G.T. (1998) The Bifidogenic nature of chicory inulin and its hydrolysis products. *Journal of Nutrition* **128**, 11-19.

Robinson R.K. and Samona, A. (1992) Health aspects of 'bifidus' products: a review. *International Journal Food Science Nutrition* **43**, 175-180.

Russell, J.B., Diez-Gonzalez, F. (1998) The effects of fermentation acids on bacterial growth. *Adv. Microbial Physiol.* **39**, 205-234.

Salminen, S. and Salminen, E. (1997) Lactulose, lactic acid bacteria, intestinal microecology and mucosal protection. *Scandinavian Journal of Gastroenterology Supplement* **222**, 45-48.

Sghir, A., Chow, J.M. and Mackie, R.I. (1998) Continuous culture selection of bifidobacteria and lactobacilli from human faecal samples using fructooligosaccharides as selective substrates. *Journal of Applied Microbiology* **85**, 769-777.

Shah, U. and Sanderson, I.R. (2000) Role of the intestinal lumen in the ontogeny of the gastrointestinal tract. In: *Development of the Gastrointestinal Tract* (Sanderson, I.R. and Walker, W.A., eds) B.C. Decker, Inc. Hamilton, Ontario, pp. 245-260.

Simon, G.L. and Gorbach, S.L. (1986) The human intestinal microflora. *Digestive Disease Science.* **31**, 147S-162S.

Spaeth, G., Berg, R.D., Specian, R. D and Deitch, E.A. (1990) Food without fiber promotes bacterial translocation from the gut. *Surgery* **108**, 240-247.

Swords, W.E., Wu, C.-C., Champlin, F.R. and Buddington, R.K. (1993) Postnatal changes in selected bacterial groups of the pig colonic microflora. *Biology of the Neonate* **63**, 191-200.

Teramoto, F., Rokutan, K., Kawakami, Y. Fujimura, Y., Uchida, J., Oku, K., Oka, M. and Yoneyama, M. (1996) Effect of $4^G$-$-D-galactosylsucrose (lactosucrose) on fecal microflora in patients with chronic inflammatory bowel disease. *Journal Gastroenterology* **31**,33-39.

Toskes, P.P. (1993) Bacterial overgrowth of the gastrointestinal tract. *Advances: Internal Medicine* **38**, 387-407.

Wilson, K.H. (1993) The microecology of *Clostridium difficile. Clinical Infectious Diseases* **16** (Suppl 4), S214-S218.

Zaloga, G.P., Roberts, P., Black, K.W and Prielipp, R.C. (1993) Gut bacterial translocation/dissemination explains the increased mortality produced by parenteral nutrition following methotrexate. *Circulatory Shock* **39**, 263-268.

Zhang, X.B. and Ohta, Y. (1993) Microorganisms in the gastrointestinal tract of the rat prevent absorption of the mutagen-carcinogen 3-amino-1,4-dimethyl-5H-pyrido(4,3-b)indole. *Canadian Journal Microbiology* **39**, 841-845.

**10**

# LECTIN MICROBIAL INTERACTIONS IN THE GUT

Patrick J. Naughton
Present Address: *Digestive Feed and Microbiology Group, Department of Animal Nutrition and Physiology, Danish Institute of Agricultural Sciences, Research Centre Foulum, P.O. Box 50, DK-8830, Tjele, Denmark.*

## Summary

Lectins are ubiquitious in nature. Plant lectins have been shown to interact with bacteria, fungi and viruses. Bacteria themselves have been shown to produce their own particular lectins. Plant lectins are highly resistant to proteolytic degradation *in vivo* and survive passage through the gastrointesinal tract and if appropriate carbohydrate receptors are present on gut epithelial cells, lectins can bind to them. Hence, some lectins can alter receptor expression, glycosylation of epithelial cells, gut metabolism and proliferation in the gut while others have little or no effect. These traits mean that lectins can change the character of the gastrointestinal tract both in terms of the gut epithelium and luminal components. Lectins both plant and bacterial in origin can alter the microbial ecology of the gut. The search for more economic yet balanced ingredients for animal rations has led to consideration of secondary plant products such as lectins. The advent of transgenic plants expressing lectins means that the gut may be exposed to new lectins or combinations of lectins. Thus, lectins have the potential for either beneficial or detrimental effects in new scenarios of gut interactions.

## Introduction

The widespread presence of lectins in feed and foodstuffs has prompted a number of investigators to examine their potential effects on body metabolism and they have been the subject of numerous books (Pusztai, 1991; Van Damme, Peumans, Pusztai and Bardocz 1998) and reviews (Grant, 1999; Woodley, 2000). There are several reports of human intoxication associated with the consumption of beans in which lectins appear to have been the causative agents (Liener and Hasdai, 1986). Lectins have been found to be resistant to proteolytic digestion. e.g WGA (Brady,

Vannier and Banwell,1978), tomato lectin (Nachbar, Oppenheim and Thomas, 1980), kidney beans lectin (Pusztai, Clarke and King, 1979) and have therefore been recovered intact from stool (Coffey, Uebersax, Hosfield and Brunner, 1985). A number of lectins of differing carbohydrate specificity have been shown to bind to bacteria and other microorganisms (Pistole, 1981). Furthermore, the inclusion of raw kidney bean or its lectin components in animal diets reduced the growth rate and sometimes even caused death (Liener, 1974) and some lectins can also render epithelial cells less protected (Ovelgonne, Koninkx, Pusztai, Bardocz, Kok, Ewen, Hendricks and van Dijk, 2000). Lectins cause these effects because they can severely interfere with or alter the metabolism of a wide range of tissues. In particular, exposure of the small intestine to lectins can greatly alter the microenvironment of the mucosal surface and induce major physiological and structural changes in the mucosa (Pusztai, Ewen, Grant, Peumans, Van Damme, Rubio and Bardocz, 1990a).

The enterocyte brush border can be damaged as a result of high intakes of raw kidney bean or lectins, resulting in abnormal development of microvilli, intestinal growth, increased cell turnover and disruption of the villi (Wilson, King, Clarke and Pusztai, 1980). Simultaneously, a dramatic overgrowth of *Escherichia coli* in the small intestine can occur. At low to moderate dietary lectin concentrations, small intestinal growth and increased cell turnover are evident but there is no significant overgrowth in the gut by *E. coli* (Pusztai, Grant, Spencer, Duguid, Brown, Ewen, Peumans, Van Damme and Bardocz, 1993). However, a proportion of enterocytes on the villous surface is immature (Pusztai *et al.*, 1993)

Bacteria can also express an array of adhesins (lectins) on their surface. Adherence via these adhesins is believed to play an important role in bacterial colonisation (Melhem and LeVerde, 1984), and the abundance of surface saccharides in various forms on animal cells provides a spectrum of possible attachment points for the bacterial lectins (Karlsson, Ångström, Bergström and Lanne, 1992; Sharon, 1993). Alternatively carbohydrate-binding proteins (animal lectins) on mammalian cells may also act as attachment points for microorganisms carrying the appropriate saccharides on their surface (Sheriff, Chang and Ezekowitz, 1994). This mechanism is utilised by macrophages for non-opsonic phagocytosis, during clearance of microorganisms in several tissues (Ofek, Rest and Sharon, 1992). Similar lectins as constituents of the cell surface in a variety of tissues (Sharon, 1989) are involved in cell-to-cell attachment and/or signalling.

## Effects of plant lectins on the gut

Plant lectins are highly resistant to proteolytic degradation *in vivo*. Functional PNA (peanut lectin; *Arachis hypogaea*) has been recovered from human faeces

(Ryder, Jacyna, Levi, Rizzi and Rhodes, 1998) and intact soybean lectin has been recovered after passage through sheep rumen (Baintner, Duncan, Stewart and Pusztai, 1993). In general, lectins of complex carbohydrate specificity bind to the intestinal epithelium of the mature rat gut after first exposure whilst galactose-specific lectins attach to a much lesser extent (Pusztai, Ewen, Grant, Peumans, Van Damme, Coates and Bardocz, 1995). However, glucose/mannose or mannose specific lectins generally have limited activity with the gut (Pusztai *et al.*, 1995). Cumulative dietary exposure to lectins such as GNA can lead to changes in the binding characteristics of the gut. (Pusztai *et al.*, 1995). Other lectins can also change the glycosylation pattern of the gut and thus its reactivity to lectins (Pusztai *et al.*, 1995). A proportion of cell-bound lectin can be endocytosed and released systemically (Bardocz, Ewen, Grant and Pusztai, 1995). The extent of initial binding and uptake will depend on the bacterial status of the animals and the specificity of the lectin. For example systemic uptake of PHA is extensive in conventional rats but occurs only to a limited extent in germ free rats (Pusztai, 1991) and binding of Con A is decreased in germ-free rats (Pusztai *et al.*, 1995). Galactose specific lectins and glucose/mannose lectins are also taken up into circulation but in far lower amounts than PHA (Wang, Yu, Campbell, Milton and Rhodes, 1998).

Some lectins have damaging effects on the gut by binding to carbohydrate structures present on the brush border membrane of the enterocyte (Weiser and Douglas, 1976) and inducing alterations to membrane structure and function. Metabolic processes may also be impaired and the microenvironment altered; all these processes can promote bacterial colonisation and proliferation. For example, Con A is resistant to gut proteolysis (Nakata and Kimura, 1985), interferes with reformation of brush border membranes (Nakata and Kimura, 1986) and causes some cytotoxic effects (Lorenz-Meyer, Roth, Elsasser and Hahn, 1985) particularly in young animals (Weaver and Bailey, 1987). However, all of these effects can be reversed by the use of high concentrations of mannose. Despite their drawbacks lectins have possible beneficial uses in chemical probiosis (Pusztai *et al.*, 1993), drug delivery (Lavelle, Grant, Pusztai, Pfüller and O'Hagan, 2000; Kilpatrick, 1999; Woodley, 2000), total parentral nutrition (Jordinson, Goodlad, Brynes, Bliss, Ghatei, Bloom, Fitzgerald, Grant, Bardocz, Pusztai, Pignatelli and Calam, 1999) and genetically modified crops (Down, Ford, Woodhouse, Raemaekers, Leitch, Gatehouse and Gatehouse, 2000).

## CON A

Seeds of jack bean (*Canavalia ensiformis*) contain a haemagglutinating lectin (Concanavalin A; Con A). It is mannose/glucose specific but exhibits greatest affinity for D-mannose and its glycosides in α-anomeric form. In oligo- and polysaccharides the reactivity of the lectin is strongest with residues containing non-reducing terminal α-linked mannose (Goldstein and Poretz, 1986). It also reacts with terminal α-linked glucose and N-acetylglucosamine but with less affinity (Goldstein and Poretz, 1986). At neutral pH values the lectin is composed of four non-glycosylated subunits of 26.5 kDa, some of which are fragmented and held together by non-covalent, forces (Wang, Cunningham and Edelman, 1971). Below pH 5.6 the lectin is a dimer of 52 kDa comprising two subunits; above this pH it associates to the tetramer form (Goldstein and Poretz, 1986).

Con A can induce or inhibit cell-mediated lympholysis in murine lymphocytes (Sitkovsky, Pasternack and Eisen, 1982) and can activate macrophages (Maldonado, Porras, Fernandez, Vazquez and Zenteno, 1994). This property of Con A can have many applications; for example facilitating the clearance by macrophages of *Candida albicans* from tissues (Felipe, Bim and Somensi, 1995). Summer and Howell (1936) showed that Con A agglutinated bacteria from the genera *Mycobacterium* and *Actinomyces* and this property of the lectin has been repeatedly confirmed (Pistole, 1981). It also binds to viruses such as Newcastle disease V4 strain (Rehmani and Spradbrow, 1995) and has recently been shown to inhibit attachment of *S. pullorum* to chicken gut (Zhou, Deng and Ding, 1995) and block attachment of *Giardia lamblia* trophozoites to Caco-2 cells (Katelaris, Naeem and Farthing, 1995).

Con A has however been shown to promote the adherence of various strains of non-fimbriated *S. typhimurium* to isolated viable intestinal cells (Linquist, Lebenthal, Lee, Stinson and Merrick, 1989). Furthermore bacterial binding was increased in Con A-treated intestinal loops (Abud, Lindquist, Ernst, Merrick, Lebenthal and Lee, 1989). This suggested that this lectin might possibly promote bacterial adherence to the small intestine *in vivo* and thereby facilitate colonisation and infection. Indeed, Naughton, Grant, Bardocz and Pusztai (2000) have shown that inclusion of Con A in the diet significantly increased the numbers of *Salmonella typhimurium* in the small and large intestine of rats.

Con A can activate basophil cells (Siraganian and Siraganian, 1974), cause morphological changes in hamster mast cells and stimulate histamine release leading to inflammation (Wyczolkowska, Rydzynski and Prouvost-Danon, 1992). It can also bind to the brush borders *in vitro* (Etzler and Branstrator, 1974) and *in vivo* leading to increased shedding of brush border membranes, accelerated cell loss and slight villus atrophy (Lorenzsonn and Olsen, 1982). Thus, Con A can potentially modulate many of the metabolic responses observed during infection by *Salmonella*, notably histamine release and activation of epidermal growth factor (EGF). However, in the absence of bacteria, Con A alone exhibits little effect on the rat gut (Pusztai *et al.*, 1995). Hence, when Con A and *Salmonella* are given together, it is likely *Salmonella* will have the primary role in the infection system with Con A compounding the effects of the bacteria.

Con A can bind to the EGF receptor on mammalian cells *in vitro* (Carpenter and Cohen, 1977) and inhibit the dimerisation and tyrosine phosphorylation of the receptor leading to inhibition of mitogenicity of EGF (Hazan, Krushel and Crossing, 1995). The adherence of *S. typhimurium* to epithelial cells leads to the activation of the EGF receptor (Galán, Pace and Hayman, 1992), and the internalisation of the bacterium. Con A may therefore promote these processes. Con A can also have post-receptor effects by interfering with the lateral movement of membrane receptors and also inhibition of DNA synthesis. Again, these may facilitate *Salmonella* uptake. Con A has been shown to activate $Ca^{2+}$ entry in human neutrophils. Neutrophils play an important role in host defence against bacterial infections and in tissue destruction (Weiss, 1989). As a result of activation, neutrophils generate superoxide anions and undergo exocytosis (Seifert and Schultz, 1991). Impairment of neutrophil function by Con A may serve to facilitate the increase *Salmonella* numbers in the GI tract. Alternatively, the increased bacterial numbers *in vivo* may be the result of Con A mimicking the action of bacterial adhesins by acting as a link between the bacterium and the cell and thereby promoting increased adherence of the bacteria. Studies *in vitro* have shown that Con A will bind both *S. enteritidis* and *S. typhimurium* (Naughton *et al* 2000). Bar-Shavit and Goldman (1976) showed that Con A mediated attachment and ingestion of yeast cells by macrophages. Gallily, Vary, Stain and Sharon (1984) showed the wheat germ agglutinin mediated uptake of bacteria by murine peritoneal macrophages.

## GNA

The snowdrop lectin, GNA, belongs to a group of mannose-specific lectins obtained from species of the plant family Amaryllidaceae (Van Damme, Allen and Peumans, 1987). The lectin GNA from *Galanthus nivalis* is contained in the bulbs of the plant and has a selective specificity for terminal mannose structures at the non-reducing ends of glycans, with the highest affinity for a 1,3- linked mannosyl terminals. It is a tetramer (50 kDa) composed of four 12.5 kDa subunits and occurs as a natural mixture of isolectins.

GNA has been shown to prevent or reduce *Escherichia coli* overgrowth in the small intestine. Thus, orally administered GNA inhibited kidney bean lectin-induced *E. coli* overgrowth in the rat small intestine *in vivo* (Pusztai *et al.*, 1993). However, GNA had little or no effect on the intestinal metabolism itself (Pusztai *et al.*, 1995). It has therefore been suggested that GNA may be useful for blocking the proliferation of bacteria expressing type 1 fimbriae in the digestive tract [Chemical probiosis] (Pusztai *et al.*, 1993). It has also recently been shown that GNA reduces the numbers of *Salmonella typhimurium* in the small and large intestine of rats (Naughton *et al.*, 2000).There are several possible mechanisms by which GNA could prevent or decrease the infection by *S. typhimurium*. One explanation is that the lectin could be cytotoxic to the bacterium. A second possibility is that GNA can agglutinate *Salmonella* and in so doing, prevent them from attaching to the substratum. This would thus prevent colonisation. High-mannose glycans are ubiquitous components of bacterial pathogens, parasites, yeasts and some viruses (Ezekowitz and Stahl, 1988), and are also present in other cells particularly immature or damaged cells. However, GNA does not bind to or agglutinate *S. typhimurium in vitro*. Therefore, the ability of GNA to decrease the numbers of *Salmonella* present in the terminal ileum and large intestine seems unlikely to be due to the aggregation of bacteria. It is unclear why GNA fails to aggregate *S. typhimurium* although numerous GNA binding sites (*i.e.* mannose residues) are present on the surface of the bacteria. One possible reason is that the mannose residues are not exposed and therefore binding and cross-linking of adjacent organisms does not occur.

GNA may bind to gut surface glycoproteins that are used by *Salmonella* for attachment to the gut. This may prevent adherence and colonisation by the bacteria. Alternatively, GNA may alter cellular metabolism in such a manner as to reduce the level of expression on the gut of glyconjugates essential for adherence. *S. typhimurium* causes major changes to gut epithelium. In particular it triggers high rates of epithelial cell division and turnover, which can facilitate infection by the bacteria (Naughton, Grant, Ewen, Spencer Brown, Pusztai and Bardocz, 1995). If GNA slowed down the rate of cell turnover, this would oppose the damaging changes of *S. typhimurium* by reducing the numbers of immature cells reaching the villus surface and hence the numbers of potential binding sites for *Salmonella*.

## Plant lectin -fungal interactions

Much of the early work investigating fungi and lectins involved Con A. The major binding site for Con A in yeast or fungi is mannan, in particular the α-linked D-Man residues. Con A agglutinates Saccharomyces cells without pretreatment, indicating that the ligands for this lectin are available on the surface. Although most studies on lectin-Saccharomyces interactions have used Con A, at least one report indicates that WGA also binds to these yeast cells (Horisberger and Rosset 1976). Con A binds to *Candida albicans* (Janson and Paktor, 1977*) Candida utilis* (Horisberger and Vonlanthen, 1977) and other *Candidia* spp (Janson and Paktor, 1977) via the mannan located in the cell walls of these microorganisms, Con A also agglutinates *Aspergillus* spp and *Penicillium* spp (Barkai-Golan, Mirelman and Sharon, 1978). Such reactions are not universal among fungi, however, since no reaction was seen with species of *Schizosacchoromyces* and

*hodotúrula* (Tkacz, Cybulska and Lampen, 1971). In such species the mannan
may exist in ß-linkages and would thus be a poor ligand for Con A. Alternatively,
by overlying ß-glucans or chitin (Barkai-Golan *et al.*, 1978) the mannan may be
masked. Wheat germ agglutinin (WGA) has been used in a number of studies in
fungal cell surfaces. It is specific for oligosaccharides of N-acetylglucosamine
GlcNAc; Goldstein and Hayes, 1978) and as such binds to the polymer of this
sugar, chitin. *Phytophthora ciliophthora*, whose cell wall is devoid of chitin,
does not bind WGA (Barkai-Golan *et al.*, 1978). Soya bean agglutinin (SBA), a
lectin with specificity for GalNAc and, to a lesser extent, D-Gal (Goldstein and
Hayes, 1978) bound to all species of *Penicillium* and *Aspergillus* examined (Barkai-
Golan *et al.*, 1978). Like SBA, peanut lectin (PNA) has been found to bind to
species of *Penicillium* and *Aspergillus* (Barkai-Golan *et al.*, 1978).

## Plant lectin-viral interactions

Lectins may also have a role in protection against viruses (Bliah, 1988). Con A
can inhibit infectivity of herpes simplex virus type 1(Ito and Barron, 1974).
Moreover, phytohaemagglutin-P, ConA, *Ricinus communis* agglutinin and WGA
can effectively inhibit growth of Sindbis virus and vaccinia virus in chick embryo
and Vero-cells (Finkelstein and McWilliams, 1976). Con A can prevent the
replication of mature vesicular stomatitis virus and this appears to be due to the
blockage of the glycoprotein receptor sites on the cell by the lectin (Cartwright,
1977). Possible explanations for the observed inhibitory effects of the lectins are:
(a) binding to the virons resulting in the agglutination of virus particles which prevents
the penetration of cells, (b) binding to the cell surface thereby blocking virus receptor
sites or (c) modification of the cellular membrane in a manner that prevents the
release of viral replicates. Lectins may also interfere with the intracellular replication
of viruses.

## Bacterial lectins

Microbial cells produce a wide range of carbohydrate binding proteins such as
lectins, sugar-specific enzymes, sugar transport proteins and toxins. The central
role of the lectins (adhesins) in the interaction of bacteria with mammalian cells, is
well-recognised (Duguid, Clegg and Wilson, 1978). The lectins are not confined to
a single site in the organism and can appear on the cell surface, on bacterial
fimbriae or on intercellular membranes. In addition, there may be more than one
type of fimbrial adhesin agglutinin on the cell's surface, each having different
carbohydrate specifies. Many *Escherichia coli* and *Salmonella* strains produce

more than one type of fimbriae (Thorns, 1995) under different growth conditions. The location of the microbial lectin is important since it determines the likely role. The agglutinin may be on the cell surface and thus possibly involved in cell-cell or cell-matrix recognition and adhesion or it may be intracellular and perhaps has cell regulatory or modulator functions (Ofek and Beachey 1980). It has been shown that type 1 fimbriae of *S. enteritidis* (SEF) are expressed and associate with the rat gut *in vivo* (Ewen, Naughton, Grant, Sojka, Allen-Vercoe, Bardocz, Thorns and Pusztai, 1997).

## Chemical probiosis

Novel approaches to modulate bacterial interactions with the gut and infection include "chemical probiosis". This has been defined as "a process designed to modify the structure and function of the absorptive surface of the small intestine through the using of natural feed additives such as appropriate lectins and/or glycoconjugates (usually of plant origin) which, through competition with bacterial adhesins or by changing the expression of surface receptors for bacterial adhesion, reduce the numbers of harmful bacteria to a minimum whilst promoting the proliferation of potentially useful strains" (Pusztai, Grant, King and Clarke, 1990b)

UEA-1 (*Ulex europaeus*) has been used for the inhibition of Streptococcal adhesion to HEP-2 cells (Stinson and Wang, 1998). Preincubation of live and fixed Caco-2 cells with peanut agglutinin (PNA) inhibited the binding of *Salmonella typhimurium* (Giannasca, Giannasca and Neutra, 1996). GNA inhibited the binding of *Chlamydia trachomatis* to McCoy cells *in vitro* (Amin, Beillevarie, Mahmoud, Hammar, Mardh and Froman, 1995). Feed lectins with the same carbohydrate-recognising specificity as the bacteria may inhibit the attachment and subsequent proliferation of bacteria. In this context, it has been demonstrated that GNA, the lectin of the snowdrop (*Galanthus nivalis*) which is highly specific for 1,3-α-linked D-mannose, prevented the proliferation of type 1 fimbriated *E. coli* in rat small intestine by blocking the adhesion sites of the fimbriae on the intestinal epithelium (Pusztai *et al.*, 1993). In addition, gerbils were protected from amoebic liver abscess by immunisation with the galactose-specific adherence lectin of *Entamoeba histolytica*, an enteric protozoan causing disease in humans (Soong, Kain, Abd-Alla, Jackson and Ravdin, 1995). Con A was able to inhibit the attachment of *S. pullorum* to chicken gut (Zhou *et al.*,1995) and block the attachment of *Giardia lamblia* trophozoites to Caco2 cells (Katelaris *et al.*, 1995). Wheat germ agglutinin (WGA) reversibly inhibited the growth of *Giardis lamblia in vitro*, and reduced the extent of infection by *G. muris* in the adult mouse model of giardiasis (Ortega-Barria, Ward, Keusch, Pereira, 1994). The lesions occurring in highly susceptible BALB/c mice infected by *Leishmania amazonensis* can be appreciably reduced by *in vivo* administration of *Canavalia brasiliensis* lectin (Barral-Netto, Von Sohsten, Teixeria, Conrado dos Santos, Pomperay, Moreira, Oliveira, Cavada, Falcoff and Barral, 1996).

## Future perspectives

The most important developments in genetic modification now means that it is possible to include lectin genes in crop plants in which they were not previously expressed. Higher levels of lectins will mean increased potential for interactions with the microorganisms in the gut. It remains to be seen whether these interactions will be detrimental or beneficial for the animal. Whatever the case, it promises to be an exciting area of research for the future.

## Acknowledgements

The author is a Senior Scientist funded by the Danish Ministry of Food, Agriculture and Fisheries, The Research Secretariat and the National Committee for Pig Breeding, Health and Production, and The Federation of Danish Pig Producers and Slaughterhouses. Thanks to B.B. Jensen (DIAS) and G. Grant (RRI) for helpful discussions.

## References

Abud, R.L., Lindquist, B.L., Ernst, R.K., Merrick, J.M., Lebenthal, E. and Lee, P.C. (1989) Concanavalin A promotes adherence of *Salmonella typhimurium* to small intestinal mucosa of rats. *Proceedings of the Society for Experimental Biology and Medicine*, **192**, 81-86.

Amin, K., Beillevarie, D., Mahmoud, E., Hammar, L., Mardh, P-A. and Froman, G. (1995) Binding of *Galanthus nivalis* lectin to *Chlamydia trachomatis* and inhibition of *in vitro* infection. *Acta Pathologica, Microbiologica et Immunologica Scandinavica*, **103**, 714-720.

Baintner, K., Duncan, S.H., Stewart, C.S. and Pusztai, A. (1993). Binding and degradation of lectins by components of rumen liquor. *Journal of Applied Bacteriology*, **74**, 29-35.

Bardocz, S., Ewen, S.W.B., Grant, G. and Pusztai, A. (1995) Lectins as growth factors for the small intestine and the gut. In: *Lectins: Biomedical Perspectives* pp 103-116. (Pusztai, A. and Bardocz, S eds) Taylor & Francis, London.

Bar-Shavit, Z. and Goldman, R. (1976) Concanavalin A-mediated attachment and ingestion of yeast cells by macrophages. *Experimental Cell Research*, **99**, 221-236.

Barkai-Golan, R., Mirelman, D. and Sharon, N. (1978) Studies on growth inhibition by lectins of Penicillia and Aspergilli. *Archives in Microbiology*, **116**, 119-124.

Barral-Netto, M., Von Sohsten, R.L., Teixeria, M., Conrado dos Santos, W.L., Pomperay, M.L., Moreira, R.A., Oliveira, J.T.A., Cavada, B.S., Falcoff, E. and Barral, A. (1996) In vivo protective effect of lectin from Canavalia brasiliensis on BALB/c mice infected by Leishmania amazonensis. *Acta Tropica*, **60**, 237-250.

Bliah, M.A.M. (1988) Methods and compositions for inhibiting the infectious activity of viruses. US PATENT 4,742,046.

Brady, P.G., Vannier, A.M. and Banwell, J.G. (1978) Identification of the dietary lectin, wheat germ agglutinin in human intestinal contents. *Gastroenterology*, **75**, 236-239.

Cartwright, B. (1977) Effect of concanavalin A on vesicular stomatitis virus maturation. *Journal of General Virology*, **34**, 249-256.

Carpenter, G. and Cohen, S. (1977) Influence of lectins on the binding of 125I-labelled EGF to human fibroblasts. *Biochemistry Biophysics Research Communications*, **79**, 545-552.

Coffey, D.G., Uebersax, M.A., Hosfield, G.L. and Brunner, J.R. (1985) Evaluation of the hemagglutinating activity of low temperature cooked kidney beans. *Food Science*, **50**, 78-81.

Down, S., Ford, R.E., Woodhouse, L., Raemaekers, S.D., Leitch, B., Gatehouse, J.A. and Gatehouse, A.M.R. (2000) Snowdrop lectin (GNA) has no acute toxic effects on a beneficial insect predator, the 2-spot ladybird (Adalia bipunctata L.) *Journal of Insect Physiology*, **46**, 379-391.

Duguid, J.P., Clegg, S. and Wilson, M.I. (1978) The fimbrial and non-fimbrial agglutinins of *Escherichia coli*. *Journal of Medical Microbiology*, **12**, 213-227.

Etzler, M.E. and Branstrator, M.L. (1974) Differential localization of cell surface and secretory components in rat intestinal epithelium by use of lectins. *Journal of Cell Biology*, **62**, 329-343.

Ewen, S.W.B., Naughton, P.J., Grant, G., Sojka, M., Allen-Vercoe, E., Bardocz, S., Thorns, C.J. and Pusztai, A. (1997) *Salmonella enterica* var Typhimurium and *Salmonella enterica* var Enteritidis express type 1 fimbriae in the rat *in vivo*. *FEMS Immunology and Medical Microbiology*, **18**, 185-192.

Ezekowitz, R.A.B. and Stahl, P.D. (1988) The structure and function of vertebrate mannose lectin-like proteins. *Journal Cell Science*, **9**, 121-133.

Felipe, I., Bim, S. and Somensi, C.C. (1995) Increased clearance of *Candida albicans* from the peritoneal-cavity of mice pretreated with Concanavalin A or jacalin. *Brazilian Journal Medical Biology Research*, **28**, 477-483.

Finkelstein, M.S. and McWilliams, M. (1976) Effects of plant lectins on virus growth in nonlymphoid cells. *Virology*, **69**, 570-586

Galán, J.E., Pace, J. and Hayman, M.J. (1992) Involvement of the epidermal growth factor receptor in the invasion of cultured mammalian cells by *Salmonella typhimurium*. *Nature*, **357**, 588-589.

Gallily, R., Vary, B., Stain, I. and Sharon, N. (1984) Wheat germ agglutinin potentiates uptake of bacteria by murine peritoneal macrophages. *Immunology*, **52**, 679-686.

Giannasca, K.T., Giannasca, P.J. and Neutra, M. (1996). Adherence of *Salmonella typhimurium* to Caco-2 Cells: Identification of a glycoconjugate receptor. *Infection and Immunity*, **64**, 135-145.

Goldstein, I.J. and Hayes, C.E., (1978) The lectins: carbohydrate-binding proteins of plants and animals. *Advances in Carbohydrate Chemistry and Biochemistry*, **35**, 127-340.

Goldstein, I.J. and Poretz, R.D. (1986) Isolation, physicochemical characterisation, and carbohydrate-binding specificity of lectins. In: Liener IE, Sharon N, Goldstein IJ (eds.), The lectins: Properties, Functions, and applications in Biology and Medicine. Orlando, USA: Academic Press, pp. 33-247.

Grant, G. *Plant lectins*. In: Caygill, J.C. and Mueller-Harvey, I (eds) Secondary plant products; antinutritional and benefical actions in animal feeding. Nottingham Universiry Press, Nottingham, UK, pp 87-110.

Hazan, R., Krushel, L. and Crossing, K.L. (1995) EGF receptor-mediated signals are differentially modulated by Concanavalin A. *Journal of Cellular Physiology*, **162**, 74-85.

Horisberger, M. and Rosset, J.(1976) Localization of wheat germ agglutinin receptor sites on yeast cells by scanning electron microscopy. *Experimentia*, **32**, 998-1000.

Horisberger, M. and Vonlanthen, M. (1977) Location of mannan and chitin on thin sections of budding yeasts with gold markers. *Archives in Microbiology*, **115**, 1-7.

Ito, M. and Barron, A.L. (1974) Inactivation of herpes simplex virus by concanavalin A. *Journal of Virology*, **13**, 1312-1318.

Janson, V.K. and Paktor, J.A. (1977) The effect of temperature on concanavalin A-mediated agglutinin of cells with rigid receptors. *Biocheim Biophysics Acta*, **467**, 321-326.

Jordinson M, Goodlad, R.A., Brynes, A., Bliss, P., Ghatei, M.A., Bloom, S.R., Fitzgerald, A., Grant, G., Bardocz,S., Pusztai, A., Pignatelli, M. and Calam, J. (1999).Gastrointestinal responses to a panel of lectins in rats maintained on total parenteral nutrition. *American Journal of Physiology*, **276**, G1235-G1242.

Karlsson, K.A., Ångström, J., Bergström, J. and Lanne, B. (1992) Microbial interaction with cell surface. *Acta Pathologica, Microbiologica et Immunologica Scandinavica*, **100**, 71-83.

Katelaris, P.H., Naeem, A. and Farthing, M.J.G. (1995) Attachment of *Giardia lamblia* trophozoites to a cultured human intestinal-cell line. *Gut*, **37**, 512-518.

Kilpatrick, D.C. (1999) Immunological aspects of the potential role of dietary carbohydrates and lectins in human health. *European Journal of Nutrition*, **38**, 107-117.

Lavelle, EC. (2000) Targeted mucosal delivery of drugs and vaccines. *Expert Opinion in Therapeutics and Patents*, **10**, 179-190.

Lavelle, E.C., Grant, G., Pusztai, A., Pfüller, U. and O'Hagan, D.T. (2000) Mucosal immunogenicity of plant lectins in mice. *Immunology*, **99**, 30-37.

Liener, I.E., (1974) Phytohemagglutinins: Their nutritional significance. *Journal of Agriculture and Food Chemistry*, **22**, 17 .

Liener, I.E. (1976) Phytohemagglutinins. *Annual Review Plant Physiology*, **27**, 291-319.

Liener, I.E. and Hasdai, A. (1986). The effect of the long-term feeding of raw soy flour on the pancreas of the mouse and hamster. *Advances in Experimental Medicine and Biology*, **199**, 189-197.

Linquist, B.L., Lebenthal, E., Lee, P.C., Stinson, M.W. and Merrick, J.M. (1987) Adherence of *Salmonella typhimurium* to small-intestinal enetrocytes of the rat. *Infection and Immunity*, **55**, 3044-3050.

Lorenz-Meyer, H., Roth, P., Elsasser, P. and Hahn, U. (1985) Cytotoxicity of lectins on rat intestinal mucosa is enhanced by neuraminidase. *European Journal of Clinical Investigation*, **15**, 227-234.

Lorenzsonn, V. and Olsen, W.A. (1982) *In vivo* responses of rat intestinal epithelium to intraluminal dietary lectins. *Gastroenterology*, **82**, 838-848.

Maldonado, G., Porras, F., Fernandez, L., Vazquez, L. and Zenteno, E. (1994) Effect of lectins on mouse peritoneal macrophage phagocytic-activity. *Immunology Investigation*, **23**, 429-436.

Melhem, R.F. and LeVerde, P.T. (1984) Mechanism of interaction of *Salmonella* and *Schistoma* species. *Infection and Immunity*, **44**, 274-281

Nachbar, M.S., Oppenheim, J.D. and Thomas, J.O. (1980). Lectins in the U.S. diet: Isolation and characterisation of a lectin from the tomato (*Lycopersicon esculentum*). *Journal of Biological Chemistry*, **255**, 2056-2061.

Nakata, S. and Kimura, T. (1985) Effect of ingested toxic bean lectins on the gastrointestinal tract in the rat. *Journal of Nutrition*, **115**, 1621-1629.

Nakata, S. and Kimura, T. (1986) Behaviour of ingested concanavalin A in the gastrointestinal tract of the rat. *Agriculture Biological Chemistry*, 50, 645-649.

Naughton, P.J., Grant, G., Ewen, S.W.B., Spencer R.J., Brown, D.S., Pusztai, A. and Bardocz, S. (1995) *Salmonella typhimurium* and *Salmonella enteritidis* induce gut growth and increase the polyamine content of the rat small intestine in vivo. *FEMS Immunology and Medical Microbiology*, 12, 251-258.

Naughton, P.J., Grant, G., Bardocz, S. and Pusztai, A. (2000) Modulation of Salmonella infection by the lectins of Canavalia ensiformis (ConA) and Galanthus nivalis (GNA) in a rat model *in vivo*. *Journal of Applied Microbiology*, 88, 720-727.

Ofek, I., Rest, R. and Sharon, N. (1992) Nonopsonic phagocytosis of microorganisms; phagocytes use several molecular mechanisms to recognise, bind and eventually kill microorganisms. *American Society of Microbiology News*, 58, 429-435.

Ofek, I., Beachey, E.H. (1980) Bacterial adherence, Receptors and Recognition, London: Chapman and Hall.

Ortega-Barria, E., Ward, H.D., Keusch, G.T. and Pereira, M.E. (1994) Growth inhibition of the intestinal parasite *Giardia lamblia* by the dietary lectin associated with arrest of the cell cycle. *Clinical Investigaton*, 94, 2283-2288.

Ovelgonne, J.H., Koninkx, J.F., Pusztai, A., Bardocz, S., Kok, W., Ewen, S.W.B., Hendricks, H.G. and van Dijk, J.E. (2000) Decreased levels of heat shock proteins in gut epithelial cells after exposure to plant lectins. *Gut*, 46, 680-688.

Pistole, T.G. (1981) Interaction of Bacteria and Fungi with lectins and lectin-like substances. *Annual Review of Microbiology*, 35, 85-112.

Poschet, J.F. and Fairclough, P.D. (1999) Effect of lectins on *Salmonella typhimurium* invasion in cultured human intestinal cells. *Gut*, 44, No.S1, pW252.

Pusztai, A., Ewen, S.W.B., Grant, G., Peumans, W.J., Van Damme, E.J.M., Coates, M.E. and Bardocz, S. (1995) Lectins and also bacteria modify the glycosylation of gut surface receptors in the rat. *Glyconjugate Journal*, 12, 22-35.

Pusztai, A. (1991). Plant Lectins, University Press, Cambridge.

Pusztai, A., Ewen, S.W.B., Grant, G., Peumans, W.J., Van Damme, E.J.M., Rubio, L. and Bardocz, S. (1990a) The relationship between survival and binding of plant lectins during small intestinal passage and their effectiveness as growth factors. *Digestion*, 46, 308-316.

Pusztai, A., Grant, G., King, T.P. and Clarke, E.M.W. (1990b) Chemical probiosis. In *Recent Advances in Animal Nutrition* ed. Haresign, W. and Cole, D.J.A. pp. 47-60. London: Butterworth Scientific Press.

Pusztai, A., Clarke, E.M. and King, T.P. (1979) The nutritional toxicity of *Phaseolus vulgaris* lectins. *Proceedings of the Nutrition Society*, **38**, 115-120.

Pusztai, A., Grant, G., Spencer, R.J., Duguid, T.J., Brown, D.S., Ewen, S.W.B., Peumans, W.J., Van Damme, E.J.M. and Bardocz, S. (1993) Kidney bean lectin-induced *Escherichia coli* overgrowth in the small intestine is blocked by GNA, a mannose specific lectin. *Journal of Applied Bacteriology*, **75**, 360-368.

Ryder, S.D., Jacyna, M.R., Levi, A.J., Rizzi, P.M. and Rhodes, J.M. (1998) Peanut ingestion increases rectal proliferation in individuals with mucosal expression of peanut lectin receptor. *Gastroenterology*, **114**, 44-49.

Rehmani, S.F. and Spradbrow, P.B. (1995) The contribution of lectins to the interaction between oral Newcastle disease vaccine and grains. *Veterinary Microbiology*, **46**, 55-62.

Seifert, R., and Schultz, G. (1991) The superoxide-forming NADPH oxidase of phagocytes. An enzyme system regulated by multiple mechanisms. *Reviews in Physiology Biochemistry and Pharmacology*, **117**, 1-338.

Sharon, N. (1993) Lectin-carbohydrate complexes of plants and animals: an atomic view. *Trends in Biochemical Science*, **18**, 221-226.

Sharon, N. and Lis, H. (1989) Lectins as cell recognition molecules. *Science*, **246**, 227-234.

Sheriff, S., Chang, C.Y.Y. and Ezekowitz, R.A.B. (1994) The structure of mouse mannose binding protein. *Nature Structural Biology*, **1**, 789-794.

Siraganian, P.A. and Siraganian, R.P. (1974) Basophil activation by concanavalin A. Characteristics of the reaction. *Journal of Immunology*, **112**, 2117-2125.

Sitkovsky, M.V., Pasternack, M.S. and Eisen, H.N. (1982) Inhibition of cytotoxic T lymphocyte activity by concanavalin A. *Journal of Immunology*, **129**, 1372-1376.

Soong, C.J., Kain, K.C., Abd-Alla, M., Jackson, T.F. and Ravdin, J.I. (1995) A recombinant cysteine-rich section of the Entamoeba histolytica galactose-inhibitable lectin is efficacious as a subunit vaccine in the gerbil model of amebic liver abscess. *Journal of Infectious Diseases*, **171**, 645-651.

Stinson, M.W. and Wang, J.R. (1998) Lectin inhibition of bacterial adhesion to Animal cells. In: Rhodes, J.M. and Milton, J.D. (eds.)Lectin methods and protocols. Humana Press, Totowa, NJ, USA.pp 529-538.

Summer, J.B. and Howell, S.F. (1936) The identification of the hemagglutinin of the jack bean with Concanavalin A. *Journal of Bacteriology*, **32**, 227-237.

Thorns, C.J. (1995) Salmonella fimbriae: novel antigens in the detection and control of *Salmonella* infections. *British Veterinary Journal*, **151**, 643-658.

Tkacz, J.D., Cybulska, E.B. and Lampen, J.O. (1971) Specific staining of wall mannan in yeast cells with fluorescein-conjugated concanavalin A. *Journal of Bacteriology*, **105**, 1-5.

Van Damme, E.J.M., Allen, A.K. and Peumans, W.J. (1987) Isolation and characterisation of a lectin with exclusive specificity towards mannose from snowdrop (*Galanthus nivalis*) bulbs. *FEBS Letters*, **215**, 140-144.

Van Damme, E.J.M., Peumans, W.J., Pusztai, A and Bardocz, S. (1998) Plant lectins: a special class of plant proteins. In: handbook of Plant lectins:Properties and Biomedical applications (eds E.J.M. Van Damme, W.J. Peumans, A. Pusztai and S. Bardocz) John Wiley and Sons, Chichester, UK.

Wang, J.L., Cunningham, B.A. and Edelman, G.M. (1971) Unusual fragments in the subunit structure of concanavalin A. *Proceedings of the National Academy of Sciences USA*, **68**, 1130-1134.

Wang, Q., Yu, L.G., Campbell, B.J., Milton, J.D. and Rhodes, J.M. (1998) Identification of intact peanut lecin in peripheral venous blood. *Lancet*, **352**, 1831-1832.

Weiss, A.A. and Goodwin, M.S. (1989) Lethal infection by *Bordetella pertussis* mutants in the infant mouse model. *Infection and Immunity*, **57**, 3757-3764.

Wilson, A.B., King, T.P., Clarke, E.M.W. and Pusztai, A. (1980) Kidney bean (*Phaseolus vulgaris*) lectin induced lesions in the small intestine.II. Microbiological studies. *Comparative Pathology*, **90**, 597-602.

Weiser, M.M. and Douglas, A,P. (1976) An alternative mechanism for gluten toxicity in coeliac disease. *Lancet*, **1**, 567-569.

Woodley, J.F. (2000) Lectins for gastrointestinal targeting-15 years on. *Journal of Drug Targeting*, **7**, 325-333.

Wyczolkowska, J., Rydzynski, K. and Prouvost-Danon, A. (1992) Concanavalin A induced activation of hamster mast-cells- Morphological changes and histamine-secretion. *International Archives of Allergy and Immunology*, **97**, 167-172.

Weaver, L.T. and Bailey, D.S. (1987) Effect of lectin concanavalin A on the neonatal guinea pig gastrointestinal mucosa *in vivo*. *Journal of Pediatric Gastroenterology and Nutrition*, **6**, 445-453.

Zhou, Z.X., Deng, Z.P. and Ding, J.Y. (1995) Role of glycoconjugates in adherence of *Salmonella pullorum* to the intestinal epithelium of chicks. *British Poultry Science*, **36**, 79-86.

**11**

# MODULATION OF THE GUT MICROFLORA BY ENZYME ADDITION

Andrew Chesson and Colin S. Stewart
*Rowett Research Institute, Bucksburn, Aberdeen AB21 9SB, UK*

## Summary

The present market for feed enzymes in Europe is stagnant and attempts to broaden their application have met with only limited success. The known ability of enzymes to release oligosaccharides from dietary polysaccharides *in situ* as a means of selectively stimulating the growth or activity of sections of the gut flora or supporting the colonisation of added microbial strains is one application that has not been seriously considered. A very limited range of oligosaccharides is produced commercially for use in human food, and feeding trials suggest that these may also be of value in animal nutrition. However the capacity of cloned single enzyme activities when coupled with different polysaccharide structures to produce an almost unlimited range of oligomer mixtures appears not to be fully appreciated. In addition, molecular methods of community analysis enable all changes to the flora, including those organisms not amenable to cultivation, to be monitored and related to any host response. This paper brings together data from a number of disparate sources to suggest that *in situ* generation of oligosaccharides by exogenous enzymes might offer a means of manipulating the gut flora to the benefit of the host.

## Introduction

Despite the widespread acceptance of feed enzymes as "natural" agents with an established role in animal production, they remain niche products with applications that have consolidated around their use in improving the utilisation of cereal-based diets by broilers and, to a lesser extent, piglets. In this respect, their apparent value to the feed industry has extended little from that established in the earliest days of use when bulk enzymes first became available in volumes and at a price which allowed their use in animal feeds. As a consequence, markets for feed enzyme have tended to stagnate in many industrialised countries because of a static demand for manufactured pig and poultry feed.

Considerable efforts have been made to extend the role of enzymes beyond the confines of their established use with cereal-based diets. These have primarily focussed on extending the range of target species or category of livestock, on the use of enzymes with maize and/or soybean and on the reformulation of pig and poultry diets using cheaper alternative ingredients. Environmental and welfare benefits have also been a consideration. There have been notable successes: the development of recombinant phytase to aid control of phosphorus excretion or improvements to the shelf-life of products and their survival during feed processing for example. Nonetheless, the totality of this work has yet to significantly influence the way in which enzymes are perceived and used by the feed industry.

The absence of a sound theoretical basis for an intended mode of action is a key reason why some applications have failed to materialise. Feed enzymes are most beneficial when they provide a unique (or at least the most convenient) solution to a defined problem such as the reduction in digesta viscosity or the sparing of phosphorus. They have proved least effective when the justification for enzyme addition is ill-defined or inappropriate. The plant cell wall (fibre) has often been perceived as an appropriate target. Initially this was seen as a possible source of otherwise unavailable carbohydrate and latterly more as a means of liberating nutrients trapped within a cell wall matrix. In the former case, studies have shown that, within the context of the digestive tract, added enzymes are relatively ineffective against an insoluble and impermeable substrate such as the plant cell wall. In the second case, enzymes at best act to correct an inadequacy of feed processing which is better tackled by altering the processing conditions.

Feed enzymes have proved most effective against readily accessible, often water-soluble, substrates. The action of mixed-linked glucanase and xylanases against the glucans and xylans released from grain endosperm walls within the relatively short time allowed by gut transit is the best documented example (Bedford, 1995). However, these enzymes are effective not only because of the availability of the substrate, but because only limited catalytic action is required to fragment the substrate and destroy the physical properties thought to contribute to their anti-nutritional effects. It is not necessary for the polysaccharide to be hydrolysed to its component monosaccharides to obtain a beneficial effect. In practice, added enzymes rarely if ever effect a total hydrolysis of the target substrate and as a result, in non-ruminants, most carbohydrate passing the ileal-ceacal junction is in the form of oligosaccharides.

## Dietary oligosaccharides

Addition to diets of a variety of oligosaccharides, has been shown to selectively favour the growth of single bacterial strains or groups of related strains occurring within the normal commensal flora of humans (Gibson, Rastall and Roberfroid, 1999) and livestock (Orban, Patterson, Adeola, Sutton and Richards, 1997). First recognised as a stimulant for bifidobacteria, such oligosaccharides were initially referred to as "bifidus-factors". However, as further work showed that other groups of bacteria could also be selectively stimulated by dietary means, oligosaccharides were recognised as part of a more general phenomenon and the term "prebiotic" (analogous to probiotic) was introduced (Gibson and Roberfroid, 1995). Although increased numbers of some lactic acid and other bacteria are generally believed to contribute to long-term health, this has proved difficult to establish conclusively for humans. Evidence of shorter-term benefits to the health and development of livestock has proved easier to obtain (Monsan and Paul, 1995) but often not in a predictable or reproducible manner.

Fructooligosaccharides (fos) are the most extensively studied of the oligosaccharides used for food and feed purposes. They are produced either by extraction from food sources (onion, artichoke), controlled hydrolysis of naturally occurring fructans such as inulin (De Leenheer, 1966) or by the transglycosylation of sucrose by fructosyltransferase (Hidaka and Hirayama, 1991). This interest, in part, reflected the ease of commercial availability and low cost of fos. However, other carbohydrate oligomers are produced in commercial amounts (Table 1) either by partial hydrolysis of an appropriate polysaccharide or by an enzyme-catalysed transglycosylation reaction.

## Effects of oligosaccharides on the mammalian flora

Determining how the diet affects the gut microflora depends upon precise measurement of the species diversity of the flora. In the past, this relied on culture methods made even more laborious by the necessity to maintain anaerobic conditions. In this way, the human faecal flora was described by, among others, Moore and Holdeman (1974) and Moore and Moore (1995), and the faecal and caecal microflora of pigs were described by Robinson, Allison and Bucklin (1981) and Moore, Moore, Cato, Wilkins and Kornegay (1987). However, the advent of molecular techniques for assessing microbial community diversity, particularly involving the use of PCR, has shown that the classical cultivation studies omit a significant proportion of the bacterial types actually present. Following rDNA sequence analysis, Wilson and Blitchington (1996) suggested that the human faecal flora was more diverse than was represented by the bacteria that could be grown in culture. Pryde, Richardson, Stewart and Flint (1999) isolated random clones of 16S rDNA genes from total bacterial genomic DNA in samples of the pig large intestine and compared these with cultivated bacteria isolated from the same samples. Almost 60% of the rDNA sequences showed less than 95% similarity to

Table 1. Commercial and other sources of oligosaccharides used to manipulate the mammalian gut flora (updated from Chesson, 1994).

| Oligosaccharide | Method of manufacture | Trade names | Ref. |
|---|---|---|---|
| *Produced in commercial quantities* | | | |
| ß-fructooligosaccharides | Hydrolysis of inulin (ex chicory) | Raftilose Fibruline | 1 |
| | Transfructosylation of sucrose | Neosugar Actilight, Nutraflora | 2, 3 |
| α-galactooligosaccharides | Extracted from legumes | Soy-oligo | 4 |
| | Transgalactosylation of sucrose | | 5 |
| ß-galactooligosaccharides | Transgalactosylation of lactose | Oligomate Oligostroop | 6, 7 |
| α-glucooligosaccharides (isomaltooligosaccharides) | Hydrolysis of starch | Isomalto-900 | 8 |
| | Transglucosylation of maltose | Panorup Biotose | 9 |
| Mannooligosaccharides | Hydrolysis of yeast cell wall | Bio-MOS | 10 |
| Xylooligosaccharides | Hydrolysis of xylans | Xylo-oligo | 4, 11 |
| *Produced in experimental quantities* | | | |
| ß-glucooligosaccharides | Transglucosylation of cellobiose, gentiobiose or laminaribiose | | 12 |

References: 1, De Leenheer, 1966; 2, Hidaka and Hirayama, 1991; 3, Yun, 1966; 4, Crittenden and Playne, 1996; 5, Van den Broek, Ton, Verdoes, Van Laere, Voragen and Beldman, 1999; 6, Fujii and Komoto, 1991; 7, Cruz, Cruz, Belote, Khenayfes, Dorta, Oliveira, Ardiles and Galli, 1999; 8, Amarkone, Ishigami and Kainuma, 1984; 9, Yoneyama, Shibuya and Miyake, 1992; 10, Newman, 1994; 11, Kontula, Suihko, Suortti, Tenkanen, Mattila-Sandholm and von Wright, 2000; 12, Nakakuki, Kalnuma, Unno and Okada, 1990.

known bacteria. Furthermore, although over 50% of the cultivated isolates from the colon wall were related to known species of lactic-acid bacteria, this accounted for only around one-third of the sequence variation obtained by random cloning. Although potential pitfalls exist in the molecular analysis of microbial communities such as the differential amplification of some sequences (Wilson and Blitchington, 1996), the further development of molecular methods will provide means to assess the effects of dietary manipulations much more accurately than previously has been possible.

In the colon, bacteria utilise dietary carbohydrates that have escaped digestion in the upper GI tract as a carbon source. Some growth may also occur on proteins and amino acids and endogenous carbohydrates. Feeding oligosaccharides has been shown to affect the faecal microflora of humans in ways that are presumed to be beneficial, most notably by the stimulation of the growth of bifidobacteria. The chain length of these oligosaccharides may affect the rate of fermentation. While both inulin and oligofructose were rapidly metabolised in simulations of the human colonic fermentation, the rate of degradation of oligomers with DP <10 was approximately double that of larger molecules (Roberfroid, Van Loo and Gibson, 1998). Human volunteers fed different amounts of synthetic fructo-oligosaccharides showed increased numbers of bifidobacteria in their faeces, the greatest increase in numbers of these bacteria tending to occur in individuals with low initial counts of bifidobacteria, irrespective of the dose of fructo-oligosaccharide ingested. More recently, Olano-Martin, Mountzouris, Gibson and Rastall (2000) described oligodextrans with similar bifidogenic activity to fos, although feeding trials have not yet been reported.

A study of the potential for the use of bifidogenic oligosaccharides in young pigs was performed by Maxwell (1994). A total of 45 *Bifidobacterium* species were isolated from pigs, including *B. boum*, *B. thermophilum*, *B. choerinum*, *B. suis*, *B. pseudolongum* and *B. globosum*. Selected strains were tested for their ability to grow on a range of commercial oligosaccharides. These tests were facilitated by the use of microtitre plates in an improved version of the method described by Roy and Ward (1990). The plates, when used in an anaerobic growth chamber, allowed growth of the strains comparable to that achieved in anaerobic culture tubes, despite the periodic need to remove plates from the chamber to read culture absorbance values. When growth (maximum culture absorbance at 595 nm) was compared with that on glucose or fructose (depending on which monosaccharide supported maximal growth of the individual strains), the substrates tested could be ranked for their bifidogenic potential. The best growth of the range of 27 selected bifidobacteria tested was obtained with Actilight P (fos), onion extract and Trouw fos (Table 2). Considerable inter-strain variation was found however, and representatives of some species seemed best adapted to growth on certain substrates. Thus *B. boum* strain U4+16 grew best on Profeed G and Actilight G, whereas *B. boum* strain T8B4 grew best on Actilight P and Trouw fos. Such studies could enable the matching of appropriate probiotic strains with the prebiotics of choice. Feeding experiments remain to be done.

## Oligosaccharides as growth promotors

Agents that act to modify the gastro-intestinal flora can do so in a manner that reduces the need of the host to defend its tissues against bacterial overgrowth and invasion. Any response to an additive will depend on the initial health status of the

**Table 2.** Bifidogenic potential of oligosaccharides for *Bifidobacterium* strains isolated from pigs.

| Oligosaccharide | Average growth* | Range | Best strain |
|---|---|---|---|
| Actilight P fos | 39 | 0-88 | *B. boum* T8B4 |
| Onion extract | 39 | 0-90 | *B.thermophilum* I2+10. |
| Trouw fos | 23 | 0-100 | *B. boum* T8B4 |
| Actilight G fos | 13 | 0-39 | *B. boum* U4+16 |
| Suntory xos | 13 | 0-57 | Unidentified strain I5+10 |
| Profeed G fos | 12 | 0-42 | *B. boum* U4+16 |
| Galactosnow | 4 | 0-27 | Unidentifed strain I5+10 |

* % of maximum growth on glucose or fructose

host animal or group of animals and is likely to be more evident in those facing the greatest microbial challenge. However, in the absence of any objective measure of microbial status, it is difficult to predict the host response to any additive with effects on the gut flora. In the first instance, limited changes to the flora or to immune competence in the compromised host may be detectable only in experimental animals. In production situations, particularly with young animals, the first visible and more readily detectable responses may be reduced morbidity and/or mortality (Mul and Perry, 1994). Ultimately, if the microbial challenge is lifted sufficiently, enough nutrients may be spared to allow repartitioning to occur. The digestive tract and the associated lymphoid tissue of a 25kg pig, for example, utilise around 40% of all ingested nutrients in maintaining integrity and mounting a local immune response (see Chesson, 1994). Consequently, any reduction in microbial pressure can lead to savings of both energy and protein that can be repartitioned to support lean muscle growth.

Virtually all of the trials with oligosaccharides have been made with fos and, to a lesser extent, ß-galactooligosaccharides with a variable response. Increased growth, improved efficiency of feed conversion and a reduction in diarrhoea have been reported on a number of occasions following inclusion of oligosaccharides in the diets of young pigs (Russell, Kerley and Allee, 1996). Others, however, have failed to detect improvements in performance characteristics (Farnworth, Modler, Jones, Cave, Yamazaki and Rao, 1992; Mathew, Robbins, Chattin and Quigley, 1997). Houdijk, Bosch, Verstegen and Berenpas (1998) noted that, in pig trials failing to elicit a response, diets often included soybean and suggested that the presence of soybean oligosaccharides of the raffinose family may have confounded results. However, this is to suggest that different oligosaccharides stimulate a very similar range of microbial strains which is not supported by the microbiological evidence or by the results of feeding studies with other species (see Iji and Tivey, 1998). Their own study (Houdijk *et al.*, 1998) made with nine-week old pigs fed corn based diets without soybean also failed to show a growth response to fos or to ß-galactooligosaccharide addition.

While oligosaccharide addition to diets may not always produce a response of sufficient magnitude to be recorded as an improvement in growth performance, there is evidence that other attributes may be beneficially affected. Changes to the microflora induced by oligosaccharide addition have been shown to reduce faecal shedding of salmonella in piglets (Leteleier, Messier, Lessard and Quessy, 2000), to reduce odour in pig manure (Sutton, Kephart, Verstegen, Canh and Hobbs, 1999) and, when fed in conjunction with a probiotic, to aid the establishment of the added organism in the pig digestive tract (Nemcova, Bomba, Gancarcikova, Herich and Guba, 1999).

In Europe, the best results have been achieved with piglets and rabbits. In a trial with 1500 rabbits in which fos was included in test diets, average weight gain was increased by over 6%, conversion efficiency increased by nearly 8% and the mortality rate decreased by 32% (Bastien, 1990). While benefits in growth performance have been seen with broilers and calves (Iji and Tivey, 1998; Monsan and Paul, 1995), other effects related to health may prove more valuable and provide a more consistent response. Addition of fos to calves had only a limited effect on performance, but reduced veterinary costs significantly (Monsan and Paul, 1995).

## Potential for *in situ* generation of oligosaccharides

Manufactured sources of oligosaccharides may allow dose to be more precisely defined and controlled, but only a very limited range of oligosaccharide structures is presently available. Most are linear, of short chain length and contain only one or two different sugar units. In contrast, plant and plant by-products used by the feed industry contain an almost unlimited range of polysaccharides, many of which have a storage function or are (partially) solubilised during feed manufacture and thus are available to hydrolytic enzymes (Table 3).

Unfortunately, the enzyme mixtures typical of most commercial products offer little opportunity for the control of a limited hydrolytic process. A mixed polysaccharidase preparation typically will declare up to three major activities and guarantee a minimum value for each. Other activities in the mixture are not usually identified or amounts guaranteed and may vary significantly between batches. It is often these "minor" activities which define the fine structure of the oligosaccharides released from branched-chain polysaccharides such as arabinoxylan or xyloglucan. However, the enzyme industry was amongst the first to make

Table 3. Feed sources of available polysaccharides for *in situ* generation of oligomers

| Polysaccharide type | Constituent sugars | Possible feed sources |
|---|---|---|
| Arabinan | Arabinose | Sugar beet pulp |
| (Arabino) ß-1,4 galactan | Galactose, arabinose | Lupin seedmeal, rapeseed |
| (Arabino) ß-1,6 galactan | Galactose, arabinose | Widely distributed |
| Arabinoxylan | Xylose, arabinose | Grain (wheat, rye) |
| Galactomannan | mannose, galactose, glucose | Legume seeds (soybean, field peas) |
| Galacturonan | Galacturonic acid, rhamnose, galactose, arabinose | Sugar beet pulp, citrus pulp, apple pommace, grape marc. |
| ß-glucans (mixed linked) | Glucose | Grain (barley, oat) |
| Glucomannan | Mannose, glucose | Various seeds and tubers |
| Glucuronoxylan | Xylose, glucuronic acid, arabinose | Cereal bran, lignified cell walls |
| Mannan | Mannose | Yeast, palm nut seedmeal |
| Xyloglucan | Glucose, xylose, galactose, fucose | Seedmeals (tamarind) and primary vegetative walls |

practical use of recombinant DNA technology and a number of cloned enzymes now are produced commercially free from other activities. In addition, the extensive search for novel catalytic activities or physical properties and the need to express these in "production" strains has increased dramatically the numbers of single activity enzyme preparations available for commercial development.

The polysaccharides listed in Table 3 represent general classes in which there is commonality of overall structure but often considerable variation in fine structure. The ratio of arabinose to xylose residues in arabinoxylan from various botanical sources can range from as little as one in 20 xylose units carrying an arabinose substitutent to a ratio of one to one or greater in cereal endosperm walls. Even when the source of the polysaccharide is constant, fine structure can vary with age, environmental conditions and between varieties. Hydrolysis of arabinoxylan extracted from different varieties of wheat grain using a single cloned endo-1, 4-xylanase, yielded much the same range of oligosaccharides but in significantly different proportions (Austin, Wiseman and Chesson, 1999). Any endo-acting enzyme will preferentially cleave unsubstituted regions in a polymer chain generating a series of linear oligomers which, in the case of arabinoxylan, will consist only of xylose residues. Hydrolysis is hindered by the presence of substitutent groups and so in regions of extensive substitution more complex oligosaccharide structures are generated (Figure 1). Since these structures are inherently resistant to further degradation by xylanase, they are available only to a much more limited number of gut microorganisms able to remove the substituent group(s). Consequently, it is the more complex branched oligomers that are likely to provide selectivity in modulating the gut flora.

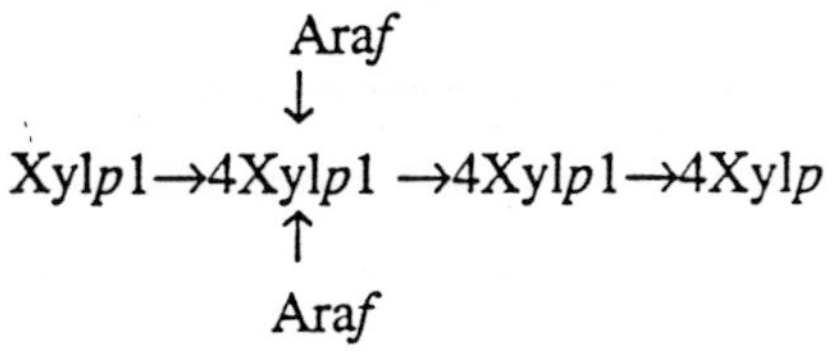

$$
\begin{array}{c}
\text{Ara}f \\
\downarrow \\
\text{Xyl}p1\rightarrow4\text{Xyl}p1\rightarrow4\text{Xyl}p1\rightarrow4\text{Xyl}p \\
\uparrow \\
\text{Ara}f
\end{array}
\qquad\qquad \text{Oligosaccharide AX6}
$$

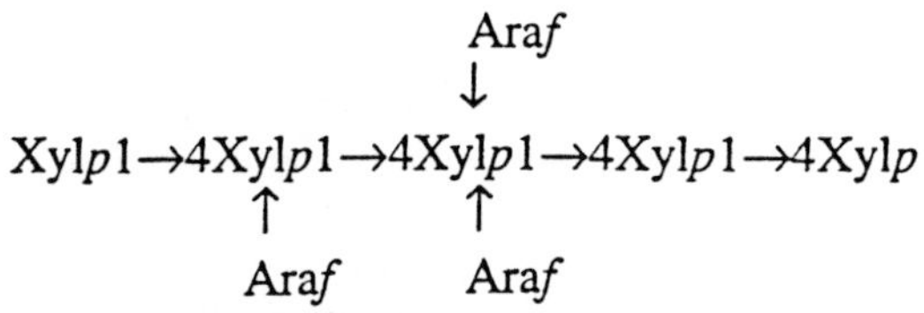

$$
\begin{array}{c}
\text{Ara}f \\
\downarrow \\
\text{Xyl}p1\rightarrow4\text{Xyl}p1\rightarrow4\text{Xyl}p1\rightarrow4\text{Xyl}p1\rightarrow4\text{Xyl}p \\
\uparrow \qquad\quad \uparrow \\
\text{Ara}f \qquad \text{Ara}f
\end{array}
\qquad \text{Oligosaccharide AX8}
$$

**Figure 1.** Two of the more common oligosaccharide structures released from wheat arabinoxylan by the action of a cloned xylanase (from Austin *et al.*, 1999). Xyl*p*, xylopyranose; ara*f*, arabinofuranose.

The use of specific enzymes, singly and in combination, against a range of polysaccharides can generate very large numbers of oligomer mixtures for testing. Using the methods described earlier it is possible to screen such mixtures against a variety of gut organisms and to monitor relative growth rates. Candidate mixtures can then be separated, oligomer structures identified by nmr (Dabrowski, 1994) and the method of generation refined to maximise production of those structures providing the desired degree of discrimination. Although it is known from studies with commercial and naturally occurring oligosaccharides that oligomers do pass the ileal-ceacal junction and can influence the gut flora, there is apparently no recorded instance where the *in situ* generation of oligosaccharides has been monitored. Nonetheless, oligosaccharides must be generated on every occasion when polysaccharide-degrading enzymes are used as feed additives. While not optimised for the purpose, if the generation of oligomers can modulate the gut flora to the benefit of the host, some evidence of this might be expected from *in vivo* trials made with feed enzymes.

## Evidence that added enzymes can produce health benefits

Use of modern methods of community analysis (Table 4) have tended to confirm earlier observations that enzyme addition to diets leads to an alteration in the microbial populations of the digestive tract, at least in poultry (Bedford, 1996). However, it is not known whether such changes arise because of a change in the flux of nutrients passing to the hindgut or whether sections of the population are selectively boosted in numbers by the presence of oligosacccharides. Xylanase addition to broilers chicks resulted in a relative increase of bifidobacteria and *Bacteroides* spp.; a response that might be expected to the presence of xylooligosaccharides. However, the proportion of lactic acid bacteria, which also might be expected to respond to xylooligosaccharides, remained unchanged (Table 4). Lactic acid bacteria are the dominant flora in chicks and, while the total proportion might be difficult to shift, substantial changes in the constituent strains are still possible.

Table 4. Changes in the fraction of total DNA contributed by the major bacterial genera found in the caeca of broiler chicks following xylanase supplementation. (from Apajalahti and Bedford, 1998)

| Bacterial group | Control birds | Xylanase birds |
| --- | --- | --- |
| Lactic acid bacteria | 0.36 | 0.37 |
| Enterobacteriaceae | 0.11 | 0.06 |
| Clostridia | 0.14 | 0.11 |
| *Bacteroides* spp. | 0.10 | 0.16 |
| Eubacteria | 0.08 | 0.10 |
| Bifidobacteria | 0.02 | 0.04 |

Although microbiological data of this type indicate that enzyme addition could contribute to the control of human enteropathogens or overgrowth by Enterobacteriaceae, very few studies have attempted to examine possible health benefits to the host animal. Where health status has been monitored, there are documented examples of a significant reduction in the frequency and severity of diarrhoea in piglets fed diets supplemented with enzyme mixtures containing polysaccharidases (Inborr and Ogle, 1988; Böhme, 1990). However, in no case was the cause of any episode of diarrhoea determined. This is important since it is necessary to distinguish between diarrhoea of dietary origin, often caused by sudden loss of water-holding capacity of dietary polysaccharides as they are degraded in the colon, from those of a bacterial aetiology which might be influenced by the presence of oligosaccharides.

Inborr and Ogle (1988) ascribed their observed reduction in the incidence of diarrhoea simply to a reduction of nutrients entering the hindgut following enzyme addition with a consequent reduction in total numbers of bacteria present. Certainly this seems to be the case for some infectious diseases, notable swine dysentery where work has shown that the spirochaete *Serpulina hyodysenteriae* can be totally excluded in animals fed a no-residue cooked rice starch diet (Pluske, Siba, Pethick, Durmic, Mullan and Hampson, 1996). However, low residue, starch-based diets do not appear to offer the same protection against post-weaning colibacillosis. It seems more likely in this case that the composition of the microbial population is of greater importance than simple numbers that fluctuate is response to the general nutrient supply.

Certain glycosidases may also have health-promoting effects suitable for commercial exploitation. For example, the release of the aglycone esculetin following the hydrolysis of the glycoside esculin by ß-glucosidases of anaerobic gut bacteria, dramatically reduces the survival of the pathogenic bacterium *Escherichia coli* O157 in mixed culture (Duncan, Flint and Stewart, 1998).

## Conclusion

This paper has sought to bring together data from a number of disparate sources to suggest that *in situ* generation of oligosaccharides by exogenous enzymes might offer a means of manipulating the gut flora to the benefit of the host. While the authors recognise that some links in their chain of reasoning are tenuous, sufficient evidence exists to suggest that this is a possibility worth pursuing. The availability of single enzyme activities and a wide range of feed ingredients containing polysaccharides of known structure and the development of modern methods of microbial community analysis make feasible what would have been technically difficult a few years ago. The phasing out of antibiotics for growth promotion purposes and the pressure to reduce veterinary prescriptions leaves the opening in livestock production that would provide a ready market for any "natural" system able to offer a measure of control over the gut flora.

## Acknowledgement

The authors acknowledge the financial support provided for this work by the Scottish Executive Rural Affairs Department (SERAD).

## References

Amarkone, S.P., Ishigami, H. and Kainuma, K. (1984) Conversion of oligo-saccharides formed during starch hydrolysis by a dual enzyme system. *Denpun Kagaku*, **31**, 1-7.

Apajalahti, J. and Bedford, M.R. (1998) Nutrition effects on the microflora of the GI tract. *In Proceedings of the 19th Western Nutrition Conference*, pp.61-68. Saskatoon, Canada.

Austin, S.C., Wiseman, J. and Chesson, A. (1999) Influence of non-starch polysaccharide structure on the metabolisable energy of U.K. wheat fed to poultry. *Journal of Cereal Science*, 29, 77-88

Bastien, R. (1990) Nouveaux régulateurs de flore. *La Revue de L'Alimentation Animale* 434, 56-57.

Bedford, M.R. (1995) Mechanism of action and potential enviromental benefits from the use of feed enzymes. *Animal Feed Science and Technology*, 53, 145-155.

Bedford, M.R. (1996) Interaction between ingested feed and the digestive system in poultry. *Journal of Applied Poultry Research*, 5, 86-95.

Böhme, H. (1990) Experiments on the effect of enzyme supplements as a growth promotor for piglets. *Landbauforschung Völkenrode*, 40, 213-217.

Chesson, A. (1994) Probiotics and other intestinal mediators. *In Principles of Pig Science*, pp. 197-214. Edited by D.J.A. Cole, J. Wiseman, and M.A. Varley. Nottingham University Press, Nottingham.

Crittenden, R.G and Playne, M.G (1996) Production, properties and applications of food-grade oligosaccharides. *Trends in Food Science and Technology*, 7, 353-360.

Cruz, R., Cruz, V.D., Belote, J.G., Khenayfes, M.D., Dorta, C., Oliveira, L.H.D., Ardiles, E. and Galli, A. (1999) Production of transgalactosylated oligosacchrides (TOS) by galactosyltransferase activity from *Penicillium simplicissimum*. *Bioresource Technology*, 70, 165-171.

Dabrowski, J. (1994) Two-dimensional and related NMR methods in the structural analysis of oligosaccharides and polysaccharides. *In Two-Dimensional NMR Spectroscopy. Applications for Chemists and Biochemists 2nd edition.* Edited by W.R Croasmun and R.M.K. Carlson, VCH Publisher Inc. New York.

De Leenheer, L. (1966) Production and use of inulin: industrial reality with a promising future. *In Carbohydrates as Organic Raw Materials Vol III.* pp 67-92. Edited by H. Van Beckkun, H. Roper and F. Voragen. Academic Press, New York.

Duncan, S.H., Flint, H.J. and Stewart, C.S. (1998) Inhibitory activity of gut bacteria against *Escherichia coli* 0157 mediated by dietary plant metabolites. *FEMS Microbiology Letters*, 164, 283-288.

Farnworth, E.R., Modler, H.W., Jones, J.D., Cave, N., Yamazaki, H. and Rao, A.V. (1992) Feeding Jerusalem artichoke flour rich in fructo-oligosaccharides to weaning pigs. *Canadian Journal of Animal Science*, 72, 977-980.

Fujii, S. and Komoto, M. (1991) Novel carbohydrate sweeteners in Japan. *Zuckerindustrie*, **116**, 197-200.

Gibson, G.R. and Roberfroid, M.B. (1995) Dietary modulation of the human colonic microbiota: introducing the concept of prebiotics. *Journal of Nutrition*, **125**, 1401-1412.

Gibson, G.R., Rastall, R.A. and Roberfroid, M.B. (1999) Prebiotics. *In Colonic Microbiota, Nutrition and Health*. Edited by Gibson, G.R. and M.B. Roberfroid, Kluwer Academic, Dordrecht, The Netherlands.

Hidaka, H. and Hirayama, M. (1991) Useful characteristics and commercial applications of fructooligosaccharides. *Transactions of the Biochemical Society*, **19**, 561-565.

Houdijk, J.G.M., Bosch, M.W., Verstegen, M.W.A. and Berenpas, H.J. (1998) Effects of dietary oligosaccharides on the growth performance and faecal characteristics of young growing pigs. *Animal Feed Science and Technology*, **71**, 35-48.

Iji, P.A. and Tivey, D.R. (1998) Natural and synthetic oligosaccharides in broiler chicken diets. *Worlds Poultry Science Journal*, **54**, 129-143.

Inborr, J. and Ogle, B. (1988) Effect of enzyme treatment of piglet feeds on performance and post-weaning diarrhoea. *Swedish Journal of Agricultural Research*, **18**, 129-133.

Kontula, P., Suihko, M-L., Suortti, T., Tenkanen, M., Mattila-Sandholm, T. and Von Wright, A. (2000) The isolation of lactic acid bacteria from human colonic biopsies after enrichment with lactose derivatives and rye arabinoxylo-oligosaccharides. *Food Microbiology*, **17**, 13-22.

Leteleier, A., Messier, S., Lessard, L. and Quessy, S. (2000) Assessment of various treatments to reduce carriage of salmonella in swine. *Canadian Journal of Veterinary Research*, **64**, 27-31.

Mathew, A.G., Robbins, C.M., Chattin, S.E. and Quigley, J.D. (1997) Influence of galactosyl lactose on energy and protein digestibility, enteric microflora and performance of weaning pigs. *Journal of Animal Science*, **75**, 1009-1016.

Maxwell, F.J. (1994) Characterisation of bifidobacteria from the pig gut and selection of strains for probiosis. PhD thesis. University of Aberdeen

Monsan, P.F. and Paul, F. (1995) Oligosaccharide feed additives. *In Biotechnology in Animal Feeds and Animal Feeding*, pp 233-245. Edited by R.J. Wallace and A. Chesson. VCH Publishers, Weinheim, Germany.

Moore, W.E.C and Holdeman, L.V. (1974) Human fecal flora: the normal flora of 20 Japanese Hawaiians. *Applied and Environmental Microbiology*, **27**, 961-979.

Moore, W.E.C. and Moore, L.V.H. (1995) Intestinal floras of populations that have a high risk of colon cancer. *Applied and Environmental Microbiology*, **61**, 3202-3207.

Moore, W.E.C., Moore, L.V.H., Cato, E.P., Wilkins, T.D. and Kornegay, E.T. (1987) Effect of high fiber and high-oil diets on the fecal flora of swine. *Applied and Environmental Microbiology*, **53**, 1638-1644.

Nakakuki, T., Kalnuma, S., Unno, T. and Okada, G. (1990) European Patent 0 415 720 A2.

Nemcova, R., Bomba, A., Gancarcikova, S., Herich, R. and Guba, P. (1999) Study of the effect of *Lactobacillus paracasei* and fructooligosaccharides on the faecal microflora in weaning piglets. *Berliner und Muchener Tierarzliche Wochenschrift*, **112**, 225-228.

Newman, K. (1994) Mannan-oligosaccharides: natural polymers with significant impact on the gastrointestinal microflora and the immune system. *In Biotechnology in the Feed Industry*, pp167-174. Edited by T.P. Lyons and K.A. Jacques. Nottingham University Press, Nottingham.

Olano-Martin, E., Mountzouris, K.C., Gibson, G.R. and Rastall, R.A. (2000) *In vitro* fermentability of dextran, oligodextran and maltodextrin by human gut bacteria. *British Journal of Nutrition*, **83**, 247-255

Orban, J.I., Patterson, J.A., Adeola, O., Sutton, A.L. and Richards, G.N. (1997) Growth performance and intestinal microbial populations of growing pigs fed diets containing sucrose thermal oligosaccharide caramel. *Journal of Animal Science*, **75**, 170-175.

Pluske, J.R., Siba, P.M., Pethick, D.W., Durmic, Z., Mullan, B.P. and Hampson, D.J. (1996) The incidence of swine dysentery in pigs can be reduced by feeding diets that limit fermentation in the large intestine. *Journal of Nutrition*, **126**, 2920-2933.

Pryde, S.E., Richardson, A.J., Stewart, C.S. and Flint, H.J. (1999) Molecular analysis of the microbial diversity present in the colonic wall, colonic lumen and caecal lumen of a pig. *Applied and Environmental Microbiology*, **65**, 5372-5377

Roberfroid, M.B., Van Loo, J.A.E. and Gibson, G.R. (1998) The bifidogenic nature of Chicory inulin and its hydrolysis products. *Journal of Nutrition*, **128**, 11-19

Robinson, I.M., Allison, M.J. and Bucklin, J.A. (1981) Characterisation of the cecal bacteria of normal pigs. *Applied and Environmental Microbiology*, **41**, 950-955.

Roy, D. and Ward, P. (1990) Evaluation of rapid methods for differentiation of *Bifidobacterium* species. *Journal of Applied Bacteriology*, **69**, 739-749.

Russell, T.J., Kerley, M.S. and Allee, G.L. (1996) Effect of fructooligosaccharides on growth performance of the weaned pig. *Journal of Animal Science*, **74** (Suppl. 1), 61.

Sutton, A.L., Kephart, K.B., Verstegen, M.W.A., Canh, T.T. and Hobbs, P.J. (1999) Potential for reduction of odorous compounds in swine manure through diet modification. *Journal of Animal Science*, **77**, 430-439.

Van den Broek, L.A.M., Ton, J., Verdoes, J.C., Van Laere, K.M.J., Voragen, A.G.J. and Beldman, G. (1999) Synthesis of a-galacto-oligosacchides by a cloned α-galactosidase from *Bifidobacterium adolescentis*. *Biotechnology Letters*, **21**, 441-445.

Wilson, K.H. and Blitchington, R.B. (1996) Human colonic biota studied by ribosomal DNA sequence analysis. *Applied and Environmental Microbiology*, **62**, 2273-2278.

Yoneyama, M., Shibuya, T. and Miyake, T. (1992) Saccharides sous forme de poudre, préparation et utilisation. French Patent 2,667, 359.

Yun, J.W. (1966) Fructooligosaccharide - occurrence, preparation, and application. *Enzyme and Microbial Technology*, **19**, 107-117.

# 12

# POSSIBLE WAYS OF MODIFYING TYPE AND AMOUNT OF PRODUCTS FROM MICROBIAL FERMENTATION IN THE GUT

Bent Borg Jensen
*Department of Animal Nutrition and Physiology, Danish Institute of Agricultural Sciences, Research Centre Foulum, DK-8830, Tjele, Denmark.*

## Summary

The diverse collection of microorganisms colonising the healthy gastrointestinal tract of pigs plays an essential role not only for the well being of the animal, but also for animal nutrition and performance and for the quality of animal products. A number of naturally occurring and artificial factors have been shown to affect the composition and activity of the microbiota in the gastrointestinal tract of pigs. These include: diet composition, feed processing, growth promoting antibiotics, copper, organic acids and fermented feed. A substantial microbial activity takes place in the stomach and the last third of the small intestine. It is generally accepted that the microbiota in the small intestine competes with the host animal for easily digestible nutrients and at the same time produces toxic compounds. Experiments have shown that as much as 6% of the net energy in the pig diet could be lost due to microbial fermentation in the small intestine. On the other hand, it has been shown that on a normal Danish pig diet, 16.4% of the total energy supply for the pig is achieved from microbial fermentation in the large intestine.

The most dominating cultivable bacteria species in the stomach and small intestine are *Enterobacteria*, *Streptococci*, *Clostridia* and *Lactobacilli*. The diversity of bacteria in the hindgut is much higher than in the small intestine. The predominant bacterial groups are *Prevotella*, *Streptococci*, *Lactobacillus*, *Sellenomona*, *Mitsuokella*, *Megasphera*, *Acidaminococci*, *Clostridia*, *Fusobacteria* and *Eubacteria*. Use of classical anaerobic cultivating techniques as well as new molecular methodologies has revealed that our understanding of this complex microbial ecosystem is still far from complete. However, it is well known that the microbiota takes part in several activities of importance for the host animal including: carbohydrate and protein fermentation, production of vitamins, degradation of bile acids, production of polyamines, metabolism of phytoestrogens, sulphate and nitrate reduction, methanogenesis and phytate degradation.

Two approaches are useful to quantify microbial fermentation in the gastrointestinal tract: use of *in vitro* fermentation studies and use of pigs fitted with cannulas in the portal vein to measure net portal absorption. An integrated *in vivo in vitro* technique based on cannulated pigs and a standardised *in vitro* fermentation system is especially a valuable technique to predict colonic fermentation *in vivo*.

The single most important control for microbial fermentation in the gastrointestinal tract is the amount and type of substrate available to the microbiota. This enables a direct control over the processes of fermentation in the gastrointestinal tract through feed composition. In particular, non-starch polysaccharides are important energy substrate for microbial fermentation, and the amounts as well as the chemical and structural composition of the carbohydrate are important factors for the microbial activity in the digestive tract. Also the processing of the feed has shown to affect the microbial activity in the gastrointestinal tract.

## Composition of the microflora in various regions of the gastrointestinal tract

The distribution of the microbiota within the gastrointestinal tract differs between animal species. Investigations of the intestinal bacteria have concentrated on studies of the human intestine and the rumen. However, although slowly, our knowledge of the components of the gut microbiota of pig is continuously increasing.

The population level of the microbiota in various regions of the gastrointestinal tract of monogastric animal, depends on the doubling time of the microorganism under the physico-chemical conditions in the part of the gastrointestinal tract under investigation, and the emptying rhythm of the particular part (reservoir). The stomach is the first reservoir where the digesta spend some time, and where the microflora may multiply. In contrast to humans, pigs and fowl harbour a permanent microflora in the proximal regions of the digestive tract, consisting of *Lactobacilli* and *Streptococci*. These permanent populations can be achieved in the proximal part of the digestive tract of pigs and fowl because the bacteria associate with the stratified squamous epithelial surface lining that part of the digestive tract of these animal species (Tannock, 1990). The crop of fowl and the *pars oseophageus* of pigs have this type of epithelium.

In contrast to the stomach, the upper part of the small intestine is no place for bacterial proliferation in healthy animals, simply because the intestinal transit is too rapid to allow time for microbial division. Proliferation occurs in the upper part of the small intestine only when there is adhesion to the gut wall, or mechanical obstruction lead to stasis of digesta, with pathological consequences.

Alimentary stasis is the rule in the lower part of the small intestine (ileum) and in the large intestine (caecum, colon and rectum) and all gut bacteria have sufficient time to multiply there, resulting in a large microbial population. This rich and diverse population of anaerobic bacteria carries out the hydrolytic digestive function in the large intestine of pigs. The density of the microbial population in the caecum and colon amounts to $10^{10}$ - $10^{11}$ viable bacteria per gram digesta, comprising more than 500 different species, of which only a few have been described in full. As pointed out by Moore, Moore, Cato, Wilkins and Kornega (1987) it looks like each animal species carries a microbiota distinct from that found in other animals species, with little overlap in flora composition. A recent experiment carried out in the author's laboratory has shown that eight out of eighteen of the most frequently isolated bacteria from the pig gut could not be assigned to known species. Characterisation of the intestinal microbiota of pigs has been done by anaerobe culturing techniques, and several studies have shown that the predominant bacterial groups in the intestine are *Streptococci, Lactobacilli, Prevotella, Selenomona, Mitsuokella, Megasphera, Clostridia, Eubacteria, Fusobacteria, Acidodaminococci*, and the *Enterobacteria* (Jensen,B.B. unpublished, this paper Table 1; Salanitro, Blake and Muirhead, 1977; Allison, Robinson, Bucklin and Booth, 1979; Robinson, Allison and Bucklin, 1981; Moore *et al.* 1987). However, these studies have shown that the media used for culturing of the microorganism, although intended to be non-selective, are indeed somehow selective for certain bacterial groups, and thus the outcome of the analysis is biased by the choice of media. Further, it has been postulated that only a fraction of the total number of bacteria present in the sample can be cultured. However, recovery-rates of bacteria by the culturing method compared to direct microscopic counts in the range of 30% (Salanitro *et al*, 1997) to 56% (Russel, 1979) have been reported. Since direct microscopic counts are known to overestimate the number of viable bacteria, a recovery-rate of 80 to 90% is probably more realistic. Although this is a high recovery compared to e.g. soil systems, and although most larger bacterial populations are probably represented, small populations performing key ecological functions may escape detection. Use of molecular methods, in particular the 16S rRNA-based analysis of microbial communities has provided unknown insight into the diversity and the population dynamics of bacterial communities in several microbial ecosystems (soils, seawater, rumen etc.). Newer data using this techniques on pig samples has indicated that the diversity of the microbiota in the pig gut also is high (Pryde, Richardson, Stewart and Flint, 1999). These results strongly support the finding of Moore *et al.* (1987) and the results presented in Table 1 in this paper that many of the bacterial species occupying the pig gut belong to unknown species.

## Microbial fermentation

It is generally accepted that the microbiota in the small intestine competes with

Table 1. Predominant cultivable bacteria from the pig gut (total isolates 1679)

| No Isolate | Total | SI | CAE | COL | Known bacteria species |
|---|---|---|---|---|---|
| | *Proportion of isolates % Similarity* | | | | |
| 1  Escherichia coli | 22.0 | 49.0 | 9.6 | 5.5 | *E. coli (99.8%)* |
| 2  Streptococcus alactolyticus | 13.5 | 18.2 | 10.7 | 8.4 | *Strep alactolyticus (99.8%)* |
| 3  Prevotella sp.1 | 10.0 | 0.0 | 17.0 | 1.0 | **UB adh 94 (98.1%)** |
| 4  Streptococcus hyointestinalis | 9.5 | 11.8 | 8.1 | 6.3 | *Strep hyointestinalis (100%)* |
| 5  Prevotella sp 1a | 2.9 | 0.0 | 6.3 | 4.8 | **Prevotella oulora (92.4%)** |
| 6  Lactobacillus acidophilus/ jonsonii | 2.2 | 0.0 | 3.2 | 3.6 | *Lact jonsonii (99.7%)* |
| 7  Lactobacillus sp 2 | 2.0 | 0.3 | 1.5 | 2.2 | **L.vitulinus (93.9%)** |
| 8  Selenomonas sp 1. | 1.9 | 0.0 | 2.3 | 3.6 | **Selenomonas ruminantum (94.7%)** |
| 9  Mitsuokella sp | 1.7 | 0.7 | 1.9 | 2.7 | *Mitsuokella multiacidicus (97.8%)* |
| 10  Megasphera sp. | 1.7 | 0.0 | 1.3 | 3.9 | **Megasphera elsdenii (93.7%)** |
| 11  Acidaminococcus fermentans | 1.5 | 0.3 | 4.2 | 1.5 | *Acidaminococcus fermentans (99.4%)* |
| 12  Clostridium perfrigens | 1.5 | 2.7 | 1.5 | 0.4 | *Clostridium perfrigens 99.7%* |
| 13  Eubacterium sp. a | 1.1 | 0.0 | 1.3 | 1.4 | **Butyrate prod bacteria (96.6 %)** |
| 14  Prevotella sp 13 | 1.1 | 0.0 | 0.0 | 1.3 | **Not known (<97%)** |
| 15  Bacteroides sp 1 | 1.0 | 0.2 | 2.7 | 0.0 | *Bacteroides vulgatus (99.5%)* |
| 16  Megasphera elsdenii | 1.0 | 0.0 | 2.5 | 0.4 | Did not survive freezing |
| 17  Fusobacterium mortiferum | 1.0 | 2.9 | 0.0 | 0.0 | *Fusobacterium mortiferum (99.9%)* |
| 18  Eubacterium sp. b | 0.4 | 0.0 | 1.0 | 0.9 | **UB adh 420 (95.6%)** |

SI: Small intestine (579 isolates), CAE: Caecum (529 isolates), COL; Colon (571 isolates).
The isolates in bold could not be assigned to any known species.
UB: uncultured bacteria

the host animal for easily digestible nutrients and at the same time produces toxic compounds. Experiments have shown that as much as 6% of the net energy in the pig diet could be lost due to microbial fermentation in the small intestine (Vervaeke, Decuypere, Dierick and Hendrickx, 1979). On the other hand the microbiota in the hindgut is believed to have a beneficial effect on the host animal since it produces energy from feed material that has not been digested in the small intestine.

The principal substrates available for microbial fermentation in the large intestine include a wider variety of dietary residues that have escaped digestion in the small intestine, the main ones being non-stach polysaccharides (NSP), various forms of starch resistant to digestion in the small intestine, sugar alcohols and proteins. Also host produced substances such as glycoproteins, exfoliated epithelial cells and pancreatic secretions are important. In particular, NSPs are important energy substrate for large intestinal microbial fermentation, and the amounts as well as the chemical and structural composition of the carbohydrate are important factors for the microbial activity in the digestive tract (Bach Knudsen, Jensen, Andersen and Hansen, 1991; Bach Knudsen, Jensen and Hansen, 1993; Jensen, 1988; Jensen and Jørgensen, 1994; Macfarlane and Cummings, 1991).

The main products of carbohydrate fermentation in the gastrointestinal tract of all monogastric animals are short chain fatty acids (SCFA, the major ones being acetic, propionic, butyric and valeric acids), lactate and various gasses (Figure 1). The energy available to the host animal after microbial fermentation is the energy found in the SCFA.

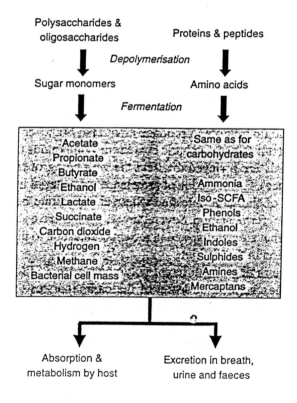

**Figure 1.** Major fermentation products formed by the microbiota in the gastrointestinal tract of pigs

According to the classical Hungate equation for carbohydrate fermentation to acetic acid, propionic acid, butyric acid, carbon dioxide and methane, 6.5% of the energy in the carbohydrates are lost as fermentation heat and 18% as fermentation gasses ($CH_4$). However, this equation is for rumen fermentation, several investigations with pigs have shown that the ratio between the fermentation products produced depends on the type of carbohydrate fermented. Further, several investigations have shown that pigs produce much less methane compared to ruminants (Jensen, 1996, Zhu, Fowler and Fuller, 1993). Apart from the energy lost as fermentation heat and fermentation gasses approximately 20% of the energy in carbohydrates is incorporated in the bacterial biomass; this energy will also be lost in monogastric animals. As a whole the energy available to the host animal is then about 60% of that of the substrate fermented. The SCFA produced are rapidly absorbed from the gut lumen. There is now considerable evidence that the individual SCFA may have specific roles in connection with health implications. Butyric acid is the preferred fuel for the colonic epithelial cells (Rodiger, 1980). It has also been shown that butyric acid protects these cells against agents that lead to cellular differentiation and may even inhibit tumour growth (Young and Gibson, 1994). Propionic acid is converted to glucose in the liver and may modify hepatic metabolism while acetic acid acts as an energy substrate for muscle tissue. Further, it is well known that SCFA stimulate gastric motility and gastric absorption.

Substantial quantities of proteinaceous material enter the large intestine of monogastric animals, in the form of a complex mixture of proteins and peptides of both endogenous and dietary origin. In the large intestine these substances are metabolised by the microbiota to produce ammonia, branched-chain fatty acids, indoles, phenols, amines and sulphuric containing compounds (Figure 1). Several of these compounds are believed to affect the well-being of the animal (reduce growth performance). Fermentation of proteinaceous material is most pronounced in the distal part of the large intestine where carbohydrate becomes a limiting factor for microbial fermentation. Several investigations have shown that addition of carbohydrates that are not digested in the small intestine to pig diets can reduce protein fermentation in the hindgut.

Intestinal bacteria degrade different polysaccharides at different rates. Many factors such as the chemical structure of the carbohydrates their occurrence in complexes with other material will influence their breakdown. Also their solubility in water is important, soluble carbohydrates are fermented more rapidly than non-soluble. Further, particle size of the feedstuffs affects breakdown, with fine particles being more readily digested than coarse ones.

## Possibility of manipulating the microbial activity in the gastrointestinal tract

### DIET COMPOSITION

Probably the single most important control for microbial fermentation in the gastrointestinal tract of monogastric animals is the amount and type of substrate available to the microbiota. This enables a direct control over the processes of fermentation in the gastrointestinal tract through feed composition. As already mentioned, especially the fibre content of the diet affects microbial fermentation in the hindgut. The results shown in Figure 2 clearly show that the microbial activity (measured as the ATP-concentration) in various regions of the gastrointestinal tract is affected by the amount and type of fibre in the diet. In all pigs a substantial microbial activity was found in the last third of the small intestine. Highest microbial activity was found in the caecum and the proximal part of the colon. In general, the microbial activity was low in the hindgut of the pigs fed the low fibre diet. Addition of oat bran to the low fibre diet increases the microbial activity in the last third of the small intestine and in the caecum, while addition of wheat bran to the low fibre diet increases the microbial activity in the more distal parts of the hindgut. These results are consistent with the fact that oat bran consists of dietary fibre that is easily fermentable for the microbiota while wheat bran consists of more slowly fermentable fibres.

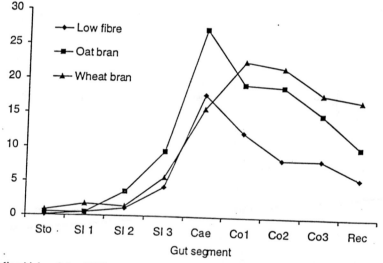

**Figure 2.** Microbial activity (ATP-concentration) in various regions of the gastrointestinal tract of pigs fed either a low fibre diet based essentially on wheat flour as carbohydrate source (56g NSP/kg feed) and two fibre enriched diets with added oat bran (93g NSP/kg feed) or wheat bran (102g NSP/kg feed): Sto, stomach; SI1, SI2; SI3, proximal, mid-, and distal third of the small intestine, Cae, caecum; CO1, CO2, CO3, proximal, mid-, and distal third of the colon; Rec, rectum.

Several investigations have shown that also the fermentation of protein in the hindgut of pigs is dependent on diet composition. Production of skatole, a volatile compound produced in the hindgut by microbial degradation of the amino acid tryptophan, which originates from feed protein, endogenous secretions or intestinal cell debris, is a good estimate of protein fermentation in the hindgut of pigs. Two alternative approaches can lead to a reduction of protein fermentation in the hindgut and thus skatole production (Jensen and Jensen, 1997). Firstly, decreasing the amount of protein reaching the hindgut will limit protein fermentation and thereby skatole production. This can be achieved by using a protein source that is easily digested in the small intestine such as casein. Secondly, if large amounts of protein reach the hindgut, the production of skatole from protein fermentation can be reduced by adding an energy source such as easily fermentable dietary fibre to the diet. This data illustrates that the factor influencing the amount of skatole produced is the availability of tryptophan. Tryptophan availability depends on both the amount of tryptophan in the intestinal contents entering the hindgut and on the proteolytic activity of the intestinal microbiota. The activity of the proteolytic bacteria can be reduced due to competition with carbohydrate fermenting bacteria for common resources. Once tryptophan is produced, it might be incorporated into bacterial protein, a process favoured by high activity of carbohydrate fermenting bacteria.

# Quantification of microbial fermentation in the gastrointestinal tract

## IN VITRO MODELS

The concentration of a given microbial metabolite in various regions of the digestive tract is not necessarily a reflection of the production of the metabolite in the respective segment, since the concentration is influenced by both production, absorption and a possible degradation. That means that measurements of metabolites in gut content provide only limited information on events occurring within the gastrointestinal tract. However, a variety of models are available that allow gastrointestinal content to be investigated under anaerobic conditions *in vitro* (Figure 3). They range from small bottles of either screw-capped or serum variety, to more complex batch and continuous culture fermentation systems (Macfarlane, Gibson and Macfarlane, 1994). Simple *in vitro* fermentation systems have been used to quantify the production of skatole in the gastrointestinal tract of pigs (Jensen and Jensen, 1993), the production af various gasses in the gastrointestinal tract (Jensen and Jørgensen, 1994) and the production of SCFA and lactate in the gastrointestinal tract (Jensen, 1998, Lærke and Jensen, 1999). An important disadvantage of simple *in vitro* fermentation study is that the pH is uncontrolled. If culture pH is not regulated, the environment in the vessel will change in a short time such that the fermentation conditions become non-representative of those occurring in the gut.Both carbohydrate fermentation (Grossklaus, Klingebel, Lorenz and Pahlke, 1984) and protein degradation (Jensen and Jensen, 1993) are known to be pH dependent. Stirred pH controlled fermentation systems can be either of the batch, semi-continuous, or continuous culture type (Macfarlane *et al.*, 1994). In general, the vessel is stirred magnetically and the pH controlled by a pH electrode and a pH controller (Macfarlane *et al.*, 1994). Jensen and Jensen (1993) has used this set up to show that the conversion of L-tryptophan to either skatole or indole in the hindgut of pigs is highly pH dependent, with an increasing amount of L-tryptophan converted to skatole with decreasing pH.

*In vitro models:*

Serum or screw -capped bottles

Stirred batch culture fermenters*

Single -stage continuous culture fermenters*

Multiple -stage continuous culture fermenter systems*

*with or without automatic pH control

*In vivo- in-vitro models:*

Integrated *in vivo - in vitro* techniques based on ileal cannulated pigs and a standardised in vitro fermentation system

*Portal absorption:*

Pigs fitted with catheters in vena porta and arteria mesenterica and fitted with an ultrasonic blood flow probe for measurement of the portal blood flow.

**Figure 3.** Useful models to quantify products from microbial fermentation in the gastrointestinal tract.

## IN VIVO-IN VITRO MODELS

A valuable technique to quantify the effect of various feed constituents on microbial fermentation in the large intestine of pigs is an integrated *in vivo – in vitro* method (McBurney and Sauer, 1993, Christensen, Knudsen, Wolstrup and Jensen, 1999). The method is especially valuable to predict the effect of dietary NSP on the amount of energy available from microbial fermentation in the hindgut. The results obtained by the method are summarised in Table 2 and Figure 4.

The results clearly show that the amount of energy obtained from microbial fermentation in the hindgut of pigs is dependent on both the type and the amount

**Table 2.** Effect of diet on SCFA produced in the hindgut measured using an integrated *in vivo - in vitro* method

| | Test meal (g) | DF content (g/kg) | Weight of pigs (kg) | SCFA produced (mmol/ kg feed) | Molar proportion | | | | Energy available from fermentation in the hindgut (%) |
|---|---|---|---|---|---|---|---|---|---|
| | | | | | Ace | Prop | But | Val | |
| **McBurney and Sauer, 1993** Control | 800 | 115 | - | 934 | 63.6 | 18.8 | 12.4 | 2.9 | 15.5 |
| Control + 5% pea fibre | 840 | 150 | - | 1265 | 64.5 | 19.1 | 12.1 | 2.9 | 21.0 |
| Control + 10% pea fibre | 880 | 186 | - | 1247 | 64.4 | 19.2 | 12.2 | 2.8 | 21.7 |
| Control + 15% pea fibre | 920 | 221 | - | 1668 | 65.6 | 18.5 | 11.3 | 2.3 | 29.5 |
| **Jensen et al., 1997** Wheat flour -soy bean | 1300 | 91 | 90.0 | 750 | 48.9 | 27.7 | 16.3 | 5.9 | 6.1 |
| Wheat flour soy bean + 10% Sugar beat pulp | 1300 | 135 | 90.0 | 1280 | 41.4 | 33.0 | 16.5 | 8.0 | 9.9 |
| Barley -wheat soy bean | 1300 | 210 | 90.0 | 1640 | 57.4 | 25.2 | 12.6 | 3.9 | 16.4 |
| **Christensen et al., 1999** Wheat flour | 510 | 63 | 59.5 | 369 | 53.6 | 27.0 | 9.6 | 5.7 | 2.4 |
| Wheat flour + oat bran | 535 | 103 | 61.5 | 850 | 48.7 | 26.0 | 14.7 | 5.6 | 6.4 |
| Wheat flour + wheat bran | 665 | 110 | 76.3 | 560 | 56.9 | 23.9 | 11.5 | 5.4 | 4.2 |
| **Monsma et al., 2000** Corn starch + oat bran | 420 | 52 | 47.6 | 509 | 69.1 | 19.1 | 11.7 | - | - |
| Corn starch + wheat bran | 420 | 62 | 52.4 | 353 | 78.1 | 7.8 | 14.1 | - | - |
| **Jiufeng and Jensen, 2000*** Boiled rice | 1000 | 43 | 60.0 | 476 | 52.0 | 23.1 | 13.4 | 6.0 | 3.7 |
| Boiled rice + 10 % potato starch Boiled rice | 1000 | 56 | 60.0 | 792 | 53.6 | 22.5 | 15.5 | 5.9 | 5.8 |
| + 12% sugar beat pulp | 1000 | 143 | 60.0 | 1202 | 59.7 | 23.7 | 12.0 | 2.6 | 8.8 |
| Boiled rice + 20% wheat bran | 1000 | 136 | 60.0 | 618 | 55.4 | 27.8 | 10.0 | 3.6 | 5.2 |

-: not given/analysed; * unpublished results

of NSP in the diet, and that the amount of energy obtained from microbial fermentation represent from 2.4 to 29.5% of the total digestible energy. Most of the diets investigated however are rather extreme pig diets. As shown by Jensen, Mikkelsen and Christensen (1998) 16.4% of the total energy supply for a pig is achieved from microbial fermentation in the hindgut for pigs fed a standard Danish pig diet based on barley and soy bean.

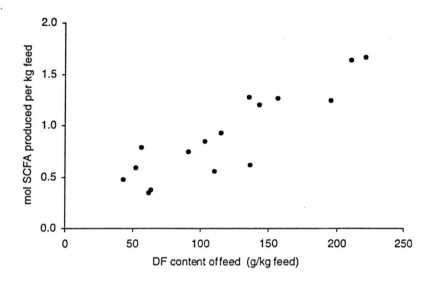

**Figure 4.** Relationship between feed dietary fibre content (g/kg feed) and the amount of SCFA produced (mmol/kg feed) in the hindgut of slaughter pigs.

## PORTAL ABSORPTION

The measurements of the portal flux of nutrients provide a rather direct estimate of the amount of nutrients available for maintenance and production after absorption from the gastrointestinal tract (Rerat, Fiszlewicz, Giusi and Vaugelade, 1987). Moreover, it can provide information of the digestive and absorptive kinetics of nutrients, and allows estimating quantitative absorption of end products from microbial fermentation in the gastrointestinal tract. The results published using this technique to quantify the absorption of SCFA produced in the gut by microbial fermentation are summarised in Table 3. As for the production results, a clear-cut effect of type and amount of dietary NSP on the amount of SCFA absorbed is evident. The values range from 210 to 1787 mmol SCFA absorbed per kg feed. Again most of the diets investigated were rather extreme pig diets. The value given by Yen, Nienaber, Hill and Pound (1991) of 1590 mmol SCFA per kg feed is probably the value most realistic to practical pig feeding. This value agrees well

**Table 3.** Effect of diet on SCFA absorption to the portal vein

| Reference | Diet | Meal size (g) | Fasting (h) | Weight of pigs (kg) | SCFA absorbed (mmol/kg feed) | Molar proportion Ace | Prop | But | Val |
|---|---|---|---|---|---|---|---|---|---|
| Yen *et al.*, 1991 | Corn-soybean | 1200 | 24 | 40 | 1590 | 42.5 | 38.0 | 14.1 | 4.0 |
| Rerat, 1987 | Barley-corn-soybean | 800 | 12 | 62 | 1450 | 52.8 | 35.4 | 8.4 | 1.8 |
|  | Barley-corn-soybean | 800 | 24 | 62 | 925 | 51.2 | 36.6 | 8.6 | 1.3 |
| Jensen and Laue, 1997 | Barley + 20%sucrose | 1100 | 12 | 70 | 1010 | 49.0 | 28.8 | 11.4 | 5.6 |
|  | Barley + 20% tagatose | 1100 | 12 | 70 | 1290 | 40.6 | 26.9 | 14.0 | 9.3 |
| Rerat, 1993 | Corn starch + 53 % malitol | 757 | 18 | 60 | 1010 | 36.9 | 49.7 | 7.8 | 3.4 |
|  | Corn starch + 53 % maltose | 757 | 18 | 60 | 375 | 73.0 | 18.6 | 5.5 | 1.1 |
| Van der Meulen *et al.*, 1997a | Corn starch | 600 | 12 | 70 | 400 | 57.3 | 29.7 | 6.5 | - |
|  | Corn starch + 35% potato starch | 600 | 12 | 70 | 1205 | 52.5 | 14.6 | 26.2 | - |
|  | 65% potato starch | 600 | 12 | 70 | 1778 | 54.5 | 12.5 | 26.7 | - |
| Bach Knudsen *et al.*, 1997 | Low fibre | 1300 | 12 | 40 | 550 | - | - | - | - |
|  | Low fibre + wheat bran | 1300 | 12 | 40 | 570 | - | - | - | - |
|  | Low fibre + oat bran | 1300 | 12 | 40 | 690 | - | - | - | - |
| Van den mulen *et al.*, 1997b | Corn starch | 800 | 12 | 42 | 210 | 69.2 | 19.7 | 5.7 | - |
|  | Pea starch | 800 | 12 | 42 | 270 | 69.3 | 20.8 | 5.4 | - |
| Giusi-Perier *et al.*, 1989 | Corn starch + 6% cellulose | 800 | 19 | 58 | 1480 | 75.9 | 18.0 | 3.8 | 0.8 |
|  | Corn starch + 16% cellulose | 800 | 19 | 58 | 1787 | 69.1 | 22.7 | 5.9 | 1.0 |
|  | Corn starch + 22 alfalfa meal | 800 | 19 | 57 | 1100 | 74.9 | 21.4 | 1.7 | 0.6 |
|  | Corn starch + 22% lactose | 800 | 19 | 57 | 1475 | 72.7 | 21.6 | 3.3 | 1.2 |
| Jansman *et al.*, 2000 | Corn + corn starch | 688 | 12 | 50 | 761 | 63.0 | 29.0 | 8.0 | - |
|  | Corn + 15% sugar beat pulp + 15% wheat bran | 784 | 12 | 50 | 1365 | 62.0 | 31.0 | 7.0 | - |

with the value of 1640 mmol per kg diet found by Jensen *et al.*, (1998) for microbial production of SCFA in the gut on a standard Danish pig diet.

## CORRELATION BETWEEN SCFA PRODUCED AND SCFA ABSORBED

Compared to the production data given in Table 2 the absorption data indicates that the molar proportion of butyric acid of the total SCFA is low compared to the molar proportion of butyric acid produced. An explanation of that may be that part of the butyric acid is metabolised by the gastrointestinal epithelium. Unfortunately, an experiment where the production and absorption have been measured in the same experiment has never been published. However, the data in Table 4 represents unpublished results obtained in the author's lab where the production and absorption were measured in the same experiment.

**Table 4.** Amount of SCFA produced in and absorbed from the gastrointestinal tract of pigs fed a diet supplemented with 20% D-tagatose

| Acid | Produced (mmol/kg feed) | Absorbed (mmol/kg feed) |
|---|---|---|
| Formic acid | 14 | - |
| Acetic acid | 441 | 524±27 |
| Propionic acid | 339 | 348±17 |
| Iso-butyric acid | 18 | 13±8 |
| Butyric acid | 416 | 267±77 |
| Iso-valeric acid | 27 | 20±15 |
| Valeric acid | 119 | 100±40 |
| Capronic acid | 27 | - |
| Total | 1402 | 1272±160 |

-: not analysed

The pigs used in this study were twelve 4 to 6 month-old Yorkshire-Danish Landrase castrated male pigs. Four of the pigs with a mean body weight of 62.2±4.1 kg were surgically prepared with catheters in the portal vein, in a mesenteric vein and a mesenteric artery for measurements of the net portal absorption of SCFA. The net portal absorption was calculated as described by Rérat *et al.* (1987). *Para*-aminohippuric acid (PAH) was infused continuously into the mesenteric vein to determine portal vein blood flow. The experimental diet was based on barley and fishmeal supplemented with 20% D-tagatose. D-tagatose is a stereoisomer of fructose and it is poorly absorbed in the small intestine. Thus large amounts reach the hindgut supplying substrate for microbial fermentation resulting in the production of SCFA (Lærke and Jensen, 1999). The pigs were fed twice daily at 07.00 and 16.00. On the experimental day the pigs were fed at 20.00 the day before the start of the experiment and at 08.00 and 20.00 the day of blood collection. The feed intake was restricted to approximately 3% of BW per day. The water was throughly mixed with the feed at a ratio of 1: 2.5 (feed : water). After 7 days' adaptation to the experimental diet, blood samples were sampled at hourly intervals from one hour before to twelve hours after the morning feeding. Blood was collected simultaneously from *A. mesenterica, V. mesenterica* and *V. porta.*

At the end of the experiment the animals were sacrificed by a lethal injection of Sodium Pentobarbital. Immediately after slaughter, the gastrointestinal tract was taken out of the animal and divided into 8 segments by ligatures. The segments consisted of the stomach, three equal parts of the small intestine, the caecum and three equal parts of the large intestine. The luminal content of each segment was carefully collected and weighed and samples were taken for *in vitro* incubations as described by Jensen and Jensen (1993). To get a precise estimate of the amount of SCFA produced the pigs were slaughtered at different times after the morning feeding (three pigs each at 0, 3, 6 and 9 hours after the morning feeding). SCFA in blood samples were measured as described by Kristensen, Danfær, Tetens and Agergaard (1996). SCFA in gut content were measured as described by Jensen, Cox and Jensen (1995).

The production of SCFA and lactic acid in the stomach, small intestine and the large intestine is shown in Figure 5. It is evident that a pronounced microbial fermentation occurs in all three compartment of the gastrointestinal tract. In general, the production of organic acids was about twice as high in the large intestine (1400 mmol/kg feed) as in the stomach (750 mmol per kg feed) and about 4 times as high in the large intestine as that in the small intestine (350 mmol per kg feed). Further, the composition of the acids produced was very different. The principal organic acid produced in the stomach and small intestine was lactic acid, while the dominating acids produced in the large intestine were acetic, propionic and butyric acid.

As shown in Table 4 very good agreement was found between the amount of SCFA produced in the hindgut and the amount of that absorbed to the portal blood. Approximately equal amounts of propionic, iso-butyric, valeric and iso-valeric acids were produced and absorbed. The amount of acetic acid produced in the hindgut was almost 100 mmol smaller per kg feed than the amount of acetic acid absorbed to the portal blood. The reason for this difference can be explained by production of acetic acid by microbial fermentation in the stomach and small intestine. In fact, it was estimated that the amount of acetic acid produced in the stomach and small intestine was 110 mmol per kg feed. It was further estimated that 13 mmol propionic acid, 20 mmol butyric acid and 970 mmol lactic acid per kg feed were produced in the stomach and small intestine. The fact that the amount of butyric

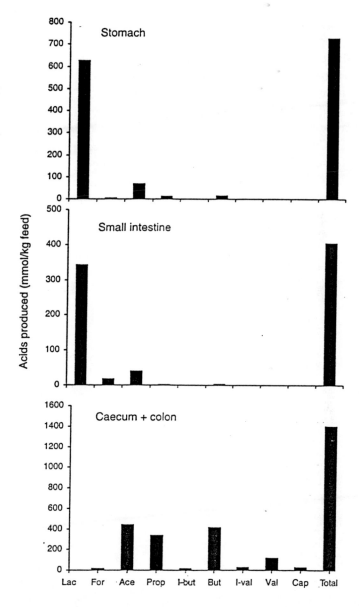

**Figure 4.** Various organic acids produced (mmol/kg feed) by microbial fermentation in stomach, small intestine and large intestine of slaughter pigs fed a diet based on barley and fishmeal supplemented with 200g/kg D-tagatose.

acid absorbed into the portal blood was significantly lower (267 mmol per kg feed) than the amount of butyric acid produced (416 mmol per kg feed) by microbial fermentation in the hindgut is probably due to metabolism of butyric acid in the intestinal epithelium, as butyric acid is known to be the preferred substrate for colonic epithelial cells (Roediger, 1980; Darcy-Vrillion, Morel, Cherbuy, Bernard, Posho, Blachier, Meslin and Duee, 1993).

That a substantial amount of lactic acid is produced by microbial fermentation in the gastrointestinal tract is supported by the results of Giusi-Perier, Fiszelewicz and Rérat (1989) and Rérat (1994). These authors found that the amount of lactic acid absorbed to the portal blood was in the same order of magnitude as the amount of SCFA absorbed. That the absorbed lactic acid especially came from microbial fermentation in the stomach and small intestine is supported by the results of Rerat (1994), which show that the absorption of lactic acid was much higher during the first hours after feeding (0-4 hours) while the SCFA absorption was highest in the period from 4 to 12 hours post feeding.

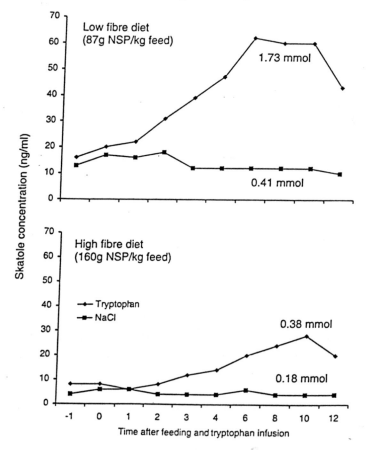

**Figure 6.** Effect of dietary fibre on portal and arterial concentrations of skatole following tryptophan (4,9 mmol) or saline infusion in the cecum. The values below the curves represent the total amount of skatole absorbed. The low fibre diet was based on barley (100g/kg feed) and wheat flour (662 g/kg feed) as carbohydrate source and soy bean meal (180g/kg feed) as protein source. The high fibre diet was similar to the low fibre diet but added 100g sugar beet pulp per kg.

## Effect of diet on skatole production and absorption

As already mentioned the production of skatole in the hindgut of pigs is dependent on the composition of the diet. This is further illustrated by a series of experiments, where the absorption of skatole to the portal blood was investigated, after tryptophan was infused into the cecum of pigs fed either a low or a high fibre diet. Figure 6 shows the absorption pattern of skatole over a period from one hour before to twelve hours after infusion of either tryptophan or saline. Both the effect of available tryptophan and the effect of fibre on skatole absorption are convincing. On the low fibre diet, the hindgut bacteria transform a substantial amount of the available tryptophan to skatole and 27% of the infused tryptophan was recovered as skatole in the portal blood. However, on the high fibre diet only 4% of the infused tryptophan was recovered as skatole in the portal blood. Also the basal skatole absorption (absorption after saline infusion) was dependent on the diet. With the high fibre diet only 0.18 mmol skatole was absorbed to the portal blood, as opposed to the situation on the low fibre diet where 0.41 mmol skatole was absorbed to the portal blood. These results strongly show the usefulness of portal absorption to study the effect of diet on the production of microbial metabolites in the gut, and confirm the important effect of diet composition on the amount of products formed by microbial fermentation in the gut. Further, the results point at the use of fibre rich diets as a relevant way to reduce boar taint (skatole) problems in practical pig production.

## References

Allison, M.J., Robinson, I.M., Bucklin, J.A. and Booth, G.D. (1979) Comparison of bacterial populations of the pig caecum and colon based upon enumeration -with specific energy sources. *Applied and Environmental Microbiology*, **37**, 1142-1151.

Bach Knudsen, K.E., Jensen, B.B, Andersen, J.O. and Hansen, I. (1991). Gastrointestinal implications in pigs of wheat and oat fractions. 2 Microbial activity in the gastrointestinal tract. *British Journal of Nutrition*, **65**, 233-248.

Bach Knudsen, K.E., Jensen, B.B. and Hansen, I. (1993). Oat bran but not a b-glucan-enriched oat fraction enhances butyrate in the large intestine of pigs. *Journal of Nutrition*, **123**, 1235-1247.

Bach Knudsen, K.E., Jørgensen, H. and Canibe, N. (1997). Quantification of the absorbtion of glucose and short chain fatty acids in experiments with catheterized pigs, p. 274-278. *In Digestive Physiology in Pigs*. Proceeding

VII[th] Symposium Digestive Physiology in Pigs, St Malo, France. Edited by J.P. Laplace, C. Février and A. Barbeau.

Christensen, D.N., Bach Knudsen, K.E., Wolstrup, J. and Jensen, B.B. (1997) Integration of ileum cannulated pigs and *in vitro* fermentation to predict the effect of diet composition on the amount of energy available from microbial fermentation in the large intestine. *Journal of the Science of Food and Agricultural*, **79**, 755-762.

Darcy-Vrillion, B., Morel, M.-T., Cherbuy, C., Bernard, F., Posho, L., Blachier, F., Meslin, J.-C. and Duée, P.-H. (1993) Metabolic characteristics of pig colonocytes after adaptation to a high fiber diet. *Journal of Nutrition*, **123**, 234-243.

Gibson G.R. and Roberfroid, M.B. (1994). Dietary modulation of the human colonic microbiota: introducing the concept of prebiotics. *Journal of Nutrition*, **125**, 1401-1412.

Grossklaus, R., Klingebel, L., Lorenz, S. and Pahlke, G. (1984) The formation of short-chain fatty acids in the caeca of non-adapted and adapted juvenile rats. *Nutrition Research*, **4**, 459-468.

Giusi-Perier, A., Fiszelewicz, M. and Rérat, A. (1989) Influence of diet composition on intestinal volatile fatty acid and nutrient absorption in unanesthetized pigs. *Journal of Animal Science*, **67**, 386-402.

Jansman, Aj.M., Bongers, L.J.G.M. and van Leeuwen, P. (2000) Effect of fermentable components in the diet on the portal flux of glucose and volatile fatty acids in growing pigs. Proceeding 8th Symposium on Digestive Physiology in Pigs. 18-22 June 2000, Uppsala, Sweden. In press.

Jensen, B.B. (1996). Methanogenesis in monogastric animals. *Environmental Monitoring and Assessment*, **42**, 99-112.

Jensen, B.B. (1998). The impact of feed additives on the microbial ecology of the gut in young pigs. *Journal of Animal Feed Science*, **7**, 45-64.

Jensen, B.B. and Jørgensen, H. (1994). Effect of dietary fibre on microbial activity and microbial gas production in various regions of the gastrointestinal tract of pigs. *Applied and Environmental Microbiology*, **60**, 1997-1904.

Jensen, B.B., Mikkelsen, L.L. and Christensen, D.N. (1998) Integration of ileum cannulated pigs and *in vitro* fermentation to quantify the effect of diet composition on microbial fermentation in the large intestine. In: NJF Rapport no, 119, p 106-110. Proceedings of NJF Seminar No 274 on energy and protein evaluation for pigs in the Nordic countries, 1998, Research Centre Foulum.

Jensen, B.B. and Jensen, M.T. (1993) In vitro measurement of microbial production of skatole in the digestive tract of pigs, p 99-105. *In Measurement and Prevention of Boar Taint in Entire Male Pigs*. Edited by M. Bonneau. INRA (Les Colloques no 60), Paris

Jensen, M.T., Cox, R.P. and Jensen, B.B. (1995). Microbial production of skatole in the hind gut of pig fed different diets and its relation to skatole deposition in back fat. *Animal Science,* **61:** 293-304.

Jensen, M.T and Jensen, B.B. (1997). Tasty meat through diet design. *Feed Mix,* **5,** 8-12.

Kristensen, N.B., Danfær, A., Tetens, V. and Agergaard, N. (1996) Portal recovery of intraruminally infused short-chain fatty acids in sheep. *Acta Agriculturica Scandinavia Section A. Animal Science,* **46,** 26-38.

Lærke, H.N. and Jensen, B.B. (1999) D-tagatose has low small intestinal digestibility but high large intestinal fermentability in pigs. *Journal of Nutrition,* **129,** 1002-1009

McBurney, M.I. and Sauer, W.C. (1993). Fiber and large bowel energy absorption: validation of the integrated ilostomy-fermentation model using pigs. *Journal of Nutrition,* **123,** 721-727.

Macfarlane, G.T.,and Cummings, J.H. (1991). The colonic flora, fermentation, and large bowel digestive function. p. 51-92. *In The large intestine: Physiology, Pathophysiology, and Disease.* Edited by S.F. Phillips, J.H. Pemberton, and R.G. Shorter. Raven Press, Ltd. New York.

Macfarlane, G.T., Gibson, G.R. and Macfarlane, S. (1994) Short chain fatty acids and lactate production by human intestinal bacteria grown in batch and continuous culture. *In Short Chain Fatty Acids –1994.* Edited by H.J. Binder, J. Cummings and K. Soergel. Kluwer Academic Publishers, London.

Monsma, D.J., Thorsen, P.T., Vollendorf, N.W., Crenshaw, T.D. and Marlett, J.A. (2000) In vitro fermentation of swine ileal digesta containing oat bran dietary fiber by rat cecal inocula adapted to the test fiber increases propionate production but fermentation of wheat bran ileal digesta dose not produce more butyrate. *Journal of Nutrition,* **130,** 585-593.

Moore, W.E.C., Moore, L.V.H., Cato, E.P., Wilkins, T.D. and Kornega, E.T. (1987). Effect of high-fiber and high-oil diets on the faecal flora of swine. *Applied and Environmental Microbiology,* **53,** 638-644.

Pryde, S.E., Richardson, A.J., Stewart, C.S. and Flint, H.J. (1999) Molecular analysis of the microbial diversity present in the colonic wall, colonic lumen, and cecal lumen of a pig. *Applied and Environmental Microbiology,* **65,** 5372-5377.

Rérat, A. (1994) Effect of the nature of ingested carbohydrates on the chronology of VFA absorption in the pig. P. 252-254. *In Digestive Physiology in Pigs.* Proceeding VI[th] Symposium Digestive Physiology in Pigs, Bad Doberan, Germany, 4-6 October, 1994. Edited by W.-B. Souffrant and H. Hagemeister.

Rerat, A., Fiszlewicz, M., Giusi, A. and Vaugelade, P. (1987) Influence of meal frequency on postprandial variations in the production and absorption of volatile fatty acids in the digestive tract of conscious pigs. *Journal of Animal Science,* **64,** 448-456.

Rérat, A., Giusi-Périer, A. and Vaissade, P. (1993) Absorption balances and kinetics of nutrients and bacterial metabolits in conscious pigs after intake of maltose- or maltitol-rich diets. *Journal of Animal Science*, 71, 2473-2488.

Robinson, I.M., Allison, M.J. and Bucklin, J.A. (1981). Characterization of the caecal bacteria from normal pigs. *Applied and Environmental Microbiology*, 41, 950-955.

Roediger, W.E.W (1980) Role of anaerobic bacteria in the metabolic welfare of the colonic mucosa in man. *Gut*, 21, 793-798.

Russell, E.G. (197) Types and distribution of anaerobic bacteria in the large intestine of pigs. *Applied and Environmental Microbiology*, 37, 187-193.

Salanitro, J.P., Blake, I.G. and Muirhead, P.A. (1977). Isolation and identification of fecal bacteria from adult swine. *Applied and Environmental microbiology*, 37, 79-84.

Tannock, G.W. (1990). The microecology of lactobacilli inhabiting the gastrointestinal tract. *Advanced Microbiological Ecology*, 11, 147-171.

van der Meulen, J., Bakker, J.G.M., Bakker, H., de Visser, H., Jongbloed, A.W. and Everts, H. (1997). Effect of resistant starch on net portal-drained viscera flux of glucose, volatile fatty acids, urea, and ammonia in growing pigs. *Journal of Animal Science*, 75, 2697-2704.

van der Meulen, J., Bakker, J.G.M., Smith, B. and de Visser, H. (1997) Effect of source of starch on net portal flux of glucose, lactate, volatile fatty acids and amino acids in the pig. *British Journal of Nutrition*, 78, 533-544.

Vervaeke, I.J., Decuypere, J.A., Dierick, N.A. and Henderickx, H.K. (1979). Quantitative *in vitro* evaluation of the energy metabolism influenced by Virginiamycin and Spiramycin used as growth promoters in pig nutrition. *Journal of Animal Science*, 49, 846-856.

Yen, J.T., Nienaber, J.A., Hill, D.A. and Pond, W.G. (1991) Potential contribution of absorbed volatile fatty acids to whole animal energy requirement in conscious swine. *Journal of Animal Science*, 69, 2001-2006.

Young, G.P. and Gibson, P.R. (1994). Butyrate and the colorectal cancer cell, pp 148-160. *In Short Chain Fatty Acids* Edited by H.J Binder, H.J., J. Cummings and K.H. Soergel. Klywer Academic Publishers, Dordrecht, Holland.

Zhu, J.Q., Fowler, V.R. and Fuller, M.F. (1993). Assessment of fermentation in growing pigs given unmolassed sugar-beet pulp: a stoichiometric aproroach. *British Journal of Nutrition*, 69, 511-525.

**13**

# ORGANIC ACIDS – THEIR EFFICACY AND MODES OF ACTION IN PIGS

Kirsi Partanen
*Agricultural Research Centre of Finland, Swine Research Station, Tervamäentie 179, FIN-05720 Hyvinkää, Finland*

## Summary

A meta-analysis of published data shows that dietary organic acids enhance the growth and feed to gain ratio of weaned piglets and fattening pigs. In weaned piglets, the improved growth performance was related to increased feed intake. Neither weaning weight, the existing level of performance nor dietary crude protein content influenced the response of weaned piglets to organic acids. In fattening pigs, the growth response increased with dietary crude protein content, whereas the existing level of performance had no effect. The performance response was greater in the growing than finishing phase. Several modes of action claimed for beneficial effects of organic acids are discussed. Improved nutrient digestibilities result from decreased microbial activity in the gut which spares nutrients from microbes to the animal and reduces microbial protein synthesis. Organic acids may also influence pancreatic exocrine secretion and gut morphology. Effects on *Escherichia coli* counts and the incidence of diarrhoea are generally inconsistent.

## Introduction

For several decades, antibiotic growth promoters have been used in diets for young and growing pigs in order to reduce the incidence of post-weaning diarrhoea and enhance performance. Because of the development of resistance in a number of pathogenic bacterial species, precautionary actions have recently been taken in Europe to exclude several antibiotics from pig diets (EC, 1998). This raises a concern for producers as any increase in the incidence of diarrhoea would increase production costs, e.g. by extending days to market. The susceptibility of weaned piglets to diarrhoea is related to several factors as was reviewed by Hampson (1994). One of those is the immaturity of digestive tract to cope with dietary changes at weaning which can lead to the proliferation of haemolytic *Escherichia coli* in the small intestine. Lactic acid formed by the bacterial fermentation of lactose in the stomach is considered important for keeping the count of *E. coli* low in suckling piglets. The first trials were carried out in the 1960s to investigate whether lactic acid added to weaner diet would have a similar effect (Burnett and Hanna, 1963). Since then numerous trials have been carried out to study effects of dietary organic acids on the performance and health of weaned piglets. Recently, an increasing number of studies has been carried out with fattening pigs as well. This paper aims to evaluate the growth promoting effect of dietary organic acids in weaned piglets and fattening pigs using meta-analysis of published data. In addition, modes of action claimed for the growth promoting effect of organic acids, e.g. increased gastric acidity, reduced coliform populations, stimulated pancreatic exocrine secretion, altered gut morphology, and improved nutrient digestibility and retention (Kirchgessner and Roth 1988; Partanen and Mroz, 1999), are discussed.

## Antibacterial activity

The antibacterial activity of organic acids is based on pH depression and the ability of acids to dissociate which is determined by the $pK_a$-value. Undissociated organic acids are lipophilic and can diffuse across the cell membrane. The lower the external pH, the more undissociated acid will cross the membrane. In the more alkaline interior acids release protons which consequently lowers internal pH. The elimination of released protons by the membrane bound ATPases has traditionally been thought to result in the dissipation of the proton-motive force which is essential for the ATP synthesis and substrate uptake into the cell (Cherrington, Hinton, Mead and Chopra, 1991). This uncoupling theory has been challenged by Russell (1992), who proposed that toxic effects of organic acids are caused by the accumulation of polar anions in the cell. This accumulation depends on the pH gradient across the membrane. Bacteria which try to resist internal pH change are more sensitive to organic acids than those which allow pH to decline (Russell and Diez-Gonzales, 1998). In addition, certain bacteria, e.g. *Salmonella* and *E. coli* have evolved complex counteractive mechanisms which allow them to cope with extreme acid conditions (Bearson, Bearson and Foster, 1997).

Organic acids are known as effective food preservatives and they can be used as an alternative to heating to control microbial contaminants, e.g. *Salmonella* in feed. In addition, they play an important role in controlling the growth of pathogens in the gastrointestinal tract (Russell and Diez-Gonzales, 1998). The rate at which organic acids kill bacteria depends on the time of exposure, the concentration of acid and the particular acid used. Gram-negative bacteria are only sensitive to acids with less than eight carbon atoms, whereas gram-positive bacteria show more sensitivity as the chain length of fatty acids increases and the molecule becomes more lipophilic (Cherrington et al., 1991). The $pK_a$ of most organic acids lies between 3 and 5, and thus ingested organic acids are expected to be most effective in acidic gastric contents. Despite absorption and metabolism, ingested organic acids are detected in the small intestine, but the high pH of intestinal contents favours the dissociated acid molecule (Thompson and Hinton, 1997).

## Absorption and metabolism

Undissociated organic acids are absorbed across intestinal epithelia by passive diffusion along a favourable electrochemical gradient. The physiological pH of intestinal contents varies between 6 and 8 and at these pH values over 94 to 99% of short chain fatty acids are dissociated. However, the existence of a constant acid microclimate at the epithelial surface makes diffusion possible (von Engelhardt, Rönnau, Rechkemmer and Sakata, 1989). Fumaric and citric acids are absorbed by a common $Na^+$-gradient mechanism specific for tri- and dicarboxylates (Wolffram, Hagemann, Grenacher and Scharrer, 1992). Absorbed short chain fatty acids, lactic, fumaric, and citric acids are eventually metabolised via the citric acid cycle to carbon dioxide and water and yield 10 to 27 moles of ATP depending on the acid (Kirchgessner and Roth, 1998). Intestinal cells can use short chain fatty acids, particularly butyrate, as an energy source (von Engelhardt et al., 1989). Sorbic acid is metabolised via ß- and ω-oxidation as are the long chain fatty acids (Sofos and Busta, 1993). Benzoic acid is primarily conjugated in the liver to the amino acid glycine and hippuric acid formed is excreted in the urine (Bridges, French, Smith and Williams, 1970). Formic acid is metabolised in the liver to carbon dioxide in a process requiring tetrahydrofolate. The pig has extremely low hepatic tetrahydrofolate levels and very low levels of the key enzyme 10-formyl tetrahydrofolate dehydrogenase in the folate pathway. Therefore, its ability to metabolise formate is limited. The accumulation of formate in the blood can lead to metabolic acidosis and ocular toxicity (Makar, Tephly, Sahin and Osweiler, 1990).

## Efficacy as growth promoters

A meta-analysis of published data was carried out to evaluate the performance response of weaned piglets and fattening pigs to dietary organic acids, and to find possible factors that may affect the response. Literature from 1970 to the current time was located from trials in which the effect of dietary organic acids on weaned piglet or fattening pig performance was studied. Trials were eligible for analysis if the following information was provided: the initial and final body weight of pigs, average daily gain, feed intake, feed to gain ratio and their standard deviations, number of observations per treatment, diet composition, crude protein content, and feed allowance (*ad libitum* or restricted). Diets which contained acid blends or antibiotic growth promoters or copper in addition to organic acids were excluded.

Response, i.e. unbiased effect size *d* was calculated on the basis of standardised mean difference adjusted for sample size as follows:

$$d \cong (1 - 3 / (4N - 9))(Y^E - Y^C) / s$$

where N is the total sample size, $Y^E$ and $Y^C$ are the respective experimental and control group means and *s* is their pooled standard deviation (Hedges and Olkin, 1985). Positive values indicate an increase and negative values a decrease in response. The effect size data were analysed by the MIXED procedure of SAS (1998) using the maximum likelihood method. In addition to the acid and its inclusion level, the influence of following factors on the response was investigated: the initial body weight of pigs, the existing level of performance, i.e. the average daily gain of control group, and dietary crude protein content. The random effect of trial was included in each model. The final models were chosen based on log likelihood ratios. Those fattening pig trials where the response was reported separately for growing and finishing phases were subjected to the repeated measures analyses using a compound symmetry covariance structure. Residuals were checked for normality and plotted against fitted values. The significance of differences between organic acids was evaluated by the *t*-test.

Forty six weaned piglet and 23 fattening pig trials from 46 published research articles satisfied the inclusion criteria. This data is the same as that used by Partanen and Mroz (1999), except that it has been updated with recent trials (Han, Roneker, Pond and Lei, 1998; Radcliffe, Zhang and Kornegay, 1998; Siljander-Rasi, Alaviuhkola and Suomi, 1998; Bosi, Jung, Han, Perini, Cacciavillani, Casini, Creston, Gremokolini and Mattuzzi, 1999; Øverland and Steien, 1999; Boling, Webel, Mavromichalis, Parsons and Baker, 2000; Partanen, unpublished). Data included several acids, i.e. formic, acetic, propionic, lactic, citric, fumaric, sorbic, tartaric and malic acid, and some of their salts. Because many of those were only studied in one or two trials, meta-analysis of weaned piglet data was restricted to formic, fumaric and citric acids and potassium diformate and that of fattening pig data to formic, propionic and fumaric acids and potassium diformate. Dietary organic acid level was restricted to ≤25 g/kg.

## WEANED PIGLETS

The effect of dietary organic acids on the performance of weaned piglets between 7 and 22 kg body weight is summarised in Table 1. The final model to analyse the effect size data of feed intake, average daily gain and feed to gain ratio included the effect of acid and its inclusion level. Formic, fumaric and citric acids and potassium diformate improved the average daily gain and feed to gain ration of weaned piglets (P < 0.05). Formic acid and potassium diformate enhanced growth more than fumaric and citric acids (P < 0.05), whereas the responses in feed to gain ratio were similar between these acids (P > 0.05). Both growth ($b = 0.026 \pm 0.010$, P < 0.05) and feed to gain ($b = -0.086 \pm 0.018$, P < 0.001) responses increased with dietary acid level. The growth promoting effect of organic acids has been similar or slightly smaller than that of in-feed antibiotics (Edmonds, Izquierdo and Baker, 1985; Øverland, Steien, Gotterbarm and Granli, 1999).

The improved average daily gain in acidified diets was related to increased feed intake ($r = 0.77$, P < 0.001). Formic acid and potassium diformate increased feed consumption (P < 0.05) whereas fumaric and citric acids had no effect (P > 0.05). The ability to maintain feed intake during the immediate post-weaning period is crucial for good growth (Pluske, Williams and Aherne, 1995). Although certain organic acids have strong odour and flavour, little attention has been paid to the acceptability of acidified diets. When offered a free choice of non-acidified and citric or fumaric acid supplemented diets, piglets have preferred the non-acidified diet (Henry, Pickard and Hughes, 1985). Diets containing formic acid or calcium formate were equally acceptable to a lactic acid supplemented diet, but less acceptable than a diet containing sodium benzoate (Partanen, unpublished).

Increased feed intake in acidified diets may result from the improved health of piglets. Reduced frequency of diarrhoea has been reported in some studies, whereas others have observed no diarrhoea or little difference in diarrhoea score (Eckel, Kirchgessner and Roth, 1992; Øverland et al., 1999). Many trials have been carried out with individually housed piglets and, therefore, risks of diarrhoea can be smaller than under practical conditions. Poor hygiene conditions increase the incidence of diarrhoea in weaned piglets and the efficacy of dietary organic acids is expected to be greater than under hygienic conditions (Ravindran and Kornegay, 1993). The growth rate of control group was used as an indicator of the existing level of performance, but it did not affect the response to organic acids (P > 0.05). Neither was the response influenced by weaning weight (P > 0.05), although it is an important risk factor associated with post-weaning diarrhoea (Skirrow, Buddle, Mercy, Madec and Nicholls, 1997).

Diet composition may be one factor influencing the response of weaned piglets to organic acids. The response has been smaller when diets with milk products have been fed to piglets compared to those without (Giesting and Easter, 1991), but not in all cases (Roth, Kirchgessner and Eidelsburger, 1993). Lactose from milk products is converted to lactic acid creating desirable changes in gastric environment and thus reducing the efficacy of acidification. Dietary buffering capacity is considered an important factor influencing the efficacy of organic acids.

Table 1. Performance response of weaned piglets to dietary formic, fumaric and citric acid and potassium diformate supplementation (≤25 g/kg feed) based on meta-analysis of published data.

| | Formic acid | Fumaric acid | Citric acid | Potassium diformate |
|---|---|---|---|---|
| Experiments | 6 | 18 | 9 | 3 |
| Observations | 10 | 27 | 19 | 13 |
| Acid levels, g/kg feed | 3 – 18 | 5 – 25 | 5 – 25 | 4 – 24 |
| Dietary CP, g/kg[1] | 234 ± 22 | 208 ± 27 | 216 ± 21 | 222 ± 5 |
| Feed intake, g/d[1] | | | | |
| Control | 667 ± 87 | 613 ± 148 | 534 ± 276 | 764 ± 9 |
| Experimental | 710 ± 75 | 614 ± 152 | 528 ± 302 | 823 ± 38 |
| Weight gain, g/d[1] | | | | |
| Control | 387 ± 65 | 358 ± 99 | 382 ± 121 | 479 ± 4 |
| Experimental | 428 ± 62 | 374 ± 101 | 396 ± 127 | 536 ± 26 |
| Feed to gain, kg/kg[1] | | | | |
| Control | 1.64 ± 0.13 | 1.59 ± 0.16 | 1.67 ± 0.25 | 1.60 ± 0.02 |
| Experimental | 1.60 ± 0.14 | 1.55 ± 0.14 | 1.60 ± 0.24 | 1.54 ± 0.04 |
| Unbiased effect size, $d$[2] | | | | |
| Feed intake | 0.46 ± 0.16[a] | -0.08 ± 0.10[b] | -0.20 ± 0.13[b] | 0.59 ± 0.14[a] |
| $P \leq$[3] | 0.01 | 0.42 | 0.14 | 0.001 |
| Weight gain | 0.77 ± 0.16[a] | 0.25 ± 0.10[b] | 0.32 ± 0.11[b] | 0.89 ± 0.15[a] |
| $P \leq$[3] | 0.001 | 0.01 | 0.01 | 0.001 |
| Feed to gain | -0.91 ± 0.36 | -0.71 ± 0.27 | -0.81 ± 0.30 | -1.04 ± 0.42 |
| $P \leq$[3] | 0.02 | 0.01 | 0.01 | 0.02 |

CP = crude protein.
[1] Mean ± standard deviation.
[2] Lsmean ± standard error of mean.
[3] Probability that the response differs from the non-acidified control diet.
[a,b] Means with different superscripts are significantly different (P < 0.05).

However, Roth and Kirchgessner (1989) found no clear relationship between piglet performance and dietary buffering capacity. Dietary buffering capacity is increased with mineral and protein content, but in this data the latter did not affect the response to organic acids (P > 0.05). In the recent trial of Paulicks, Roth and Kirchgessner (1999), the response of weaned piglets to potassium diformate was greater for wheat than maize or barley-based diets.

## FATTENING PIGS

The response of growing-finishing pigs to dietary organic acids is summarised in

Table 2. Because feed allowance was restricted in most trials, the effects on feed intake were not investigated. The final model used to analyse the effect size data of average daily gain included effects of acid, its inclusion level, their interaction and dietary crude protein content. The effect size data of feed to gain ratio was analysed by having the effect of acid and its inclusion level in the model. Formic, propionic and fumaric acids and potassium diformate improved the weight gain and feed to gain ratio of fattening pigs (P < 0.01). The responses were similar between these acids (P > 0.05). A tendency (P = 0.07) for acid/level interaction was observed for growth responses. In fattening pigs, the effect of diet composition on the efficacy of organic acids has received little attention. The literature data showed that growth response increased with dietary crude protein content ($b = 0.017 \pm 0.006$, P < 0.05). In weaned piglets, potassium diformate supplementation has resulted in greater nitrogen retention with increasing dietary lysine level (Roth, Windisch and Kirchgessner, 1998). This was explained by decreased microbial degradation of essential amino acids.

Table 2. Performance response of fattening pigs to dietary formic, propionic and fumaric acid and potassium diformate supplementation (≤25 g/kg feed) based on meta-analysis of published data.

| | Formic acid | Propionic acid | Fumaric acid | Potassium diformate |
|---|---|---|---|---|
| Experiments | 8 | 3 | 4 | 4 |
| Observations | 15 | 6 | 10 | 8 |
| Acid levels, g/kg feed | 5–16 | 5–25 | 6–25 | 6–20 |
| Dietary CP, g/kg[1] | 164±11 | 159±10 | 162±16 | 156±10 |
| Weight gain, g/d[1] | | | | |
| Control | 807±66 | 755±79 | 727±24 | 805±49 |
| Experimental | 857±62 | 784±74 | 753±28 | 842±52 |
| Feed to gain, kg/kg[1] | | | | |
| Control | 2.48±0.19 | 2.82±0.43 | 2.82±0.18 | 2.64±0.13 |
| Experimental | 2.36±0.16 | 2.71±0.43 | 2.74±0.19 | 2.59±0.14 |
| Unbiased effect size, $d^2$ | | | | |
| Weight gain | 0.84±0.15 | 0.94±0.17 | 0.67±0.15 | 0.78±0.16 |
| P ≤[3] | 0.001 | 0.001 | 0.01 | 0.001 |
| Feed to gain | -0.72±0.12 | -0.57±0.17 | -0.65±0.19 | -0.56±0.16 |
| P ≤[3] | 0.001 | 0.01 | 0.01 | 0.01 |

CP = crude protein.
[1] Mean ± standard deviation.
[2] Lsmean ± standard error of mean.
[3] Probability that the response differs from the non-acidified control diet.

Figure 1 demonstrates that responses in average daily gain and feed to gain ratio were greater in the growing than finishing phase (P < 0.05). However, the limitation of dietary acidification to piglet period has not been sufficient to maintain the performance improvement until market weight (Kirchgessner, Paulicks and Roth, 1997). The existing level of performance did not influence the response to organic acids (P > 0.05). Research at our Institute has shown that when piglets came from the same sow unit for fattening, no diarrhoea was observed and formic acid enhanced performance only in the growing period, but not during the whole fattening period (Siljander-Rasi et al., 1998). However, when piglets from different farms were brought into the same fattening unit and mixed, formic acid and formic acid-sorbate blend improved performance and reduced the frequency of diarrhoea in the growing period. Performance was improved during the whole fattening period as well (Partanen, unpublished). Compared to antibiotic growth promoters, formic acid was equally effective to carbadox and avilamycin in the growing period (Siljander-Rasi et al., 1998; Partanen, unpublished).

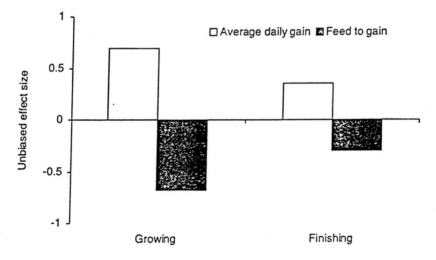

**Figure 1.** Dietary organic acids improve the performance of fattening pigs in growing and finishing phases (P < 0.05), but the response is greater in the former (P < 0.05).

## Mode of action of organic acids

The exact mechanisms regulating the growth promoting effect of organic acids remains unclear, although several hypotheses have been investigated. Because organic acids are antibacterial substances, it is likely that their growth promoting effect is primarily associated with their effect on gastrointestinal microflora. Organic acids may also have physiological effects on the host animal.

## GASTRIC ACIDITY

Lowered gastric pH is perhaps the most favoured hypothesis to explain the mode of action of dietary organic acids. Acidic gastric conditions are considered essential for the prevention of the survival of ingested pathogens in the stomach so that they do not gain access to the small intestine. However, the disease can also result from an increase in numbers of bacteria that have colonised the intestines before weaning (Hampson, 1994). Low gastric pH is also needed for the activation of gastric proteases which are secreted as zymogens (Cranwell, 1995). As reviewed by Partanen and Mroz (1999) it has been proven difficult to demonstrate *in vivo* that dietary organic acids reduce gastric pH. Acidified drinking water or liquid feed with high naturally lactic acid content can be more effective in lowering gastric pH (Jensen, 1998), simply because more acid is ingested than from dry feed. Dietary buffering capacity is considered an important factor affecting gastric pH, as diets rich in protein and minerals can resist changes in pH (Roth and Kirchgessner, 1989). It is unlikely that dietary organic acids would influence the pH of intestinal contents because of the neutralising effect of pancreatic secretions. Strongly acidic gastric conditions are not desirable because they may result in the development of gastric ulcers (Argentzio and Southworth, 1975).

The reduced rate of gastric emptying due to lower gastric pH would be desirable as it would allow more time for acids to act on pathogenic bacteria. In addition, it would prevent the small intestine from becoming overwhelmed (Ravindran and Kornegay, 1993). However, most studies have been unable to show that organic acids have any effect on stomach dry matter content which has been used as an indication of gastric emptying (Partanen and Mroz, 1999). The post-mortem techniques used may not be satisfactory to investigate such an effect.

## EFFECTS ON THE MICROFLORA

The outbreak of post-weaning diarrhoea is caused by the proliferation of enterotoxigenic bacteria, mainly *E. coli* in the small intestine and(or) fermentation of less digestible nutrients of weaner diet in the large intestine (Hampson, 1994). According to Jensen (1998) lactic acid has reduced gastric and intestinal *E. coli* populations, whereas the effect of other acids have been inconsistent. Decreased *E. coli* numbers have been reported with formate supplemented diets (Gedek, Kirchgessner, Eidelsburger, Wiehler, Bott and Roth, 1992; Øverland et al., 1999), although formates reduce lactic acid production in gastric and intestinal contents (Bolduan, Jung, Schneier, Block and Klenke, 1988; Roth, Eckel, Kirchgessner and Eidelsburger, 1992; Partanen, unpublished). Organic acids do not only act on pathogenic bacteria but also modify beneficial flora. *In vitro* gas production studies have shown that organic acids result in considerable reduction in microbial fermentation, although some acids, e.g. lactic acid may stimulate it (Piva, Biagi, Meola, Luchansky and Gatta, 1999). Reduced microbial fermentation spares fermentable carbohydrates from microbes to the animal. In the case of antibiotics, reduced microbial fermentation almost entirely accounts for the improved feed to gain ratio (Jensen, 1998). Reduced ammonia concentrations have been observed in the digesta of pigs fed formic acid supplemented diets (Roth et al., 1992).

## PANCREATIC EXOCRINE SECRETION

At weaning, the pancreas of 3 to 4 week old piglet is not prepared for the digestion of solid food (Cranwell, 1995). Impaired exocrine pancreatic secretion may result in disturbances in the performance and health of piglets after weaning. In growing pigs, exocrine secretion may limit performance (Botermans, Svendsen, Svendsen and Pierzynowski, 1999). Some results indicate that short chain fatty acids *per se* may stimulate pancreatic secretion in pigs (Harada, Kiriyama, Kobayashi and Tsuchita, 1988). In theory, this should result in larger improvements in the digestibility of poorly than highly digestible diets. Increased secretion of proteases should also result in improved true ileal amino acid digestibilities.

## GUT MORPHOLOGY

At weaning the small intestine of the piglet generally undergoes a reduction in villous height and an increase in crypt depth, changes which are associated with a decreased capacity for absorption. Similar changes are observed with a reduction in voluntary feed intake and post-weaning diarrhoea (Pluske et al., 1995). Changes in gut morphology are important as they can reduce growth rate. Short chain fatty acids produced by microbial fermentation of dietary fibre stimulate epithelial cell proliferation which should increase absorptive surface (Sakata, 1988). So far, little is known about the influence of dietary acidification on pig gut morphology. Dietary sodium butyrate has resulted in a substantial increase in the number of cells constituting microvilli and in the length of microvilli in the ileum of growing pigs (Gálfi and Bokori, 1990). Pigs also grew faster compared to the control group.

## Digestibility and retention of nutrients and energy

## PROTEIN

Several studies have reported improved apparent ileal digestibilities of both essential and nonessential amino acids when diets for weaned piglets and fattening pigs have been supplemented with organic acids. The changes in apparent ileal lysine digestibility have ranged from –3 to 8 %-units in weaned piglets and 1 to 5 %-units in fattening pigs relative to the non-acidified control diet (Partanen and Mroz, 1999). The response was negatively related to the digestibility of the basal diet ($r$ = -0.73 for crude protein and –0.65 for lysine, P < 0.001, calculated from 10 published trials). The average 3 %-unit improvement in apparent ileal lysine digestibility would increase the supply of apparent ileal digestible lysine by 0.2, 0.4, 0.5 and 0.6 g/d in 7.5, 15, 35 and 65-kg pigs, respectively.

The effects of dietary buffering capacity on the digestibility response of organic acids have been inconsistent. Neither formic acid nor dietary buffering capacity increased with calcium carbonate and dicalcium phosphate had an effect on apparent ileal amino acid digestibilities in semipurified fish meal diet (Gabert, Sauer, Schmitz, Ahrens and Mosenthin, 1995). Recently, Blank, Mosenthin, Sauer and Huang (1999) reported a decrease in apparent ileal amino acid digestibilities in diets supplemented with sodium bicarbonate. Fumaric acid improved apparent ileal amino digestibilities in low, but not high buffering capacity diets due to greater variation in digestibility coefficients. Lowering dietary buffering capacity with calcium benzoate has improved apparent ileal amino acid digestibilities, and they were further improved by organic acid supplementation (Mroz, Jongbloed, Partanen, van Diepen, Vreman and Kogut, 1998).

Recently, Partanen, Valaja, Siljander-Rasi, Jalava and Panula (1998) found that formic acid improved apparent ileal amino acid digestibilities in a complex by-product based diet but not in a simple barley-soybean meal diet fed to growing-finishing pigs. However, true ileal lysine digestibility determined using the homoarginine method was not affected. The improved apparent digestibilities were due to reduced endogenous nitrogen flow, particularly that of bacterial origin in the ileum. There is considerable microbial activity in the stomach and small intestine of growing pigs (Argentzio and Southworth, 1975) and bacterial nitrogen represent a considerable proportion (40 to 66%) of ileal nitrogen (Bartelt, Drochner, Götz, Sxakacz, Ceresnáková and Sommer, 1999). Endogenous nitrogen is an easily available nitrogen source for bacterial protein synthesis, and 89 to 98% of bacterial nitrogen is of endogenous origin. Therefore, when bacterial growth is restricted by organic acids, more endogenous nitrogen is absorbed rather than being incorporated into bacterial protein. This should result in improved nitrogen retention which has been observed in several trials (see Partanen and Mroz 1999).

## FAT AND ENERGY

Improved total tract digestibility of energy has been reported in several trials but not always (Eckel et al., 1992; Roth, Windisch and Kirchgessner, 1998). Improved energy digestibility results from improvements in apparent total tract digestibility of crude protein, fat and nitrogen free extracts. Roth et al. (1998) found no effect of potassium diformate supplementation on total tract digestibility of fat in weaned piglets. However, in growing pigs, formic acid supplementation has resulted in noticeable improvements in both ileal and total tract fat digestibility (Partanen et al., 1998). Improved fat digestibility is generally associated with reduced microbial activity in the digestive tract.

## MINERALS

Several studies indicate that organic acids may improve the apparent total tract digestibility and(or) retention of calcium and phosphorus in diets for weaned piglets or fattening pigs (Han et al., 1998; Boling et al., 2000). When phosphorus deficient diets are used, improved calcium and phosphorus digestibility naturally results in increased retention. However, improved retention has also been observed with diets containing sufficient phosphorus (Roth et al., 1998b). Young piglets have high calcium and phosphorus requirement. Dietary mineral supplements act as buffer in the stomach and can make more favourable conditions for the proliferation of *E. coli*. Dietary calcium and phosphorus content can be reduced by microbial phytase addition. However, the hypothesis that dietary organic acids may favour the action of microbial phytase has not been proven (Radcliffe et al., 1998).

## Conclusions

Meta-analysis of published data shows that dietary organic acids have a beneficial effect on the performance of weaned piglets and fattening pigs. Reduction in the incidence of diarrhoea is less evident. Quite high dietary organic acid levels are used in trials. From a practical point of view, acid levels below 10 g/kg feed should be targeted. In addition, the limitation of acidification to periods and conditions where pigs are most susceptible to diarrhoea should be considered. It seems that the growth promoting effect of organic acids is primarily associated with effects on gastrointestinal microflora. However, more detailed studies are needed to clarify the exact modes of action and quantify their effect on performance.

## References

Argentzio, R.A. and Southworth, M. (1975) Sites of organic acid production and absorption in the gastrointestinal tract of pig. *American Journal of Physiology*, **228**, 454-460.

Bartelt, J., Drochner, W., Götz, K.-P., Sxakacz, J., Ceresnáková, Z. and Sommer, A. (1999) Determination of endogenous nitrogen associated with bacteria in ileal digesta of pigs receiving cereal-based diets with or without fish meal and various fibre supplements by using a simple $^{15}$N-dilution technique. *Journal of Animal and Feed Sciences*, **8**, 425-440.

Bearson, S., Bearson, B. and Foster, J.W. (1997) Acid stress responses in enterobacteria. *FEMS Microbiology Letters*, **147**, 173-180.

Blank, R., Mosenthin, R., Sauer, W.C. and Huang, S. (1999) Effect of fumaric acid and dietary buffering capacity on ileal and fecal amino acid digestibilities in early-weaned pigs. *Journal of Animal Science*, **77** , 2974-2984.

Bolduan, G., Jung, H., Schneier, R., Block, J. and Klenke, B. (1988) Die Wirkung von Propion- und Ameisensäure in der Ferkelaufzucht. *Journal of Animal Physiology and Animal Nutrition*, **59**, 72-78.

Boling, S.D., Webel, D.M., Mavromichalis, I., Parsons, C.M. and Baker, D.H. (2000) The effects of citric acid on phytate-phosphorus utilization in young chicks and pigs. *Journal of Animal Science*, **78**, 682-689.

Bosi, P., Jung, H.J., Han, I.K., Perini, S., Cacciavillani, J.A., Casini, L., Creston, D., Gremokolini, C. and Mattuzzi, S. (1999) Effects of dietary buffering characteristics and protected or unprotected acids on piglet growth, digestibility and characteristics of gut content. *Asian-Australasian Journal of Animal Science*, **12**, 1104-1110.

Botermans, J.A.M., Svendsen, J., Svendsen, L.S. and Pierzynowski, S.G. (1999) The exocrine pancreas in pig growth and performance. *In Biology of the pancreas in the growing animal*, pp 395-408. Edited by S.G. Pierzynowski and R. Zabielski. Elsevier, Amsterdam.

Bridges, J.W., French, M.R., Smith, R.L. and Williams, R.T. (1970) The fate of benzoic acid in various species. *Biochemistry Journal*, **118**, 47-51.

Burnett, G.S. and Hanna, J. (1963) Effect of dietary calcium lactate and lactic acid on faecal *Escherichia coli* counts in pigs. *Nature*, **79**, 815.

Cherrington, C.A., Hinton, M., Mead, G.C. and Chopra, I. (1991) Organic acids: chemistry, antibacterial activity and practical applications. *Advances in Microbial Physiology*, **32**, 87-108.

Cranwell, P.D. (1995) Development of the neonatal gut and enzyme systems. *In The Neonatal Pig - Development and Survival*, pp 99-154. Edited by M.A. Varley. CAB International, Oxon.

EC (1998) Commission Regulation (EC) No 2788/98 of 22 December 1998 amending Council Directive 70/534/EEC concerning additives in feedingstuffs as regards the withdrawal of authorisation for certain growth promoters. *Official Journal of European Commission*, **L347**, 31-32.

Eckel, B., Kirchgessner, M. and Roth, F.X. (1992) Zum Einfluss von Ameisensäure auf tägliche Zunahmen, Futteraufnahme, Futterverwertung und

Verdaulichkeit. *Journal of Animal Physiology and Animal Nutrition,* **67,** 93-100.

Edmonds, M.S., Izquierdo, O.A. and Baker, D.H. (1985) Feed additive studies with newly weaned pigs: Efficacy of supplemental copper, antibiotics and organic acids. *Journal of Animal Science,* **60,** 462-469.

Gabert, V.M., Sauer, W.C., Schmitz, M., Ahrens, F. and Mosenthin, R. (1995) The effect of formic acid and buffering capacity on the ileal digestibilities of amino acids and bacterial populations and metabolites in the small intestine of weanling pigs fed semipurified fish meal diets. *Canadian Journal of Animal Science,* **75,** 615-623.

Gálfi, P. and Bokori, J. (1990) Feeding trial in pigs with a diet containing sodium *n*-butyrate. *Acta Veterinaria Hungarica,* **38,** 3-17.

Gedek, B., Kirchgessner, M., Eidelsburger, U., Wiehler, S., Bott, A. and Roth, F.X. (1992) Zum Einfluss von Ameisensäure auf die Keimzahlen der Mikroflora und deren Zusammensetzung in verschiedenen Segmenten des Gastrointestinaltraktes. *Journal of Animal Physiology and Animal Nutrition,* **67,** 206-214.

Giesting, D.W. and Easter, R.A. (1991) Effect of protein source and fumaric acid supplementation on apparent ileal digestibility of nutrients by young pigs. *Journal of Animal Science,* **69,** 2497-2503.

Hampson, D.J. (1994) Postweaning *Escherichia coli* diarrhoea in pigs. *In Escherichia coli in domestic animals and humans,* pp 171-191. Edited by C.L. Gyles. CAB International, Oxon.

Han, Y.M., Roneker, K.R., Pond, W.G. and Lei, X.G. (1998) Adding wheat middlings, microbial phytase, and citric acid to corn-soybean meal diets for growing pigs may replace inorganic phosphorus supplementation. *Journal of Animal Science,* **76,** 2649-2656.

Harada, E., Kiriyama, H., Kobayashi, E. and Tsuchita, H. (1988) Postnatal development of biliary and pancreatic exocrine secretion in piglets. *Comparative Biochemistry and Physiology,* **91A,** 43-51.

Hedges, L.V. and Olkin, I. (1985) Statistical methods for meta-analysis. Academic Press, San Diego.

Henry, R.W., Pickard, D.W. and Hughes, P.E. (1985) Citric acid and fumaric acid as food additives for early-weaned piglets. *Animal Production,* **40,** 505-509.

Jensen, B.B. (1998) The impact of feed additives on the microbial ecology of the gut in young pigs. *Journal of Animal and Feed Sciences,* **7,** 45-64.

Kirchgessner, M., Paulicks, B.R. and Roth, F.X. (1997) Effects of supplementations of diformate complexes (Formi™ LHS) on growth and carcass performance of piglets and fattening pigs in response to application time. *Agribiological Research,* **50,** 1-7.

Kirchgessner, M. and Roth, F.X. (1988) Ergotrope Effecte durch Organische Säuren in der Ferkelaufzucht und Schweinemast. *Übersichten zur Tierernährung,* **16,** 93-108.

Makar, A.B., Tephly, T.R., Sahin, G. and Osweiler, G. (1990) Formate metabolism in young swine. *Toxicology and Applied Pharmacology,* **105,** 315-320.

Mroz, Z., Jongbloed, A.W., Partanen, K., van Diepen, J.Th.M., Vreman, K. and Kogut, J. (1998) Ileal digestibility of amino acids in pigs fed diets of different buffering capacity and with supplementary organic acids. *Journal of Animal and Feed Sciences,* **7,** 191-197.

Øverland, M. and Steien, S. H. (1999) K-diformate (Formi™LHS) in diets for pigs. *In Manipulating Pig Production VII.* pp 127. Edited by P.D. Cranwell. Australasian Pig Science Association.

Øverland, M., Steien, S. H., Gotterbarm, G., and Granli, T. (1999) Formi™LHS - An alternative to antibiotic growth promoters. 50th Annual meeting of the EAAP. 6 p.

Partanen, K. and Mroz, Z. (1999) Organic acids for performance enhancement in pig diets. *Nutrition Research Reviews,* **12,** 117-145.

Partanen, K., Valaja, J., Siljander-Rasi, H., Jalava, T. and Panula, S. (1998) Effects of carbadox or formic acid and diet type on ileal digestion of amino acids by pigs. *Journal of Animal and Feed Sciences,* **7,** 199-203.

Paulicks, B.R., Roth, F.X. and Kirchgessner, M. (1999) Nutritive Wirksamkeit eines Ameisensäure-Formiat-Komplexes (Formi™ LHS) auf die Leistung von Absetzferkeln in Abhängigkeit von der Rationszusammensetzung. *Proceedings of the Society of Nutrition and Physiology,* **8,** 127.

Piva, A., Biagi, G., Meola, E., Luchansky, J.B. & Gatta, P.P. (1999) Inhibitory/ stimulatory effect of organic acids on intestinal microflora. *Journal of Animal Science,* 77(Suppl. 1), 199 (abstract).

Pluske, J.L., Williams, I.H. and Aherne, F.X. (1995) Nutrition of the neonatal pig. *In The Neonatal Pig - Development and Survival,* pp 187-235. Edited by M.A. Varley. CAB International, Oxon.

Radcliffe, J.S., Zhang, Z. and Kornegay, E.T. (1998) The effects of microbial phytase, citric acid, and their interactions in a corn-soybean meal-based diet for weanling pigs. *Journal of Animal Science,* **76,** 1880-1886.

Ravindran, V. and Kornegay, E.T. (1993) Acidification of weaner pig diets: A review. *Journal of the Science of Food and Agriculture,* **62,** 313-322.

Roth, F.X., Eckel, B., Kirchgessner, M. and Eidelsburger, U. (1992) Zum Einfluss von Ameisensäure auf pH-Wert, Trockenmassegehalt, Konzentrationen an flüchtigen Fettsäuren und Milchsäure im Gastrointestinaltrakt. 3. Mitteilung. Untersuchungen zur nutritiven Wirksamkeit von organischen Säuern in der Ferkelaufzucht. *Journal of Animal Physiology and Animal Nutrition,* **67,** 148-156.

Roth, F.X. and Kirchgessner, M. (1989) Significance of dietary pH and buffering capacity in piglet nutrition. 1. pH and buffering capacity of diets supplemented with organic acids. *Landwirtschaftliche Forschung, 42,* 157-167.

Roth, F.X., Kirchgessner, M. and Eidelsburger, U. (1993) Zur nutritiven Wirksamkeit von Milchsäure in der Ferkelaufzucht. *Agribiological Research, 46,* 229-239.

Roth, F.X., Windisch, W. and Kirchgessner, M. (1998a) Effect of potassium diformate (Formi™ LHS) on nitrogen metabolism and nutrient digestibility in piglets at graded dietary lysine supply. *Agribiological Research, 51,* 167-175.

Roth, F.X., Windisch, W. and Kirchgessner, M. (1998b) Mineral metabolism (P, K, Ca, Mg, Zn, Mn, Cu) of piglets supplied with potassium diformate (Formi™ LHS). *Agribiological Research, 51,* 177-183.

Russell, J.B. (1992) Another explanation for the toxicity of fermentation acids at low pH: anion accumulation *versus* uncoupling. *Journal of Applied Bacteriology, 73,* 363-370.

Russell, J.B. and Diez-Gonzales, F. (1998) The effects of fermentation acids on bacterial growth. *Advances in Microbial Physiolgy, 39,* 205-234.

Sakata, T. (1988) Chemical and physical trophic effects of dietary fibre on the intestine of monogastric animals. *In Digestive Physiology in the Pig,* pp. 128-135. Edited by L. Buraczewska, S. Buraczewski, B. Pastuszewska and T. Zebrowska. Polish Academy of Sciences, Jablonna.

SAS (1998) SAS/STAT User's Guide, Release 6.03. SAS Institute, Inc., Cary, NC.

Siljander-Rasi, H., Alaviuhkola, T. and Suomi, K. (1998) Carbadox, formic acid and potato fibre as feed additives for growing pigs. *Journal of Animal and Feed Sciences, 7,* 205-209.

Skirrow, S.Z., Buddle, J.R., Mercy, A.R., Madec, F. and Nicholls, R.R. (1997) Epidemiological studies of pig diseases: 2. Post-weaning diarrhoea and performance in Western Australian pigs. *Australian Veterinary Journal, 75,* 282-288.

Sofos, J.N. and Busta, F.F. (1993) Sorbic acid and sorbates. *In Antimicrobials in foods,* pp 49-94. Edited by P.M. Davidson and A.L. Branen. Marcel Dekker, Inc., New York.

Thompson, J.L. and Hinton, M. (1997) Antibacterial activity of formic and propionic acids in the diet of hens on salmonella in the crop. *British Poultry Science, 38,* 59-65.

von Engelhardt, W., Rönnau, K., Rechkemmer, G. and Sakata, T. (1989) Absorption of short-chain fatty acids and their role in the hindgut of monogastric animals. *Animal Feed Science and Technology, 23,* 43-53.

Wolffram, S., Hagemann, C., Grenacher, B. and Scharrer, E. (1992) Characterization of the transport of tri- and dicarboxylates by intestinal brush-border membrane vesicle. *Comparative Biochemistry and Physiology,* **101A,** 759-767.

# 14

# SAFETY ASPECTS ON NON-USE OF ANTIMICROBIALS AS GROWTH PROMOTERS

Christina Greko
*Department of Antibiotics, National Veterinary Institute, Sweden*

## Summary

The use of antibiotics as growth promoters, or antimicrobial performance enhancers (APE), has been questioned ever since this practice began. The dosages used are low compared to therapeutic dosages, but for inherently susceptible bacteria they are clearly inhibitory. Emergence of resistance is an inevitable result of the selective pressure applied. Thereby, the use of APE contributes to an increase and maintenance of the pool of resistance genes in various ecosystems. Available evidence clearly indicates that resistance genes can be, and are, transferred from animal to human microbiota. Food is considered to be the main vehicle for transfer. Available data indicates that non-use of APE has been effective in reducing or preventing resistance in animal populations, thereby reducing the risk of spread of resistance through the food chain.

All food-borne diseases pose a considerable threat to human health. Therefore, possible effects of APE on colonisation and shedding of zoonotic enteric pathogens must be considered. Theoretically, APE active against Gram-negative bacteria could reduce the risk of colonisation, at least until resistance is developed in the pathogens. On the other hand, APE suppressing the Gram-positive flora could enhance this risk. A dose-dependent response, with increased salmonella shedding of chickens, has been established for avoparcin. For other APE, no dose-response studies have been found.

The disease preventing effect of antimicrobials given at dosages used for growth promotion on intestinal diseases is well documented. Experience from Sweden, and recently other countries confirm that withdrawal of APE may lead to problems with diseases such as necrotic enteritis in chickens and post-weaning diarrhoea in piglets. However, these problems may be overcome through changes in the production. With improved feed and feeding regimens, hygiene and health-orientated systems it is possible to adjust to non-use of APE.

## Introduction

The controversy concerning possible effects of the use of antimicrobials as feed additives on the selection of resistant bacteria goes back to the 50s. In 1969, a Brittish committee recommended restrictions in the use of antimicrobials for growth promotion in order to mitigate the risk of resistance (Swann Committee 1969). In Europe, this led to the withdrawal of several substances from the list of authorised additives because of a decision to restrict certain antibiotics to therapeutic use (e.g. penicillin, streptomycin and tetracyclines).

In Sweden, the intensive debate from the 60s never ceased. In the discussion, at the beginning of the 80s, a broad discussion on use of antibiotics and practices in animal production prompted the Swedish Farmers Union (LRF) to write to the Government and ask for a ban on growth promoting antibiotics. From 1986, antibiotics for animals are available on prescription only and use is restricted to preventive or therapeutic uses (i.e. use for growth promotion was banned).

During the 90s, the problems with resistance in human medicine worldwide have increased markedly. Simultaneously, use of techniques such as molecular epidemiology has provided information that helps to clarify some of the more pertinent issues. Consequently, the scientific and public debate about possible risks related to the use of antimicrobials as feed additives has been intensified. Several opinions and evaluations from different Committees have recently been made available (WHO 1997; JECATAR 1999; SSC 1999). In the European Union, this has led to the suspension of the authorisation of several antibacterial performance enhancers (APE). Furthermore, the Council of Ministers and the Commission have indicated the intention to phase out those APEs that still remain authorised.

In the current debate, the notion has been made that non-use would lead to consequences that outweigh those of resistance. Specifically, concerns relating to effects on animal health, resistance and prevalence of zoonotic pathogens are raised. In the following, some arguments will be examined on basis of the Swedish experiences.

## Use of APE and bacterial resistance

The main risk factor for increased resistance is the use of antibiotics in concentrations high enough to kill or inhibit sensitive bacteria (Levy 1996). It has been argued that the dosages used for performance enhancement are too low for any development of resistance to occur. However, the concentrations of APE in feed exceed the susceptibility ranges of naturally susceptible intestinal bacteria (SOU 1997:132 1997). An association between use of the glycopeptide avoparcin and prevalence of resistance has been clearly demonstrated (Bager, Madsen, Christensen and Aarestrup 1997).

Enterococci that are resistant to avoparcin are simultaneously resistant to other glycopeptides, notably vancomycin. Modern techniques allow not only the identification of specific resistance determinants, but also a closer scrutiny of their phylogenetic relationships. The *van*A gene cluster (mediating resistance to avoparcin-vancomycin) has been subject to several studies. It has been shown that vancomycin resistant enterococci (VRE) from different animal species and humans can contain indistinguishable genetic elements coding for resistance (Jensen, Hammerum, Aarestrup, Palepou, Adebiyi, Tremlett, Jensen and Woodford 1998; Woodford, Adebiyi, Palepou and Coockson 1998; Stobberingh, van den Bogaard, London, Driessen, Top and Willems 1999). This clearly indicates either horizontal transfer between enterococci of human and animal origins, or the existence of a common source.

Vancomycin is a glycopeptide antibiotic that is used in human medicine when other therapeutical options are limited or non-existent. Thus, the consequences of resistance in human bacteria are serious. In Europe, 2-5% of the healthy people in the community has been reported to carry VRE. It has been suggested that that transmission from animals to man via food is a major source for this community carriage (e.g. Witte 1996). Various transferable resistance genes, including *van*A-genes in enterococci have been identified in gram-positive bacteria isolated from food (Aarestrup 1995; Klare, Heier, Claus, Böhme, Marin, Seltmann, Hakenbeck, Antanassova and Witte 1995; Roberts, Facinelli, Giovanetti and Varaldo 1996; Perreten, Kollöffel and Teuber 1997; Wegener, Madsen, Nielsen and Aarestrup 1997).

Available evidence from Denmark indicates that abstention from APE has been effective in reducing the prevalence of VRE in animal populations (DANMAP 98 1999). This concurs with observations from Sweden. Glycopeptides have not been used in Swedish animal production systems since the early 80s. Contrary to the situation in other European countries, VRE of the *van*A genotype are rarely detected in samples from Swedish animals (Greko and Lindblad 1996; Quednau, Ahrné and Molin 1998; van den Bogaard, London and Stobberingh 2000). Interestingly, the prevelence of VRE in nonhospitalised Swedes also seems to be very low (Torell, Cars, Olsson-Liljequist, Hoffman, Lindbäck, Burman and The Enterococcal Study Group 1999). A plausible explanation for the absence of community carriers in Sweden is that the prevalence of VRE in food is comparatively low.

## Effects on animal health

The changes in 1986 had little or no impact on dairy, beef, calves, sheep or layers as these production sectors never or hardly used APEs. More affected were the chicken and swine industry.

## CHICKENS

Before 1986, almost all chicken feed contained both an antibacterial feed additive and a coccidiostat. The chicken producers identified the occurrence of clinical or subclinical necrotic enteritis (caused by *Clostridium perfringens*) as the main problem to tackle subsequent to the ban. It was agreed that a transition period would be necessary and that the veterinarians would prescribe virginiamycin as prophylaxis during this period. Field experience and more formal research confirmed the construction and climate of stables, hygiene, management and feed composition all contributed to the disease. Further, it was found that coccidiostats of the ionophore type also prevent necrotic enteritis (Elwinger, Schneitz, Berndtson, Fossum, Teglöf and Engsröm 1992; Elwinger, Engström, Fossum, Hassan and Teglöf 1994).

Already in 1988, all prophylactic medications were abandoned. Strong emphasis was placed on improving animal environment, measures that could be foreseen to prevent other diseases as well. A special bonus was given for good animal management and care, which also led to improvements in the total level of quality of the production. The most important changes related to feed involved a reduction of protein content, a higher fibre content and supplementation with enzymes. Ionophores are used as coccidiostats for conventionally reared chickens.

## PIGS

Before 1986, practically all piglets were given antibacterial feed additives (olaquindox or carbadox), from weaning until delivery to the finishing units at the age of 10-12 weeks. Slaughter pigs were, to a lesser extent, given antibacterial feed additives (avoparcin or virginiamycin) until slaughter.

The most notable problems that were observed arose in weaner pigs. In a comparison of production averages from 220 piglet producing herds from the years 1985 and 1986, Robertsson and Lundeheim (1994) reported that post-weaning mortality was about 1.5 percentage units higher the year after the ban and an the time from birth to 25kg was increased. A comparison of the average values for 1994-1995 and 1986-1987 reveals that post-weaning mortality to has now decreased with 0.9 percentage units and the age at 25 kg to have been reduced by 1-2 days (Wierup 1996).

Since the ban of antibacterial feed additives numerous measures have been, and are continuously, undertaken to optimise rearing and production systems and to employ available techniques (e.g. sectioning of buildings, age segregation, planned production). The ban also stimulated a development towards new rearing systems. Today, around 40% of piglet production in Sweden use age-segregated systems. The most prominent changes in feed composition have been a lowering of the protein content, use of water soluble fibres and supplementing amino acids (Göransson, Lange and Lonnroth 1995).

In 1992, zinc oxide was approved for incorporation into piglet feed at 2000 ppm of zinc as an aid to prevent weaning diarrhoea. Zinc oxide is presently licensed for sale as a pharmaceutical subject to veterinary prescription. Clearly, the use of zinc oxide is not desirable for environmental reasons. A strategy including education and prescription-only policies for phasing-out the use of zinc has therefore been agreed and successfully implemented. In 1998, the sale of medicated feed with zinc oxide was around 12% of the maximum figures from 1995.

The ban of antibacterial feed additives did not create obvious clinical problems for growing or finishing pigs. However, the use of pharmaceuticals with swine dysentery as main indication increased in the end of the 80s (see below). It is unclear whether this is a sequel to the ban or merely a result of a spread of more virulent strains across the country. The production results from this sector are comparable to those from, for example, the Danish production (source: Advisory Service Optima).

## WHAT HAPPENED WITH THE CONSUMPTION OF ANTIMICROBIALS?

From the above, it is clear that the use of antibiotics at dosages used for growth promotion had a preventive effect on certain enteric diseases in animal production. In evaluating the effects of the ban, it is therefore of interest to study the effects on the usage of antibiotics for therapy. The total use of antimicrobials for use in animals has been studied in detail (Wierup, Löwenhielm, Wold-Troell and Agenäs 1987; Wierup, Wold-Troell, Franklin 1989; Björnerot, Franklin and Tysen 1996; Odensvik and Greko 1998). The statistics are based on sales figures from Apoteket AB (the National Corporation of Swedish Pharmacies) and show the total amount of antimicrobials sold by pharmacies or delivered by feed mills during the specified time period. Thus, the figures include antimicrobials for all animal species (food animals, fish, pets and horses).

In table 1, data on sales statistics for antimicrobials from 1980-1999 are presented. As the substances in question are not equal in their biological activity per weight unit, total figures might be misleading (i.e. if a substance requiring high dosages for full efficacy is replaced by a more active substance, a false impression of a reduction could be given). Therefore, each substance group should be assessed separately for trends.

Of special interest in relation to feed additives is the consumption of antimicrobials intended for group or flock medication. In Sweden, these are the tetracyclines, macrolides, quinoxalines, streptogramins, pleuromutilins and nitroimidazoles. The remaining groups are mainly or only used for medication of individual animals. Trends in the use of the latter group are largely unrelated to the ban on feed additives.

Table 1. Total quantity of antibacterial substances (kg active substance) for treatment of animals based on sales statistics from Apoteket AB (National Corporation of Pharmacies) (from SOU 1997 and Odensvik, 2000)

| Substance group[1] | | | Year | | | |
|---|---|---|---|---|---|---|
| | 1980 | 1984 | 1988 | 1992 | 1996 | 1999 |
| Tetracyclines | 9819 | 12955 | 4691 | 8023 | 2698 | 2251 |
| Chloramphenicol | 47 | 49 | 35 | | | |
| G-and V penicillins[2] | 3222 | 4786 | 7143 | 7446 | 8818 | 8692 |
| Aminopenicillins | 60 | 714 | 655 | 837 | 835 | 809 |
| Other betalactam-antibiotics | 9 | 2 | | | | 245 |
| Aminoglycosides | 5274 | 5608 | 3194 | 2139 | 1164 | 846 |
| Sulphonamides | 6600 | 4325 | 3072 | 2362 | 2198 | 2403 |
| Trimetoprim and derivatives | 134 | 186 | 250 | 284 | 339 | 397 |
| Macrolides and lincosamides | 603 | 887 | 1205 | 1710 | 1649 | 1467 |
| Fluoroquinolones | | | | 147 | 173 | 155 |
| Pleuromutilins | | | 124 | 268 | 1142 | 847 |
| Other substances[3] | 861 | 1637 | 1567 | 1634 | | |
| Quinoxalines | 6250 | 9900 | 7164 | 4917 | 1098 | |
| Streptogramins | | 8800 | 1088 | 1275 | 525 | 125 |
| Antibacterial performance enhancers | 8380 | 700 | | | | |
| Total | 41259 | 50549 | 30189 | 31043 | 20639 | 18237 |

[1] Susbtance groups given in bold characters are mainly used for groups or flock medication (i.e. feed or water)
[2] Calculated to equivalents of benzyl penicillin.
[3] Mainly nitroimidazoles

After the ban, a decrease in use of tetracyclines was noted. However, between 1988 and 1993, an increase was again noted. As this could not be connected to an altered disease situation, investigations were initiated. It was found that the increase could almost entirely be explained by the prescriptions of one veterinarian to one herd. The veterinarian was reported and the cause corrected. The total tetracycline consumption is now less than a quarter of that before 1986.

The observed increase over time of macrolides, and that of the pleuromutilins introduced in 1988, is believed to reflect an increase in the incidence of swine dysentery (the major indication for these drugs) (Wallgren 1998). It has been estimated that today, around 10% of the slaughter pigs are treated for swine dysentery (Wallgren 1998).

The consumption of substances formerly approved as feed additives and subsequent to the ban approved as therapeuticals (quinoxalines and streptogramins) has decreased substantially in spite of higher doses being given for therapy than for growth promotion. The major quinoxaline, olaquindox, was exclusively used in pigs. After the ban, the use decreased sharply. In 1988, the use as veterinary medicine for prevention of weaning diarrhoea had increased to levels approaching those pre-ban. However, as the dosage used was three times higher than before, fewer animals were exposed. After this, the use decreased gradually and from July 1997 olaquindox is no longer available in Sweden. As mentioned, zinc oxide has been used as prophylaxis for weaning diarrhoea during the 90s. This practice is now under phasing out and the consumption has recently declined to 12% of its maximum amount.

## Effects on resistance

Unfortunately, there are no systematic studies on resistance in bacteria of animal origin from Sweden that are relevant for the APE discussion from the time before withdrawal of growth promoting antibiotics. Proper monitoring for resistance has only been conducted for salmonellae. The results from that programme show that since 1978, resistance in salmonellae has decreased and today, the situation is very favourable compared to most European countries. However, this can hardly be taken as a direct effect of the ban since few antibiotics active against salmonellae (and thus with potential to select for such resistance) were used as APEs

For lack of historical data, observations on effects rely on comparisons with other countries. A comparison of the prevalence of resistance in faecal indicator bacteria (*E. coli* and enterococci) of pigs in Netherlands and Sweden has been published (van den Bogaard, London and Stobberingh 2000). The data show significantly lower prevalences of resistance to APEs, but also to therapeuticals, in Swedish samples. For VRE, the authors report 39% positive samples from the Netherlands and none from Sweden. The finding of a very low prevalence of VRE in Swedish animals is also supported by other investigations. The authors concluded that the Swedish ban on antibacterial feed additives is effective in reducing the degree of resistance. They also considered that their data indicate that the prohibition has not led to an increase in the use of therapeuticals to such extent that the selection pressure is higher than in countries using antibiotics for growth promotion.

## Effects on the occurence of zoonotic pathogens

The protective effect of the normal microflora against salmonella infection was demonstrated by Nurmi and Rantala in the early 70s (Nurmi and Rantala 1973). As most APE that have been used in Europe recently are not active against salmonella, their presence in the intestine would be expected to favour rather than disfavour salmonella colonisation. However, the quinoxalines and perhaps flavomycin are active against Gram-negative bacteria. For these APEs, a prevention of intestinal colonisation by sensitive Gram-negative zoonotic pathogens could occur.

A substantial amount of studies have been performed on the effects of APE on salmonella colonisation (for a review see SOU 1997:132 1997). Most of these studies are, however, inconclusive and while some are excellent, many have considerable shortcomings regarding study design and conclusions drawn. The interest has mainly been focused on prevalence and duration of salmonella shedding in experimentally infected animals. Most studies have been conducted for 40-50 days and evaluated at the end of the study period. Roughly, 18 experiments show non-significant results, 14 experiments indicate an increase in prevalence/duration of salmonella shedding among medicated animals, and 4 trials indicate a decrease in shedding by medicated animals (SOU 1997:132 1997).

Titration of infectious dose and establishment of dose-response relationships is an essential part of risk assessment. This type of investigation is crucial when determining causal relationships and also for explaining the seemingly conflicting results obtained in different studies. If the doses used are close to the threshold value of response/no response, different studies are bound to show equivocal results. In all dose-response experiments, Barrow (1989) found significant increases in salmonella shedding by chickens in all groups receiving concentrations of avoparcin from 15 ppm. For lower concentrations, variable results were obtained. This explains the contradictory results obtained in studies where 10 ppm has been used. Regarding changes in the infectious dose, or increased susceptibility of infected animals, the prevalence of salmonella in the different experimental groups shortly after infection may give a hint. One study, by Smith and Tucker (1980) clearly showed, by dose-titration, a decrease (from $10^4$ to $10^3$) in the infectious dose necessary for colonising avoparcin-fed birds as compared to non-medicated birds.

Colonisation of the animals with other zoonotic pathogens could also be affected. No studies on the effects of APE on colonisation with pathogens such as *Campylobacter* spp., *Yersinia* spp., or verotoxin-producing *Escherichia coli* have been found. Increased presence in the animal intestine of these bacteria could have serious consequences for either human or animal health. No studies specifically addressing this topic have been found.

## Concluding remarks

The use of APE contributes to the increase and maintenance of a pool of resistance genes in animal microbiota. Resistance genes can be, and are, transferred between animal and human microbes. Available evidence indicates that non-use of APE has been effective in reducing or preventing resistance in animal populations, thereby reducing the risk of spread of resistance through the food chain.

Data from the literature does not indicate that non-use of APE would have any negative effects on the occurence of zoonotic pathogens. On the contrary, the few studies using a dose-response design indicate that at least use avoparcin could have such effects.

The disease preventing effect of antimicrobials given at dosages used for growth promotion on intestinal diseases is well documented. Experience from Sweden, and recently other countries confirm that withdrawal of APE may lead to problems with diseases such as necrotic enteritis in chickens and post-weaning diarrhoea in piglets. However, these problems may be overcome through changes in the production. With improved feed and feeding regimens, hygiene and health-orientated systems it is possible to adjust to non-use of APE. Further, the non-use of APE has not had any appreciable negative effects on bacterial resistance to therapeutic antimicrobials. On the contrary, the situation in Sweden seems favourable in comparison with other countries.

## References

Aarestrup, F.M. (1995) Occurence of glycopeptide resistance among *Enterococcus faecium* isolates from conventional and ecological poultry farms. *Microbial Drug Resisatance*, 1, 255-257.

Bager, F., Madsen, M., Christensen, J. and Aarestrup, F.M. (1997) Avoparcin used as a growth promoter is associated with the occurrence of vancomycin-resistant *Enterococcus facecium* on Danish poultry and pig farms. *Preventive Veterinary Medicine*, 31, 95-112.

Barrow, P.A. (1989) Further observations on the effect of feeding diets containing avoparcin on the excretion of salmonellas by experimentally infected chickens. *Epidemiology and Infection*, 102, 239-252.

Björnerot, L., Franklin, A. and Tysen, E. (1996) Usage of antibacterial and antiparasitic drugs in animals in Sweden between 1988 and 1993. *Veterinary record*, 139, 282-286.

DANMAP 98 (1999) Consumption of antimicrobial agents and occurrence of antimicrobial resistance in bacteria from food animals, food and humans in Denmark. Copenhagen, DANMAP.

Elwinger, K., Engström, B., Fossum, O., Hassan, S. and Teglöf, B. (1994) Effect of coccidiostats on necrotic enteritis and performance in broiler chickens. *Swedish Journal of Agriultural Research,* 24, 39-44.

Elwinger, K., Schneitz, C., Berndtson, E., Fossum, O., Teglöf, B. and Engsröm B. (1992) Factors affecting the incidence of necrotic enteritis, caecal carriage of *Clostridium perfringens* and bird performance in broiler chickens. *Acta Veterinaria Scandinavica,* 33, 361-370.

Greko, C. and Lindblad, J. (1996) *Vancomycin sensitivity of enterococci from Swedish poultry and pigs.* Symposium: Food Associated Pathogens, Uppsala, Dept. of Food Hygiene, SLU, Uppsala.

Göransson, L., Lange, S. and Lonnroth, I. (1995) Post weaning diarrhoea: focus on diet. *Pig News and Information,* 16, 89N-91N.

JECATAR (1999) The use of antibiotics in food producing animals: antibiotic resistant bacteria in animals and humans. Report of the Joint Expert Committee on Antibiotic Resistance. Canberra, Commonwealth Department of Health and Aged Care and Department of Agriculture, Fisheries and Forestry, Australia.

Jensen, L.B., Hammerum, A.M., Aarestrup, F.M., van den Bogaard, A.E. and Stobbering, E.E. (1998) Occurrence of *sat*A and *vgb* genes in streptogramin-resistant *Enterococcus faecium* isolates of animal and human origin in the Netherlands. *Antimicrobial Agents and Chemotherapy,* 42, 3330-3331.

Klare, I., Heier, H., Claus, H., Böhme, G., Marin, S., Seltmann, G., Hakenbeck, R., Antanassova, V. and Witte, W. (1995) *Enterococcus faecium* strains with *van*A-mediated high level glycopeptide resistance isolated from animal food-stuffs and faecal samples of humans in the community. *Microbial Drug Resisatance,* 1, 265-272.

Levy, S. (1996) *Antibiotic resistance: an ecological imbalance.* Antibiotic resistance: origins, evolution, selection and spread, London, Whiley, Chichester (Ciba Foundation Symposium 207).

Nurmi, E. and Rantala, M. (1973) New aspects of *Salmonella* infection in broiler production. *Nature,* 241, 210-211.

Odensvik, K. (2000) Försäljning av antibakteriella och antiparasitära läkemedel för djur — 1999 års siffror. *Svensk veterinärtidning,* 52, 445-449.

Odensvik, K. and Greko, C. (1998) Antibakteriella läkemedel för djur - en uppdatering. *Svensk veterinärtidning,* 50, 313-316.

Palepou, M.-F.I., Adebiyi, A.-M.A., Tremlett, C.H., Jensen, L.B. and Woodford N. (1998) Molecular analysis of diverse elements mediating VanA glycopeptide resistance in enterococci. *Journal of Clinical Microbiology,* 42, 605-612.

Perreten, V., Kollöffel, B. and Teuber, M. (1997) Conjugal transfer of the Tn*916*-like transposon TnFO1 from *Enterococcus faecalis* isolated from cheese to other gram-positive bacteria. *Systematic Applied Microbiology*, **20**, 27-38.

Quednau, M., Ahrné, S. and Molin, G. (1998) Antibiotic resistant strains of *Enterococcus* isolated from Swedish and Danish retailed chicken and pork. *Journal of Applied Bacteriology*, **84**, 1163-1170.

Roberts, M.C., Facinelli, B., Giovanetti, E. and Varaldo, P.E. (1996) Transferable erythromycin resistance in *Listeria* spp. isolated from food. *Applied and Environmental Microbiology*, **62**, 269-270.

Robertsson, J.Å. and Lundeheim, N. (1994) Prohibited use of antibiotics as a feed additive for growth promotion - effect on piglet health and production parameters. 13th IPVS Congress, Bangkok.

Smith, W.H. and Tucker, J.F. (1980) Further observations on the effect of feeding diets containing avoparcin, bacitracin and sodium arsenilate on the colonization of the alimentary tract of poultry by salmonella organisms. *Journal of Hygiene*, **84**, 137-150.

SOU 1997:132 (1997) Antimicrobial feed additives. Report from the commission on antimicrobial feed additives. Stockholm.

SSC (1999) Opinion of the Scientific Steering Committee on Antimicrobial Resistance. Brussels, European Commission, Directorate-General DGXXIV.

Stobberingh, E., van den Bogaard, A., London, N., Driessen, C., Top, J. and Willems, R. (1999) Enterococci with glycopeptide resistance in turkeys, turkey farmers, turkey slaughterers, and (sub)urban residents in the south of the Netherlands: evidence for transmission of vancomycin resistance from animals to humans? *Antimicrobial Agents and Chemotherapy*, **43**, 2215-2221.

Swann Committee (1969) Joint Committee on the use of antibiotics in animal husbandry and veterinary medicine. London, Her majestys stationery office: pp. 83.

Torell, E., O Cars, B. Olsson-Liljequist, B.-M. Hoffman, J. Lindbäck, L.G. Burman and The Enterococcal Study Group (1999) Near absence of vancomycin-resistant enterococci but high carriage rates of quinolone-resistant ampicillin-resistant enterococci among hospitalised patients and nonhospitalised individuals in Sweden. *Journal of Clinical Microbiology*, **37**, 3509-3513.

Wallgren, P. (1998) Anvendelse af antibiotika i Sverige. Den Danske Dyrlaegeforeningens Årsmode, sektion svin, Hotel Nyborg Strand.

van den Bogaard, A., London, N. and Stobberingh, E. (2000) Antimicrobial resistance in pig faecal samples from the netherlands (five abbatoirs) and Sweden. *Journal of Antimicrobial Chemotherapy*, **45**, 663-671.

Wegener, H.C., Madsen, M., Nielsen, N. and Aarestrup, F.M. (1997) Isolation of vancomycin resistant *Enterococcus faecium* from food. *International journal of Food Microbiology*, **35**, 57-66.

WHO (1997) The medical impact of the use of antibiotics in food animals. Reprt of a WHO meeting. Berlin.

Wierup, M. Wold-Troell, M., and Franklin A. (1989) Antibiotikaförbrukning hos djur i Sverige under perioden 1980-1987. *Svensk Veterinärtidning*, **41**, 299-311.

Wierup, M. (1996) Sverige förbjöd antibiotika i tillväxtbefrämjande syfte 1986 - vad hände med djurhälsan och hur löstes problemen? *Kungliga Skogs- och Lantbruksakademiens Tidskrift*, **135**, 69-78.

Wierup, M., Löwenhielm, C., Wold-Troell M. and Agenäs, I. (1987) Animal consumption of antibiotic and chemotherapeutic drugs in Sweden during 1980, 1982 and 1984. *Veterinary research communications*, **11**, 397-405.

Witte, W. (1996) *Impact of antibiotic use in animal feeding on resistance of bacterial pathogens in humans*. Antibiotic resistance: origins, evolution, selection and spread, London, Whiley, Chichester (Ciba Foundation Symposium 207).

Woodford, N., Adebiyi, A.M.A., Palepou, M.F.I. and Coockson, B.D. (1998) Diversity of vanA glycopeptide resistance elements in enterococci from humans and nonhuman sources. *Antimicrobial Agents and Chemoterapy*, **42**, 502-508.

**15**

# CURRENT STATUS AND FUTURE PERSPECTIVES IN E.U. FOR ANTIBIOTICS, PROBIOTICS, ENZYMES AND ORGANIC ACIDS IN ANIMAL NUTRITION

M.Vanbelle

*Past-Chairman of SCAN, Vice-Chairman of the S.S.C., Laboratory of Biochemistry and Nutrition, University of Louvain-La-Neuve, Belgium.*

## Summary

Antibiotics as feed additives have proven during more than 35 years to be effective means of improving weight gain and feed conversion and to reduce environmental pollution. The progressive increase of antibiotic resistance among pathogen microorganisms has questioned the prophylactic use of these feed additives. For this reason E.U. has banned the most of them. Only four remain authorised at this moment: Flavophospholipol, Monensin sodium, Salinomycin sodium and Avilamycin. There is an urgent request for the development of new alternatives. Several options have been proposed, and the state of art is discussed in this paper for probiotics, enzymes and organic acids.

The results reported for probiotics in the literature are often contradictory and conflicting regarding their efficacy. Their status in the E.U. is discussed as well as perspectives to increase their efficacy. Enzymes are not really alternatives to growth-promoters , but do fit the literal definition of digestive enhancement in that they enable more efficient use of existing and new raw materials. Enzymes appear to be particularly beneficial to monogastric animals and especially for poultry and to a lesser degree for pigs. The status of enzymes at the E.U.-level is briefly discussed. Fourty seven enzyme-products are provisionally authorised on a Community level.

For decades, organic acids have been used to improve feed hygiene especially for weaner pigs. Their possible mode of action is outlined.

At the moment no alternatives reach the efficiency of the antibiotic growth-promoters, and stronger attention should be focused to the nutritional and hygienic aspects of animal husbandry.

## Introduction

Has there been an abuse of feed antibiotics? What is their future in view of an increasingly strong consumer lobby? Will all the feed antibiotics be banned in the E.U.? Do we have alternatives for feed-additives? These questions are currently being addressed in virtually every country.

In order to increase animal production and to reduce costs, feed additives have been used for more than 40 years and sanctioned in the EEC countries by Directive 70/524 (1970), updated by Directive 87/153 (1987), Directive 93/113 and consolidated by Directive 94/40 of 22nd July, 1994 including micro-organisms and enzymes. The Directive 96/51/EC, better known as the fifth amendment can be summarised as following: Community authorisation of an additive is given only if *inter alia* it affects favourably the characteristics of feedingstuffs or of animal products and satisfies the nutritional needs of animals, or improves animal production. Further conditions are that an additive may not adversely affect human or animal health or the environment nor harm the consumer by altering the characteristics of livestock products, that its presence can be monitored, that at the level permitted, treatment or prevention of animal disease is excluded(this condition does not apply to additives belonging to the group of coccidiostats and other medicinal substances). An additive may not be authorised, if for serious reasons concerning human or animal health its use must be restricted to medical or veterinary purposes. Provisional authorisation may be given for the use of a new additive or a new use of an additive already authorised, provided that the above mentioned conditions are met but the effectiveness of the additive has not yet been demonstrated. Until 30 September 1999 Member States where free to authorise or not to authorise on a national level provisionally authorised additives (listed in Annex 2). As from 1 October 1999 the provisional authorisations are valid in the whole Community but limited in time, up to a maximum of four years. Fifteen categories of feed additives are listed by Directive 70/524

## The use of antibiotics as feed additives: their future

Additives belonging to the group of antibiotics, coccidiostats and other medicinal products, and growth promoters authorised before 1 January 1988 are provisionally authorised as from 1 April 1998 and will be re-evaluated. After the re-evaluation they will, no later than 1 October 2003, be linked to a person responsible for putting them into circulation for a period of 10 years. For antibiotics, coccidiostats and other medicinal products, and growth promoters authorised after 31 December 1987, such a re-evaluation procedure is not foreseen. For them "brand specific" authorisations will be granted already before 1 October 1999 for a period of 10 years.

The last directive 96/51 contains two annexes. Annex 1 lists the additives authorised in all the EEC- countries and annex 2 gives the products provisionally authorised in all the Member States for maximum 4 years, pending establishments of the dossiers, in agreement with the guidelines published by the Commission. Nine antibiotics and 2 growth promoters were approved as feed additives in annex 1 till October1995 with 4 antibiotics in annex II. On the other side 20 products were listed as Coccidiostats and medicinal substances in annex I until February 1997. Four products were at that moment provisionally listed in annex II. Many antibiotic feed additives still authorised in the U.S., are not allowed in the E.U.

Efficacy of the subtherapeutic use of antibiotics in food producing animals was summarised by Hays (1991) in the US and confirms the European results. The effects are greater in very young animals than in older animals, probably because the younger animals have a less well-developed immune system. The effects are also smaller when animals are exposed to environmental conditions which minimise exposure to pathogenic bacteria or which minimise stress (Beermann, 1995). The control and inhibited growth of harmful bacteria seems to be the major benefit from the subtherapeutic use of antibiotics. Nutrients sparing effects and some metabolic effects are also evoked as mode of action of the antibiotic feed additives. Furthermore, the antibiotic feed additives by improving efficacy of growth and feed efficiency exert a positive and substantial contribution to the reduction of the environmental pollution especially for nitrogen and phosphate.

## HISTORICAL EVOLUTION OF THE USE OF ANTIBIOTICS AS FEED-ADDITIVES SINCE 1970 TILL 1995

An old storm is brewing a new in the E.U. related to the famous problem of resistance building of strains of micro-organisms in the gut of animals treated with antibiotics. This is an old story going back to the famous Swan Report (1969) from which it was concluded in 1974 by the EEC authorities to ban all the antimicrobials exercising a selective pressure for resistance in the Enterobacteriae and other micro-organisms. The guiding principle of the Swan report was to separate antimicrobials into "feed" and "therapeutic" categories. The latter were to be available only on prescription, and the former legally sold without prescription. "On the grounds that resistance development as a consequence of antibiotic use in animals might endanger human health, the Swan report recommendations have led to a drastic restriction or even prohibition of the use of certain antibiotics as growth promoting agents in animal production in many countries of the world in order to attempt to decrease resistance to drugs which are reserved exclusively for therapeutic and prophylactic use" (Gedek, 1981). This same theory surfaced in the New England Journal of Medicine in the US. In an epidemiological study, researchers found a direct relationship between the use of antibiotics in beef cattle feeds and the appearance of 18 cases of severe Salmonella poisoning in man. They recommended to ban, just as the EEC did in 1974, the use of tetracyclins and penicillins. Still, the fundamental question remains: after 30 years of banning these antibiotics in animal feeds, is there any reduction in bacterial resistance against these products?

Several reports (Linton, 1981; Gedek, 1981; Anon, 1988) state clearly that there was no evidence in the EEC countries and the US that the use of subtherapeutic levels of antibiotics has led to an increase in multiple resistance in Salmonellae, E. Coli and other Enterobacteriae. As stated by Gedek (1981), the R-plasmids are so widely spread that one must always anticipate their appearance. They occur in the intestinal microflora of humans and animals without the selective pressure of antibiotic treatment. Chromosome related resistance must not be neglected but seems to be less pathogenic (Gedek, 1981). A similar conclusion was drawn in a study published in 1980 by the National Academy of Sciences who conducted a large study on the use of subtherapeutic doses of antimicrobials in animal feeds and found no evidence of their contribution to the increased pool of bacterial resistance. On the contrary, they emphasised the positive contribution of the therapeutic doses used in human and veterinary medicine.

Since 1981, there are a lot of publications demonstrating the positive relationship between the prophylactic and therapeutic use of antibiotics in humans and animals and the emergence and spread of antibiotic resistant bacteria (Baquero, Martinez and Loza, 1991; Endzt, Rijs, Van Klingem, Jansen, Van der Reyden and Mouton, 1991; D'Aoust, Sewell, Daley and Creco, 1992; Jones, Kerhrberg, Erwin and Anderson, 1994; Murray, 1992; Anon, 1995; Swartz, 1994; Murray, 1995). Contrary to earlier reports, however, it seems that the continuous use of subtherapeutic antibiotics may also exert a pressure to select resistance building of pathogens in animals (ASM report, 1995) (SSC report 1999). In the ASM report, it is stated that " the laws of evolution dictate that microbes will eventually develop resistance to practically any antibiotics".

Gedek (1981) in a report "10 years on from Swan" stressed that since R-plasmid prevalence is clearly related to antibiotic use, the less antibiotics are employed in treatment, the lower will be the selection pressure for plasmid carriage. As R-plasmids often carry multiple resistance this will favour selection of linked resistant genes. Clearly the presence or absence of certain strains of resistant bacteria is too simple a criteria upon which to base use or banning antibiotics. What will the future look like?

# EVOLUTION OF THE ANTIBIOTIC FEED ADDITIVES USE SINCE 1995

In the middle of 1995 (21st of May) the Danes issued an outright ban against the inclusion of a single glycopeptide antibiotic, Avoparcin, in pig and chicken diets. This antibiotic has been accepted and approved for pigs and chickens since 1979. The Danish government invoked the clause of safeguard in order to ban the additive, for Danish producers by saying that there is evidence that in pigs and chicken herds given feeds containing this antibiotic, the appearance of Avoparcin resistant Enterococci strains has increased. These strains harboured the van A gene (a jumping gene) and are simultaneously resistant to Vancomycin (a glycopeptide used in human therapy against infectious Enterococci) and Teicoplanin (another glycopeptide drug). This cross-resistance among animal Enterococci strains raises the question whether these strains constitute a risk to human health. Can they be transferred to humans? This central major question opened a new debate, a very serious and emerging scientific debate and DG IV and SCAN were aware of the complexity and the possible consequences of the problem and all the necessary measures have been taken to prepare appropriate advice based on the actual scientific knowledge, the necessary epidemiological data in Europe, as well as the most specialised scientific expert opinions from Europe and elsewhere.

It is interesting to note that the Danish government asked their producers also to exclude all feed additives of an antibiotic or chemotherapeutic nature from diets fed to pigs after 30 kg liveweight and this voluntary ban has been accepted by the commercial feed manufacturers. The Danish National Institute of Animal Science calculated that the removal of these growth promoters would cost producers about 1 US dollar per pig in lost growth and higher feed conversion rates. Sweden has prohibited feed additive antibiotics for pigs, since 1986. In contrast with the total ban on non-therapeutic feed-grade antibiotics in Sweden, the Danes have recognised the value of antibiotic growth promoters in weaning and starter pig feeds. It is acknowledged in Denmark that the voluntary exclusion of feed-grade growth promoters is more based on sales image than on scientific evidence. Also in Germany, a temporary ban of 6 months was issued on Avoparcin use for all domestic species (January 19 th, 1996).

What happened since then? In view of the above, the Commission consulted the Scientific Committee on Animal Nutrition,(SCAN) which concluded in its opinion expressed on 21 May 1996, that in the absence of further scientific information, there are insufficient data to establish conclusively the risk of transfer of resistance invoked by Germany and Denmark but also that the available evidence does not allow the risk to be excluded with certainty. It also concluded that because of the absence of elements critical to establishing cause and effect with regard to a role for glycopeptide resistant organisms of animal origin (Enterococci) or their genes in human disease, it is not necessary to reserve the use of glycopeptides exclusively for human medicine. However, the Committee accepted that the reports raise serious questions, and it would propose that the feed-additive use of Avoparcin be reconsidered at once should it be shown that transfer of resistance were possible from animal to man. Moreover, as a precautionary measure, the Committee recommends that no further glycopeptide sharing the same site and mechanism of antibiotic action as Avoparcin should be approved until it is satisfied with the results of research still to be carried out.

The SCAN suggested that various investigations should be undertaken to pinpoint the problem of possible resistance to antibiotics induced by the use of antibiotic additives in animal feed and proposed a scheme for the surveillance of microbial resistance in animals which receive antibiotics. On December 19th 1996, the Commission proposed the Standing Committee for Animal Feedingstuffs the prohibition of the use of Avoparcin, as an *ad interim* protective measure taken as a precaution, which could, if necessary, be reconsidered were the doubts expressed about the additive are dissipated in the light of the investigations which will have been carried out and of a surveillance program which will have to established.

Article 2 of these Commission Directive 97/6/EC amending Council Directive 70/524/EEC, concerning additives in feedstuffs, which received a majority favourable vote at the Standing Committee meeting of 19 December 1996, establishes that the Commission should re-examine before 31 December 1998, the provisions of the present Directive on the basis of the results given by the different investigations concerning the development of resistances by the use of antibiotics in particular the glycopeptides, and the surveillance program of microbial resistance in animals which have received antibiotics, to be carried out in particular by the persons responsible for putting the concerned additives into circulation. This re-examination never took place and the use of the glycopeptide antibiotic Avoparcin was prohibited by Directive 97/6 EC, with effect from 1 April 1997.

The animal health and nutrition industry is collaborating with DG.VI, per Directive 96/7, per protocol confirmed by the Director General DG VI, in a surveillance program on feed additive antibiotics. Under the program, 14,000 samples are being taken relative to the use of six feed antibiotics in Europe. The first 2000 samples have been collected. The withdrawal of these products will invalidate the scientific basis of the study that is to be completed by early 2000. Financial resources have been allocated to this.

In June 1997 the SCAN was requested to examine the scientific information provided by the Republic of Finland, concerning the use of macrolides Tylosin and Spiramycin as feed additives and expresses its opinion on the following question: should the use of Tylosin and Spiramycin for serious reason concerning animal and public health be restricted to controlled veterinary therapeutic use? The primary conclusion expressed on 05 February 1997 by SCAN was as following : "The laboratory data and the literature cited do not provide sufficient evidence that the use of macrolides as feed additives presents a significant risk to human or animal health. It is presumptuous to claim that any risk from allowing macrolides as feed additives have been proven. In the absence of sufficient research data on the epidemiology and spread of macrolide resistance, both among farm animals and from them to man, there is no reason for a general ban on the use of macrolides as feed additives".

In June 1998 Denmark invoked the clause of safeguard to ban Virginiamycin as feed additive and SCAN was requested to give an opinion on whether the use of Virginiamycin as a growth promoter for pigs and broilers selects for Virginiamycin resistant Enterococcus faecium and that Pristinamycin and Synercid used for human therapy etc. and that Virginiamycin resistant E. faecium were detected in food and in faecal samples from healthy humans and that Virginiamycin resistant E. faecium can be transmitted from animals to man and whether or not Streptogramin resistant E. faecium and Staphylococci selected by the use of Virginiamycin as a growth promoter constitute a public health risk at present, or could they constitute such a risk if Streptogramins take a pivotal role for treatment of serious human infections in the future, notably infections with Vancomycin resistant E.faecium and multiresistant Staphylococci. Having considered the evidence provided by the Danish Government in support of their action taken under the safeguard clause against Virginiamycin SCAN (Dec '98) concludes that: "No new evidence has been provided to substantiate the transfer of a Streptogramin or Vancomycin resistance from micro-organisms of animal origin to those resident in the human digestive tract and so compromise the future use of therapeutics in human medicine". In summary, for different reasons SCAN concludes that the use of Virginiamycin as a growth promoter does not constitute an immediate risk to public health in Denmark.

Increasing human resistance to antibiotics is rising to the top of agenda for many health - care regulators at both Member States and EC level. By the end of 1998 ; the Commission was under pressure to take action. On 14 December 1998, 12 of the EC's 15 agriculture ministers voted to ban 4 antibiotics used since years as growth-promoters in animal feed. These products were Spiramycin, Tylosin, Phosphate, Virginiamycin and Bacitracin-zinc. Reactions on this decision came from industry saying that the ban has no scientific justification, but EC. Agriculture Commissioner Franz Fishler says that these products should be banned because either they, or closely related products have important human medical applications. The Commission applies the precautionary principle. Mr. Fishler also ordered in December 1998 an investigation into four other antibiotics growth promoter substances: Flavophospholipol, Avilamycin, Monensin Sodium and Salinomycin, which have so far escaped the ban because they do not belong to antibiotic families used in human medicine. The escalation is further reinforced by the fact that the

EC. Feedstuffs Standing Committee, on request of Denmark, unanimously voted at the end of December 1998 not to renew the licences of three animal feed additives after their current licences expire on 30 th. September. A ban came into force on 1st. October 1999. The products involved are Aprinocide, Dinitolmide, and Ipronidazole, classed as "coccidiostats" and other medicinal substances.

Already in February 1997 the Federal Republic of Germany invited the services of the Commission to re-evaluate the authorisation of the N-Dioxides Carbadox and Olaquindox concerning the possible risk for consumers, operators and animals due to their use as feed additives (Growth promoters). Also the Kingdom of the Netherlands prohibited the use on its territory of Carbadox in feedingstuffs on September 6, 1997, on grounds that Carbadox has been found to be genotoxic and carcinogenic and poses risk for workers in the feed industry. Under pressure, the Commission consulted SCAN and this Committee noted in its opinion issued on July 10 1998 that it was maintaining its previous opinion on the acceptability of the Quinoxaline-N-Dioxides Carbadox and Olaquindox, within their previously defined conditions of use, but acknowledged that Carbadox was genotoxic and carcinogenic to rodents, and that Olaquindox was genotoxic and tumorigeneic for rodents. SCAN recognises the exposure of workers is a possible risk through the skin or by inhalation of the parent substances. The Commission banned the 2 N-Dioxides Carbadox and Olaquindox on December 22-1998. The regulation N° 2788-98 shall apply from January 1st. 1999, but Member States could authorise their use until August 31-1999. Finally,but probably not the end of the escalation is the request of Sweden (January 1999) for a general ban of antibiotics, coccidiostats, and other medicinal substances and growth promoters as feed additives, but become under veterinary prescription. Is this the end of the antibiotics as feed additives?

In order to have a global approach of the problem a working group has been created by the S.S.C. on his meeting of 16-17 April 1998. The prevalence and development of antimicrobial resistance and its implications for human and animal health particularly with regard to the development and management of infections, is a complex and multidisciplinary problem (human food consumption, animal nutrition, pharmaceuticals and medicine). The group evaluates the factors contributing to the aetiology of the present situation, examines means of influencing or controlling the development of antimicrobial resistance and makes recommendations based on scientific evidence. It advises on the means of monitoring the outcome of measures that it might recommend and considers the implications of its advice. In particular the following elements have been considered:

- Use/misuse in human and veterinary medicine (prophylactic, therapeutic and including over- prescription).
- Poor compliance of patients with the prescribed treatment (e.g. using lower dosage or interrupting therapy as soon as the symptoms disappear)

- Poor compliance of the dosage regime by animal owners.
- Nosocomial infections (hospitals!)
- Use/misuse of feed additives.
- Use/misuse for phytosanitary purposes.
- Presence of antibiotic resistant genes in GMO's
- Prevention of zoonoses food safety.
- Resistant/multiresistant microbials.
- Microbial ecology (changes in normal flora in particular environment e.g. in hospitals due to frequent use of desinfectants.)
- Identification of the factors involved in the increase of antimicrobial resistance.
- Promotion of alternative preventive methods.

The opinion of the Scientific Steering Committee has been adopted on 28 of May 1999, with the following recommendations for the antibiotics used as feed-additives: "The use of agents from classes which are or may be used in human or veterinary medicine (i.e. where there is a risk of selecting for cross-resistance to drugs used to treat bacterial infections) should be phased out as soon as possible and ultimately abolished. Efforts should also be made to replace those antimicrobials promoting growth with no known risk of influencing intestinal bacterial infections by non-antimicrobial alternatives. It is essential that these actions are paralleled by the introduction of changes in animal husbandry practices which will maintain animal health and welfare during the phase-out process. Thus, the phase-out process must be planned and co-ordinated since precipitous actions could have repercussions for animal health. Meanwhile, it should be re-iterated to manufacturers and farmers that the continuous feeding of AMGPs to food animals for the purpose of disease prevention is a contravention of E.U. regulations and represents misuse; more effective enforcement measures should be adopted." The future of growth promoters and antibiotics, however, will probably not rest with the Scientific Community but with the consumer lobby. This lobby is growing increasingly strong. Consumers will scrutinise the use of antibiotics as therapeutic and prophylactic agents and evaluate the new growth promoters that will be presented in the future. Could we have a world without use of antibiotics as growth promoters? First of all we must point out that antibiotics like Virginiamycin, Bacitracin, Flavomycin, Carbadox, Olaquindox and others have proven to be effective means of improving weight gain and feed conversion. Moreover, their effectiveness in growth promotion has not declined during some thirty-five years of use.

The antibiotic feed additives are undergoing re-assessment, to be completed by 2003. This reassessment will require that these products meet the highest safety, quality and efficacy standards (Directive 96/51). The actual guidelines (EEC Directive 87/153) reviewed and consolidated for the inclusion of enzymes and probiotics (EEC Directive 94/40) will be submitted as a new change and will impose more stringent requirements.The toxicological implications of residues in meat and other animal products will be evaluated with more precision by introducing the notion of MRL (Maximum Residue Limits) and more specific details will be introduced in each chapter of the guidelines. SCAN adopted on 22 October 1999 the revision of the guidelines. These new guidelines will be submitted for comments to the Member States. The conclusion is that for all feed additives used in the E.U., the most important item is safety for the consumer, safety for the animals and safety for the environment. The ongoing revision of the new guidelines is based only on safety and new knowledge in this field

At the moment only four remaining antibiotics are still authorised in the E.U.: Flavophospholipol, Monensin Sodium, Salinomycin Sodium and Avilamycin. The Commission has now to examine the scientific grounds cited by Sweden and to decide, whether to invite Sweden to lift its ban or to withdraw the Community authorisations. It appears that the use of antibiotics as feed additives will be increasingly criticised by politicians and if the probable ban in the E.U. is maintained for anabolic agents and for the natural and recombinant growth hormone (PST and BST) , till the year 2000 , than the question is raised about the possible alternatives in order to maintain animal production along the best lines. Can the new additives such as living yeasts, probiotics and enzymes, organic acids or combinations of these additives, help us in these areas?

## Probiotics as feed additives

### MICROORGANISMS AS PROBIOTICS

Probiotics are defined as "a live microbial feed supplement which beneficially affects the host animal by improving its intestinal microbial balance" (Fuller, 1989; 1992). Probiotics, appropriate strains of viable lactic acid bacteria and Bacillus strains are able to improve performance in calves, pigs and domestic birds (Vanbelle, Teller and Focant, 1989; Teller and Vanbelle, 1991). Clinical signs of disease are generally reduced as is morbidity and mortality, but the results reported in the literature in relation to efficacy are often contradictory and conflicting (Thomke and Elwinger 1998). We summarise the main reasons for these indifferent results:

- Nature of the strains used, viability during production and storage.
- Technology of distribution (stability)
- Ignorance of the equilibrium in the diets and the presence or absence of other additives.
- Absence of information about the physiological state of the animals and the sanitary conditions in which they are kept.

- Ignorance of the exact mechanism of action in the gut.

The different dossiers of microbial strains presented to the SCAN in 1996 raise a lot of questions (see SCAN report from 4 June 1998), especially in relation to the safety of these strains for the animal species under the conditions proposed. Safety problems would only be expected from Bacillus and Enterococcus strains which belong to facultatively pathogenic genera. Under the proposed conditions the Saccharomyces strains and Lactobacillus strains are acceptable as probiotics, provided they do not carry transferable resistance genes. The use of Enterococcus and Bacillus strains should be accepted only for clearly defined strains which have been tested negative for toxicity and pathogeneicity *in vitro* and *in vivo*.

In June 1999 Denmark drew the attention of the Commission on the detection of toxigeneic strains of Bacillus cereus and other Bacillus species. SCAN was requested to reassess the safety of these bacteria as probiotics in animal nutrition. SCAN came to a lot of new conclusions and recommendations. The most important can be summarised as following:

- The incidence of food poisoning involving strains of the B. cereus taxonomic group is common.
- The majority, if not all, strains of Bacillus cereus and closely related species produce toxins that may be damaging to human health.
- SCAN recommends that the use of strains from the B. cereus taxonomic group should be strongly discouraged in the future as feed additives.
- For additives of this taxonomic group with an existing history of use, or for new products the best available methods should be used to demonstrate the absence of toxin production.
- The risk posed by strains of Bacillus other than those from the B. cereus taxonomic group are less severe and that with the exception of strains from the B. subtilis group, detection of toxin-production is the exception, and these strains could be considered safe for use.

SCAN (1999) was also requested to give an opinion and to answer the following questions:

1. What is the most appropriate way to assess the efficacy of micro-organisms used as feed additives in animal nutrition in order to improve animal production?
2. When the product contains several different strains of micro-organisms, what data are necessary to justify the presence of each active component of the additive?

As far as the first question is concerned, SCAN (18/02/00) agrees that to assess the efficacy, 3 studies at $P < 0,05$ are necessary. These studies, with the lowest application rate claimed , should be carried out in different locations.All data of all trials should be presented and evidence that these trials have been properly conducted (best practice) should be provided. Consideration should be given to a sufficient numbers of animals and to the use of a replicated block-design or equivalent for performance trials. For example : for piglets the 3 studies should be performed from birth till weaning time (creep feed) , or from weaning to 25 kg (or according to local custom). For pigs for fattening during the growing or fattening period until slaughter; and for sows during at least 2 reproduction cycles. Animal performance can be expressed in terms of an improvement in the efficiency of nutrient utilisation, or animal growth, or in the quality and yield or animal products, or improved animal welfare. Other beneficial effects, such as reduced morbidity or mortality, can be used as further evidence of the practical value of the probiotic used (for more details see SCAN report expressed on 18 February 2000).

Probiotics are often used to reinforce or re-establish the microbial balance, to correct the disturbance of the gut microflora and doing so to re-inforce the homogeneity of a herd. SCAN specifies also "that in contrary to veterinary medicine they are not disease specific pathogens and it is not possible to treat a disease with probiotics". Thus they don't need a veterinary prescription. It is also noticed by SCAN (18/02/00) "that this primary effect on the gut flora may produce a range of direct and indirect effects, including some that occur within the tissues of the host, such as a modulation of the immune response (Matsuzaki 1998 ; Dunne, Murphy, Flynn, O'Mahony, O'Halloran, Feeney, Morrissey, Thornton, Fitzgerald, Daly, Kiely, Quigley, O'Sullivan, Shannon and Collins, 1999) or control of opportunistic pathogens (Tortuero, Rioperez, Fernandez and Rodriguez, 1995) with as a consequence, reduced morbidity and mortality , especially in young piglets". Claims for microbial products can also be considered "as benefits for the consumer through improved product quality."

Concerning the second question for the justification of different components of multi-strain products, SCAN is of the opinion that: "the requirement to justify the presence of each strain in a final product containing multiple strains, based on evidence from animal trials is neither practical nor theoretically justified". SCAN questions the value of requiring a justification for the presence of each strain present in the mixture. Claims made by a manufacturer are for the mixture as a whole and not for its component parts. This means that the guidelines should be modified on this specific point. In any way, the results obtained with probiotics in monogastric animals are highly variable, often unpredictable and as shown by meta-analysis with limited positive performances; especially better for young growing pigs than in older animals.

The proposed mechanisms of beneficial and detrimental effects of LAB probiotics can be summarised as follows: (Vanbelle, Teller and Focant 1989; Nousiainen and Setälä, 1993).

- Suppression of harmful bacteria; through the production of antibacterial compounds as organic acids decreasing the pH, as well as the production of specific antimicrobials as bacteriocins and/or through the competition for nutrients and colonization sites.
- By the alteration of the microbial and host metabolism; through the production of enzymes which support digestion (e.g. lactase), through the decreased production of ammonia, amines or toxic enzymes and/or through the improved gut wall function.
- By stimulation of the immune response of the host ,through increased antibody levels (IgA, IgM, IgE) and increased macrophage activity.

As detrimental effects of LAB probiotics, we have to stress the competition for nutrients with the host (consumption of glucose, aminoacids etc.). The criteria used for screening probiotics are often based on: acid tolerance, bile tolerance, acid production, production of antimicrobial substances, adhesion to gut epithelial cells, heat tolerance, tolerance of feed antimicrobials. Piva and Rossi (1999) have published an excellent review on the performances obtained with different probiotics in monogastric animals.

## THE USE OF LIVING YEASTS AS PROBIOTICS

Since decades, living yeast cells were used in the sense of an "enteral stimulation therapy". More recent studies (Hänsel, 1988) show that living yeasts are increasing the immunological defence mechanisms (endemic as well as local) through harmless immunogenic stimuli. This has been proven in animal trials as well as in clinical studies. Especially in gastro-intestinal infectious diarrhoea (Buts, Bernasconi, van Craynest, Maldague and De Meyer, 1986; Gedek and Hagenhoff, 1988), but not all the strains of Saccharomyces cerevisiae have the same properties. Some strains like Saccharomyces CBS 5926 (S. boulardii) increase the content of vitamins and the activity of mucosal disaccharidases but also a reduction of infectious E. coli and Salmonella is achieved. The cell wall of these yeasts specifically binds the type I fimbrinated E.coli bacteria through the cell wall mannans.

Recently, the continuous feed supplementation with 50 ppm of a Sacch.cerivisiae strain (Levucell SB) on sows at farrowing (Bertin, Brault, Baud, Mercier and Tournut, 1997a; Bertin, Brault, Mercier, Baude and Tournut, 1997b) and during the gestation, has given direct positive zootechnical effects: increase of number of live piglets, increase of sow weights at weaning, reduction of weight loss between cycles, reduction of sows mortality and reduction of farrowing interval. The feed utilisation and feed digestibility are increased during lactation. Indirect positive zootechnical effects were also observed in piglets born from sows given the yeast strain. These effects were confirmed in piglets receiving the yeast strain incorporated into the prestarter feeds at 200 and 100 ppm: weight gain increases with 3.3 to 3.5 % and mortality was reduced by 2.6 %. These studies need confirmation, as well as the mechanism of action that are actually poorly understood.

It is noteworthy that living yeast is also used in ruminant feeds (10 g/day) with improved productivity due to the increased rumen bacterial viability with increased pH, decreased methane and lactate production, increased rate of cellulolysis with increased flow of microbial protein, resulting globally in increased feed intake and productivity. The removal of toxic molecules like oxygen by the yeasts, initiates probably the metabolic processes in the rumen (Wallace and Newbold,1992, 1993; Dawson, 1993; Chaucheyras, Fonty, Bertin, Gouet, 1995; Newbold, McIntosh and Wallace, 1998).

Another microbial product designed to improve the productivity of ruminants by modulating a similar rumen function as yeast , is a spent culture medium from the growth of Aspergillus species (Varel and Kreikemeier 1993 ; Yoon and Stern 1996).

The extracellular enzymes remaining in the spent medium are invoked as a possible mechanism of action. As stated by SCAN (2000) as for monogastric animals, the results obtained with yeasts and Aspergillus species for ruminants are also variable and unpredictable. Production responses of both yeast and Aspergillus products are generally greater at early rather than mid- or late lactation of dairy cows.


## Perspectives for new technologies to increase the efficacy of probiotics

### THE INTRODUCTION OF THE CONCEPT OF PREBIOTICS AND CHEMICAL PROBIOSIS

The concept of probiosis is essentially the ability of an intact gastro-intestinal flora to resist the overgrowth of any component or foreign strain (Fuller 1998). A prebiotic is a non-digestible feed or food ingredient which passes through the small intestine and is fermented by the endogeneous microflora. (Saris, Asp, Bjorck, Blaak, Bornet, Brouns, Frayn, Fürst, Ricard, Roberfroid and Vogel, 1998). Gibson and Roberfroid (1995) have given a more functional food directed definition: "a prebiotic is a non digestible food ingredient that beneficially affects the host by selectively stimulating the growth and/or activity of one or limited number of desirable bacteria in the colon". This means that if prebiotics can be used by specific probiotic strains, this microbial population may increase and in some conditions can develop a probiotic effect. Gibson and Roberfroid (1995) introduced also the concept of synbiotics: "This is the product in which both probiotic and prebiotic are combined in a single product. It is defined as a mixture of a probiotic and prebiotic that beneficially affects the host by improving the survival and implantation of live microbial dietary supplements in the gastro-intestinal tracts, by selectively stimulating the growth and/or by activating the metabolism of one or a limited number of health promoting bacteria".

The main types of indigestible carbohydrates are the non-starch polysaccharides (NSP's) , resistant starch and the so called oligosaccharides. The main NSP's are cellulose, hemicelluloses, pectins, ß- glucans, pentosans, gums, mucilages, algal polysaccharides, uronic acids and fructans. The main non-digestible carbohydrates used as prebiotics are the non digestible oligosaccharides (NDO's) and various polyols (sugar-alcohols). Especially the anaerobe Bifidobacteria are stimulated by the fructo- oligosaccharides (FOS's) as inulin and oligo-fructose, the trans-galactosyl oligosaccharides (TOS's) as raffinose, stachyose and verbascose; the galacto-oligosaccharides derived from lactose as well as some xylo oligosaccharides. Various polyols as lactitol, xylitol and the disaccharide lactulose, promote also the growth of the beneficial Bifidobacteria in the gut.

At the time being, most studies were realised with the prebiotic fructo oligosaccharide inulin and oligo fructose: they promote not only the growth of Bifidobacteria but also inhibit pathogens as Clostridia and E. Coli, as well as Bacteriodes species (Saris et al., (1998). Other potential beneficial effects include: lowering of the activity of hydrolytic and toxic reductive enzymes thought to be involved in colonic carcinogenesis (see Saris *et al.*, 1998).

Resistant starch, this means starch and hydrolysed product thereof that are not absorbed in the small intestine reaching the hind gut where they are fermented by the colonic flora with high yields of butyrate who is known for his stimulating activity for the growth of colonocytes.

It is noteworthy that short chain fatty acids (SCFA) produced in the small intestine and during colonic fermentation are increasingly discussed in relation to their systemic effects on glucose and lipid metabolism of the host (Cummings, 1997; Saris *et al.*, 1998)

Significant amounts of ingested polyols reach also the large intestine and the colon, where they are fermented by different microorganisms to $H_2$, $CO_2$ , $CH_4$ and SCFA. The latter lower the pH of the gut and may influence the composition of the colonic microflora.

## PROPHYLACTIC EXCLUSION OF ENTEROPATHOGENS OR ANTI ADHESION THERAPY

Aside the stimulation of a beneficial microflora, research is ongoing to master and inhibit the adhesion of enteropathogens on their mucosal receptors, through the oral distribution of sugars miming sugar receptors for the microbial adhesins. (fimbriae=pili) In this field the mannose- oligosaccharides of the yeast cell wall are used to exclude that the type I fimbriae of pathogens as E.Coli and Salmonella are able to find their specific receptors on the mucosa or microvilli.

Other glycans such as the oligomannoside glycopeptides of soya, glycans of plasma or mannose glycopeptides from ovalbumin are under study. (Kelly, Begbier and King, 1994)

## DISTRIBUTION OF SOLUBLE LECTINS COMPETING FOR THE GLYCOSYL BINDING SITE OF THE FIMBRIAE ADHESINS OF PATHOGENS

Here the approach is reversed, soluble lectins simulating the structure of the fimbrial adhesins of pathogens are given orally in order to occupy the gut receptors, thus preventing the attachment of real pathogens (Kelly *et al.*, 1994; Pusztai and Bardocz, 1995). Soluble lectins of the snowdrop acts as a mannose specific lectin, other lectins from garlic, shallots and bananas are under study. In summary, bacterial attachment can be blocked for combating infections. As a prelude to infection, bacterial surface proteins called fimbriae or lectins attach to surface carbohydrates on susceptible host cells. Drugs containing similar carbohydrates could prevent the attachment by binding to the lectins. Alternatively, drugs consisting of lectin like molecules could have the same effect by innocuously occupying the binding sites on the carbohydrates (Sharon and Lis, 1993).

The intestinal microecology is very complex (Gournier,Larpent, Castellanos and Larpent) (1994). The majority of bacteria are associated with the mobile viscous layer of the mucosa. They must be able to thrive in the environment and nutritional circumstances found in such habitats (Savage, 1983). This means they must also be able to digest enzymatically the mucoid glycoproteins and use the degradation products of carbohydrates as energy and nitrogen in situ. The mechanism by which microorganisms associate with the epithelia is still poorly understood. They have to overcome peristalsis in the small intestine and turnover of the epithelial cells. It is clear that research is still necessary on the mechanisms by which endogenous microorganisms colonise the gastrointestinal tracts of animals (Jensen, 1993). Much also must be learned about the capacity of microbes to bind to epithelial cells in relation to infections by the pathogenic E. Coli and Salmonella

(Onderdonk,Marshall, Cisneros and Levi, 1981). More knowledge is required about the epithelial cell receptors from normal indigenous and pathogenic microorganisms (glycolipids, mannoside binding, glucosamin, etc.) and also the chemical composition of the mucous along the gastrointestinal tract (Martin, 1994 ; Newman, 1995; Kelly *et al.* 1994). The problem is complicated by the fact that most wild strains of E. coli carry the ability to form several different adhesions preferentially expressed at different stages of the infection process. Can we master this in the future? Lactic acid bacteria are used widespread as animal probiotics (Vanbelle *et al.*, 1989 ; Nousiainen and Setälä, 1993).

They have to be given continuously at a minimum effective dosage of $10^6$- $10^7$ CFU /g feed. The probiotics that are provisionally authorised on a Community level for a period that may not exceed four years from 1 October 1999 are listed by Commission regulation n° 2293/1999 and n° 2690/1999. This list contains at the moment 16 products from which: 4 strains of Saccharomyces, 5 strains of Enterococcus, 2 strains of Bacillus cereus, 1 strain of Bacillus licheniformis, 1 strain of Bacillus subtilis, 1 strain of Pediococcus, 1 strain of Lactobacillus farciminis and 1 strain of Lactobacillus rhamnosus. This list will be regularly updated with new adopted microbial products.

## The use of enzymes as feed additives

The large scale industrial production of enzymes began in the early 1960s, but was almost applied within the food industry. The animal feed enzymes were a later development, this means during the late 1970s and especially during the last 15 years. As stated by Cowan (1995), Scandinavia has been the launching pad for the development and the first application of ß glucanases for barley use in poultry. Since 1987 there was a massive increase in the application of industrial enzymes within the feed industry in different areas and for different reasons. Compared to a few years ago , when even the role of ß-glucanases in barley was unknown , the amount of information that has been amassed concerning enzymes and their substrates in feed, is impressive. For monogastric animals, poultry and pigs a lot of reviews have been published: Vanbelle *et al.* (1989), Chesson (1987,1994), Dierick (1989), Jeroch, Dänicke and Brufau (1994), Dierick and Decuypere (1995), Bedford and Schulze (1998) and two European symposia (1993 in Switzerland and 1995 in The Netherlands) were devoted on feed enzymes.

## OPPORTUNITIES OF ENZYMES IN FEED

The use of crude enzyme preparations help to overcome poor performances through:

- Digestive help for piglets and calves. In these young animals the enzymatic digestive activity is not yet fully developed : bioavailability of polysaccharides (starch) and proteins can be increased, resulting in improved digestive capacity.
- Breaking down raw materials with specific antinutritional properties such as ß-glucans in barley and oats, water soluble pentosans in rye, crude fiber (NSP) in feeds, not usually degraded by natural enzymes in the animal , thus releasing more nutrients. (e.g., better absorption of fats etc.) with an increase in available energy.
- Re-evaluation and increased use of cheap components like brans, grain by-products, legumes, rape, sunflower, sorghum, potatoes etc., currently considered as inferior ingredients.
- Hydrolyzing phytate from cereals and concentrates reducing the phosphate excretion into the environent.
- Increase of the quality of meat products and yield in meat processing.
- Improvement of poultry welfare by avoiding sticky droppings. Increasing also the sanitary condition of piglets by avoiding diarrhea, resulting in more homogenous litter size.
- Changing the composition and content of bacteria in the small and large intestine.
- Inhibition of special germs in pig and poultry (i.e. salmonella, coli, treponema) by lysozyme, chitinases and b glucanases.
- Enzymes for silage preparations with or without LAB.

Enzymes are not really alternatives to growth promoters , but do fit the literal definition of digestive enhancement in that they enable more efficient use of feed materials.Enzymes appear to be particularly beneficial to monogastric animals (Thomke and Elwinger, 1998; Bedford and.Schulze, 1998), and especially in poultry nutrition and to a lesser degree for pigs.


## IDEAL PRODUCT PROFILE FOR FEED ENZYMES

The first crucial property is their activity. Enzymes, are proteins that catalyse a specific chemical reaction, this means : increases the rate of these reactions by decreasing the activation energy. They have to complex first their substrates who must be accessible. The knowledge of their kinetic behaviour is essential as is the effect of activators and inhibitors. The enzymes requires a conformational active state determined by the primary, secondary, tertiary and eventually quaternary structure. This means also that for each enzyme exists an optimal pH and optimal temperature in an aqueous medium.

The second practical property is the stability of enzymes during the technological manipulations of the feed. During the pelleting in relation to the addition or not of vapour, the state of dies, temperature can easily increase to 70 even 90 ° C during 20 to 30 seconds. Denaturation must also be avoided during storage, by acidic or alkaline conditions and even by the presence of heavy metals and trace elements. The stability must be maintained during the passage in the tract of the different animal species in relation to pH and transit time. Added to feed, the enzymes must express their maximum activity in the small intestine and resist to a lot of proteolytic endogenous and microbial proteases. The enzyme should be thermostable, acting rapidly (minutes and hours, not days) between pH 2 and 7. Easy for use: For the mixer in order to precisely admix to feeds (granulated particle size 0,1 mm up to 0.3 mm). The liquid form should be easy to mix and to handle. Precise and straight forward enzyme analysis (Premix and feed) must be available. Lack of dust, preferably dust free processing is to be recommended, as well as optimal flowing behaviour. Without risks for plant users: no allergy related problems for handling personnel.

## STATUS OF ENZYMES AT THE E.U. LEVEL

As for microorganisms SCAN 1996-1999 was requested to give an opinion on the safety of use of the enzymes to the target animal species under the conditions proposed, as well as to known if the toxicological studies done for each enzyme preparation allow to conclude that the proposed use does not present risks to the consumer, the user, or to the animals! SCAN considers that the majority of the enzymes examined (47 till October 1999) were safe to the corresponding animal species under the condition proposed. Moreover enzymes as such, are protein catalyst known to be widely distributed in nature and used industrially for several purposes in food processing with a long history of safe use: they have to be produced by well-known non pathogenic strains, and they are qualitatively and quantitatively analysed regarding the major catalytic activity and the absence of impurities and contaminants, including micro-organisms, mycotoxins, heavy metals and antimicrobials. The safety for animals is performed with a tolerance test. The safety for the users workers is especially addressed in relation to the ability of enzymes (foreign proteins) to induce an immune response which may cause hypersensivity (allergenic potential). Appropriate protective measures should be taken.

For enzyme production of Bacillus species which do not constitute the whole organism, the producing strain should be shown not to produce toxins under production conditions. When production strains contain antibiotic resistance marker gene, its absence in the enzyme-preparation must be verified. Concerning the assessment of the efficacy of enzymes, SCAN (1999) is of the opinion that for the enzymes which are used to improve the nutritional value of feed ingredients containing non starch polysaccharides (mainly arabinoxylans and b glucans) , the efficacy should be demonstrated using *in vivo* studies on target animals. These (dose response) studies are of two types : animal performance and balance nutritional studies. Enzymes may also be used as technological additives, in that case efficacy should be demonstrated with the appropriate technological test. At least, one experiment must be determined where animals are fed diets containing ingredients with a certain level of substrates which are sensitive to the enzyme application, reflecting the current standard animal husbandry conditions. If the company recommends a range of levels of incorporation of the enzyme preparation, at least 3 significant confirmation studies are necessary with recommended doses in target species and categories. To prove the reproducibility of the effect of efficacy, animal studies must be carried out in at least two different locations, with similar protocol design. If the company claims for nutritional benefits such as an improvement on increased nutrient digestibility and decreased excreta output (e.g. phytase), a balance study is an essential trial to support such a claim. Concerning the multienzymatic products, the evaluation of efficacy should be conducted as a single enzyme. The presence of each enzyme should be justified. The 47 enzyme products that are provisionally authorised on a Community level for a period that may not exceed four years from 1 October 1999 , are listed by Community regulation n° 2293/1999 and n° 2690/1999. They include: 3 phytases, 1 a galactosidase, 32 endo-1.3 (4) ß glucanases, 33 endo 1.4 - ß-xylanases, 6 a amylases, 4 subtilysins and 2 polygalacturonases. This list will be regularly updated with new adopted enzyme products by SCAN.

## The use of organic acids

For decades, organic acids have been used to improve feed hygiene. Especially in feed for young animals (as weaner piglets) organic acids as citric acid, fumaric acid, propionic acid, malic acid and formic acid, or mixtures of them (sometimes mixed with mineral acids as phosphoric acid) have proven to influence positively the piglet performances (Kirchgessner and Roth 1988). More recent work by the team of Kirchgessner (Roth and Kirchgessner 1995; Schöner, 2000) shows the way in which these organic acids could act. The antimicrobial effects in the feed itself, by lowering the pH, reducing the acid-binding capacity and by acting against molds and mycotoxins (i.e. propionic acid). The effects in the digestive tract especially in the piglets stomach where at that time there is still limited hydrochloric acid production. The accelerated pH value reduction for optimal activity of the pepsin enzyme (at pH 3.5), has also an inhibiting effect on micro-organisms. In the small intestine the anionic form of the organic acids acts as complexing agent for various cationic macro-and microelements, increasing the digestibility and retention of these elements in piglets. The anionic form of organic acids acts also as an antimicrobial in the small intestine especially against the accompanying flora (E. Coli, Enterococci). At the same time the ammonia concentrations are reduced. Globally the organic acids used in right concentrations (1.2 to 1.8 %) improve the feed utilisation and reduce incidence of diarrhea.Generally, the efficacy of organic acids are higher than their salts and inorganic acids. As most organic acids are containing a significant energy level, they increase also the energy content of the piglet diet. The coating of mixed organic acids could be an improvement in order to release them at the terminal ileum and reducing the pH values at that level. The choice of the appropriate acid mixture relative to both pKa and the acid delivery system is critical for its efficacy (Piva, 1998). Organic acids can also induce acid resistance e.g. for E.Coli (Guilfoyle and Hirshfield, 1996).

Negative nutritional interactions between organic acids and inorganic bases in the gut of the pig and the chicken are not excluded (Krause, Harrison and Easter, 1994), pending of the lower external pH gut values (Park, Bearson, Bang, Bang and Foster, 1996). The main results obtained with organic acids in pigs and poultry are summarised by Piva and Rossi (1999) and Schöner (2000). At the E.U. level the organic acids are classified as acidity regulators and no specific problems are encountered, aside the fact that preserving liquid acids, as formic acid, acetic acid and propionic acid are often problematic to use because of their acrid odour, their capacity for causing skin irritation and also their corrosive effect on pipes and machinery.

# References

Anonymous (1988) Human health risks with the subtherapeutic use of penicillin or tetracyclins in animal feed. Institute of Medicine, *The National Academy of Science*, Washington, DC, USA

Anonymous (1995) *Report of the ASM task force on antibiotic resistance.* Suppl. to antimicrobial agents and chemotherapy.

Baquero, F., Martinez, B.J. and Loza, E. (1991) A review of antibiotic resistance patterns of Streptococcus pneumoniae in Europe. *Journal of. Antimicrobial Chemotherapy*, **28,** Supplement C, 31-38.

Bedford, M.R. and Schulze, H. (1998) Exogenous enzymes for pigs and poultry. *Nutrition Research Reviews*, **11**, 91-114.

Beermann, D.H. (1995) Existing and emerging strategies for enhancing efficiency and composition of meat animal growth. EU meeting presentation, Dec.1995 Brussels.

Bertin, G., Brault, M., Baud, M.M., Mercier, M. and Tournut, J. (1997a) *Saccharomyces cerevisiae 1079*, microbial feed additive: zootechnical effects on piglets. Proc. VIIth Int. Symposium on Digestive Physiology in Pigs, EAAP Publication 88, St Malo, France, 446-449.

Bertin, G., Brault, M., Mercier, M., Baude, M. and Tournut, J. (1997b) Efficiency of *Saccharomyces cerevisiae* I - 1079 as a microbial feed additive in the diet of the pregnant and lactating sows. Proc. VIIth Int. Symposium on Digestive Physiology in Pigs, EAAP Publication 88 St Malo, France, 450-453.

Buts, J.P., Bernasconi, P., van Craynest, M.P., Maldague, P. and De Meyer, R. (1986) Response of human and rat small intestinal mucosa to oral administration of *Saccharomyces boulardi- Pediatric research.*, **20**, 192-196.

Chesson, A. (1987) Supplementary enzymes to improve the utilisation of pig and poultry diets. *In Recent Advances in Animal Nutrition- 1987 , pp 71-89.* Edited by W. Haresign and DJA Cole Nottingham University Press, Nottingham.

Chesson, A. (1994) Manipulation of fiber degradation: An old theme revised *In.Biotechnology. in the feed Industry.* Proceedings of Alltech's 10th annual Symposium. Edited by T.P.Lyons, KA Jacques, Nottingham University Press. pp. 83-98

Chaucheyras, F., Fonty, G., Bertin, G. and Gouet, P. (1995) Effects of live *Saccharomyces* cells on zoospore germination growth and cellulolytic activity of the rumen anaerobic fungus *Neocallimastic frontalis MCH3. Current Microbiology.*, **31**, 201-205.

Cowan, W.D; (1995) Feed enzymes: The development of the application, its current limitation and future possibilities in proceedings of ESFEZ, Noordwijkershout, The Netherlands. 25,27 october.pp.17-22

Cummings, J.H. (1997) *The large intestine in nutrition and disease* pp 155 Ed. Institut Danone, rue du Duc, 100 B. 1150 Bruxelles.

D'Aoust, J.Y., Sewell, A.M., Daley, E. and Creco, P. (1992) Antibiotic resistance of agricultural and foodborne Salmonella isolates in Canada (1986-1989) *Journal of Food Protection.*, **55**,428-434.

Dawson, K.A. (1993) Current and future role of yeast culture in animal production: a review of research over the last six years. In : *Biotechnology in the Feed Industry* (Lyons, T.P. ed) pp. 269-291. Alltech Technical Publications, Nicholsville, USA.

Dierick, N.A. (1989) Biotechnology aids to improve feed and feed digestion enzymes and fermentation. *Archives of Animal Nutrition, Berlin*, **39**, 241-249.

Dierick, N.A. and Decuypere, J. (1995) Advances in the use of supplementary enzymes in pig nutrition.In *2nd European Symposium on Feed enzymes*, pp.23-29 , Proceedings of ESFE2, Noordwijkerhoudt, The Netherlands 25-27 Oct., 1995 Ed. by Vanhartingsveldt, Hessing M, Vanderlught, JP. and Somers WAC.

Dunne, C., Murphy, L., Flynn, S., O'Mahony, L., O'Halloran, S., Feeney, M., Morrissey, D., Thornton, G., Fitzgerald, G., Daly, C., Kiely, B., Quigley, E.M.M., O'Sullivan, G.C., Shannon, F. and Collins (1999) Probiotics from myth to realty. Demonstration of functionality in animal models of disease and in human clinical trials. *Anton Leeuwenhoek. International Journal..G.*, 76, 279-292.

EEC. Directive 70/524,1970. Official J.L., 270,14,12

EEC. Directive 87/153, 1987.Official J.L., 64, 139.

EEC. Directive 93/113 ,1993.Official J.L., 334,17.

EEC. Directive 94/40, 1994. Official J.L. , 208,15.

EEC. Directive 96/51, 1996. Official J.L. , 235,39.

EEC. Directive 97/6 , 1997. Official J.L., 35, 11.

EEC. Ban regulation. 2821/1998 ,Official J.L. 17/12/98.

EEC. Ban regulation. 2788/1998 Official J.L. 347, 31.

EEC. Regulation. 2293/1999, Official J.L. 284, 1.

EEC Regulation.2690/1999, Official J.L. 326, 3

Endzt, H.P., Rijs, G.J., Van Klingem, B., Jansen, W.B., Van der Reyden, T. and Mouton, R.P. (1991) Quinolone resistance in Campylobacter isolated from man and poultry following their introduction in veterinary medicine. *Journal of Antimicrobial Chemotherapy*, 27, 199-208.

Fuller, R. (1989) Probiotics in man and animals. *Journal of. Applied Bacteriology.*, 66, 365-378.

Fuller, R. (1992) *Probiotics*. R. Fuller Edited by R. Fuller. Chapman and Hall, London.

Gedek, B. (1981) Factors influencing multiple resistance in enteric bacteria in animals. *In ten years on Swann*, AVI Symposiun London pp. 111-126. Ed. AVI.

Gedek, B. and Hagenhoff, G. (1988) Orale Verabreichung von Lebensfähigenzellen des Hefe stammes *Saccharomyces cerevisiae*. Hansen.CBS.5926. und deren Schicksal während der Magen-Darm-passage-*Therapiewoche*, 38, Sonderheft.33-40.

Gibson, G.R.and Roberfroid, M.B. (1995) Dietary modulation of the Human Colonic Microbiota: introducing the concept of prebiotics. *Journal of Nutrition*, 125, 1401-1412.

Guilfoyle, D.E. and Hirshfield, I.N. (1996) The survival benefit of short-chain fatty acids and the inducible arginine and lysine decarboxylase genes for *Escherichia coli. Letters of Applied Microbiology.*, **22**, 1-4.

Gournier,N., Larpent, J.P., Castellanos, M.I. and Larpent, J.L. (1994) *Les probiotiques en alimentation animale et humaine.*Ed. Lavoisier. Paris.

Hänsel, R. (1988) Medizinische hefen as paramunitäts.Inducer: III. Inter.Presseworkshop Paris. *Therapie Woche* **38**, Sonderheft November,pp.5-7.

Hays, V.W. (1991) Effects of antibiotics.In: *Growth regulation in farm animals.* Pearson, A.M.,Dutson,T.R. Ed.,Elsevier Publishing, Essex, England. Vol 7,Chapter **10**, pp.299-320.

Jensen, B.B. (1993) The possibility of manipulating the microbial activity in the digestive tract of monogastric animals. In *44th. Annual Meeting of the European Association for Animal Production.* Aarhus,Denmark.

Jeroch, H., Dänicke., S. and Brufau, J. (1994) Enzyme preparations in poultry feeding in *45th Annuial Meeting of the European Association for Animal Production.* Edinghburgh, Scotland, 5-8 Sept.

Jones, R.N., Kerhrberg, E.N., Erwin., M.E. and Anderson, S.C. (1994) Prevalence of important pathogens and antimicrobial activity of perenteral drugs at numerous medical centers in the US. *Diagnostic Microbial of Infectious Disease*, **19**, 203-215.

Kelly, D., Begbier, R. and King, T.P. (1994) Nutritional influences on interactions between bacteria and the small intestinal mucosa. *Nutrition Research Reviews*, **7**, 233-257.

Kirchgessner, M. and Roth, F.x. (1988) Effekte durch organische Säuren in der Ferkelaufzucht und Schweinemast.*Ubersicht Tiererernährung*, **16**, 93-108.

Krause, D.O., Harrison, P.C. and Easter, R.A. (1994) Characterization of the nutritional interactions between organic acids and inorganic bases in the pig and chick. *Journal of Animal. Science*, **72**. 1257-1262.

Linton, A.H. (1981) Has Swann failed? *Veterinary Record,* **104**, 329-335.

Martin, S.A. (1994) Potential for manipulating the gastro-intestinal flora. A review of recent progress. In *Biotechnology in the feed industry.*Alltech's 10th Annual Symposium, Lyons,T.P. (Ed)pp 155-166.

Matsuzaki, T. (1998) Immuno modulation by treatment with *Lactobacillus casei strain shirota. International Journal of Food Microbiology,* **41**, 133-140.

Murray, B.E. (1992) Problems and dilemmas of antimicrobial resistance. *Pharmacology,* **12**,86-93.

Murray, B.E. (1995) What can we do about Vancomycin resistant Enterococci? *Clinical infection Diseases*, **20**, 1134-1136.

Newbold, C.J., McIntosh, F.M. and Wallace, R.J. (1998) Changes in the microbial population of a rumen simulating fermenter in response to yeast culture.

Canadian Journal of Animal Science, 78, 241-244.

Newman, K.E. (1995) Les mannan-oligosaccharides en nutrition animale. In Alltech European Tour, pp.51.

Nousiainen, J. and Setäla, J. (1993) Lactic acid bacteria as animal probiotics.In Lactic acid bacteria. Salminen,S. and Wright,A. (Eds), Marcel Dekker Incorporation.

Onderdonk,A; Marshall, B; Cisneros,R. and Levi, S.D.,(1981) Competition between congenic Escherichia coli K-12 strains " in vivo". Infectious Immunity. 32,74-79;

Park, Y.K., Bearson, B., Bang, S.H., Bang, I.S. and Foster, J.W. (1996) Internal pH crisis,lysine decarboxylase and the acid tolerance response of Salmonella typhimurium. Molecular Microbiology, 20, 605-611.

Piva, A. (1998) Non conventional feed additives. Journal of Animal and Feed Science., 7, 143-154.

Piva, G. and Rossi,F. (1999) Future prospects for the non-therapeutic use of antibiotics.-Proceedings of the A.S.P.A. XIIIth Congress Piacenza. June 21-24.

Pusztai, A. and Bardocz, S. (1995) Lectins Biomedical Perspectives Ed. Taylor and Françis.UK.

Roth, F.X. and Kirchgessner, M. Zum Einsatz von Ameisensaure in der Tierernährung. Ludwigshafen,Germany: BASF AG, 1995: 5-20

Savage,D.C. (1983) Association of indigenous microorganisms with the gastrointestinal epithelial surfaces. In D.J.Hentges(Ed), Humans intestinal microflora and disease,Academic Press. London,pp 55-74.

SCAN. (1996) Opinion on the use of Avoparcin as feed additive. May 21.

SCAN. (1998) Opinion on the use of Macrolides as feed additive: February 5.

SCAN. (1998) Opinion on the use of Virginiamycine as feed additive: July 10

SCAN. (1998) Opinion on the use of Carbadox and Olaquindox : July 10.

SCAN. (1999) Adoption of new Guidelines :October 22.

SCAN. (1998) Draft Report on Microbial strains: Updated June 4.

SCAN. (1999) Draft Opinion on the safety of Bacillus strains.

SCAN. (2000) Report on how to assess the efficacy of probiotics:.February 18.

Saris, W.H.M., Asp, N.G.L., Bjorck, I., Blaak, E?, Bornet, F., Brouns, F., Frayn, K.N., Fürst, P., Ricard, G., Roberfroid, M. and Vogel, M. (1998) Functional food science and substrate metabolism. British Journal of Nutrition ,80, Supplement 1, 47-75.

Schöner, F.J. (2000) Nutritional effects of organic acids-In III Conference-show Feed Manufacturing in the Mediterranean region. Reus,Spain, 22-24 March.

Sharon, N.and Lis, H. (1993) Carbohydrates in cell recognition. Scientific American, January p.74

SSC. (1999) Opinion of the Scientific Steering Comittee on antimicrobial resistance EU Commission.Brussels .28 may ,pp.52.

Swann Committee Report on the use of antibiotics in animal husbandry and veterinary medicine, (1969) CMND 4190 (Ed), HMSO, London.

Swartz, M.N. (1994) Hospital acquired infections diseases with increasingly limited therapies. *Proceedings of the National Academy of Science.*, **91**, 2420-2427.

Teller, E. and Vanbelle, M. (1991) Probiotics facts and fiction. *Mededeling Faculteit Landbouw Rijksuniversiteit Gent.*, **56**, 4a, 1591-1599.

Thomke, S. and Elwinger, K. (1998) Growth promotants in feeding pigs and poultry. III Alternatives to antibiotic growth promotants. *Annales de. Zootechnie ,* **47**, 245-271.

Tortuero, F., Rioperez, J., Fernandez, E. and Rodriguez, M.L. (1995) Response of piglets to oral administration of lactic acid bacteria. *Journal of Food Protection,.* **58,** 1369-1374.

Vanbelle, M., Teller, E. and Focant, M. (1989) Probiotics in animal nutrition : A review. *Archives of Animal Nutrition*, **7**, 543-561.

Varel, V.H. and Kreikemeier, K.K. (1993) Influence of feeding *Aspergillus oryzae* fermentation extract (Amaferm) on in situ fiber degradation, ruminal parameters and bacteria in non-lactating cows fed alfalfa or bromegrass hay. Journal of Dairy Science, **71**, Supplement 1, 287.

Wallace, R.J. and Newbold, C.J. (1992) Probiotics for ruminants. In:*Scientific basis of the probiotic concept.* R. Fuller (Ed), Chapman Hall London, pp 317-353.

Wallace, R.J. and Newbold, C.J. (1993) Rumen fermentation and its manipulation. The development of yeast culture as feed additives. In: *Biotechnology in the feed Industry* (Lyons TP, Ed) Alltech Technical Publications, Kentucky, pp.173-192.

Yoon, I.K. and Stern, M.D. (1996) Effects of *Saccharomyces cerevisae* and *Aspergillus oryzae* culture on ruminal fermentation in dairy cows. *Journal of Dairy Science,* **79**, 411-417.

# INDEX